Principles of Medical Pharmacology

Principles of Medical Pharmacology

Edited by

Derek Waller
Senior Lecturer in Clinical Pharmacology
Clinical Pharmacology, Faculty of Medicine
University of Southampton, UK

and

Andrew Renwick
Reader in Clinical Pharmacology
Clinical Pharmacology, Faculty of Medicine
University of Southampton, UK

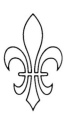

Baillière Tindall
London   Philadelphia   Toronto   Sydney   Tokyo

Baillière Tindall
W. B. Saunders Company Ltd

24–28 Oval Road
London NW1 7DX

The Curtis Center
Independence Square West
Philadelphia, PA 19106-3399, USA

Harcourt Brace & Company
55 Horner Avenue
Toronto, Ontario M8Z 4X6, Canada

Harcourt Brace & Company, Australia
30–52 Smidmore Street
Marrickville, NSW 2204, Australia

Harcourt Brace & Company, Japan
Ichibancho Central Building, 22–1 Ichibancho
Chiyoda-ku, Tokyo 102, Japan

A catalogue record for this book is available from the British Library

ISBN 0-7020-1613-6

Typeset by Alden Multimedia, Northampton, England
Printed in Great Britain by Butler and Tanner, Frome, Somerset

Contents

The Musculoskeletal System

The Gastrointestinal System

The Immune System

The Endocrine System and Metabolic Disorders

Skin Disorders

The Eye

Chemotherapy

Drug Toxicity and Abuse

Drug Prescribing

Contributors

Vivian F. Challenor DM, MRCP
Lecturer in Clinical Pharmacology, Clinical Pharmacology, Faculty of Medicine, University of Southampton, UK

Charles F. George BSc, MD, FRCP
Professor of Clinical Pharmacology, Clinical Pharmacology, Faculty of Medicine, University of Southampton, UK

Keith Hillier BSc, PhD, DSc
Senior Lecturer in Clinical Pharmacology, Clinical Pharmacology, Faculty of Medicine, University of Southampton, UK

Una Martin MB, BCh, PhD, MRCPI
Lecturer in Clinical Pharmacology, Clinical Pharmacology, Faculty of Medicine, University of Southampton, UK

J. Gavin Millar BA, BM, MSc, FRCP
Senior Lecturer in Endocrinology, Renal Medicine, Faculty of Medicine, University of Southampton, UK

Andrew G. Renwick BSc, PhD, DSc
Reader in Clinical Pharmacology, Clinical Pharmacology, Faculty of Medicine, University of Southampton, UK

Derek G. Waller BSc, DM, FRCP
Senior Lecturer in Clinical Pharmacology, Clinical Pharmacology, Faculty of Medicine, University of Southampton, UK

Introduction

Therapeutic drugs are developed for their ability to affect pathological, physiological or homeostatic mechanisms in humans. The safe and effective prescribing of modern medicines requires a knowledge and understanding of:

- The relationship between dose and effects (both beneficial and unwanted).
- The mechanism by which drugs produce their effect(s).
- Factors that may affect the response in the patient (due to altered delivery to the site of action or altered efficacy at the site of action).
- The possibility of interactions when more than one drug is given to the same patient.

Early agents were often naturally occurring inorganic salts such as mercury compounds or plant extracts containing one or more complex organic compounds. The active component of many plant-derived preparations was a nitrogen-containing organic molecule or alkaloid; laudanum, for example, is an alcohol extract of opium which contains high concentrations of the alkaloid morphine. Early therapeutic successes included the use of foxgloves (which contain cardiac glycosides) for the treatment of "dropsy" (fluid retention); however, there was also considerable toxicity since the plant preparations contained variable amounts of the active glycoside and such compounds have a narrow therapeutic index.

A major advance in the safe use of naturally derived agents was the isolation, purification and chemical characterization of the active component. This had three main advantages:

(1) The administration of controlled amounts of the active agent removed any biological variability in potency of the plant preparation — for example, due to climatic or soil conditions when the plant grew.
(2) The active component with the desired effect could be prescribed without having to give a cocktail of other unnecessary natural components. Other components may have interfered with therapy by producing unrelated and unwanted effects or possibly reduced the desired effect by blocking the mechanism of action.

(3) The identification and isolation of the active component allowed the mechanism of action to be defined leading to the synthesis and development of improved agents with the same action but with greater potency, greater selectivity, fewer side-effects, altered duration of action, greater absorption, etc.

Thus, although drug therapy has natural and humble origins, it is the application of scientific principles which has given rise to the clinical safety and efficacy of modern medicines. The aim of this book is to give the principles of clinical pharmacology and to show their relationship to the clinical use of modern therapeutic drugs.

A major advantage of modern drugs is their ability to act selectively, that is, to affect only certain specific body systems or processes. For example, a drug which lowered blood glucose but also reduced blood pressure would not be suitable for the treatment of patients with diabetes or patients with hypertension or even patients with both conditions (because different doses may be needed for each effect).

Key questions facing every prescriber are "which drug" and "how much"? A knowledge of how drugs produce their effects is central to understanding the balance between benefit and possible risk for the particular patient and the possible benefits and disadvantages of co-prescribing other drugs. The amount of drug necessary to produce the beneficial effect depends on two factors:

(1) The relationship between the concentration and effect at the site of action.
(2) The fate of the drug in the patient's body which will determine the relationship between the amount prescribed and the concentration at the site of action.

The aim of the present text is to provide a framework for such knowledge and understanding. It is not designed to be a comprehensive list of all currently available drugs, nor is it a reference source which would allow the clinician to check on all clinical aspects of any particular drug; such information is available in regularly updated form from other sources, such as the *British National Formulary*. A knowledge of mechanisms and sites of action combined with an understanding of factors influencing the delivery of drug to the site of action provides a foundation for safe and effective prescribing.

General Principles

1

Sites and Mechanisms of Drug Action

Modern clinical and biological sciences have provided a detailed understanding of the interaction of many therapeutic drugs with biological systems. A difficulty faced by many medical students is appreciating the depth of information necessary for them to use the drug effectively. Information may range from the general (e.g. it paralyses the patient) to the highly specific (e.g. it alters the quaternary structure of the receptor protein by interfering with the hydrogen bonding between certain specific amino acids). The former is totally inadequate as it allows no possibility of predicting any problems, while the latter is excessive (but may be fascinating, e.g. such detailed information could explain why some patients show abnormal responses). The depth of information necessary is that which provides:

- A suitable framework to allow comparison of the relative benefits and risks of alternative drugs (drug selection).
- An ability to predict possible problems in the particular patient due to other disease processes, other medicines, etc.

SITES OF DRUG ACTION

The sites of drug action can be divided into:

- *Specific*, that is, effects produced by interaction of the drug with a specific site(s) either on the cell membrane or inside the cell. Such sites may be specific to the cells of one particular tissue.

- *Non-specific*, where the effect is mediated via a generalized effect in many organs, and the response observed depends on the different distribution of the drug within the body or the sensitivity of the organ.

SPECIFIC SITES OF ACTION

Receptor mediated effects

A *receptor* is a specialized macromolecule which is designed to recognize certain endogenous signals or messengers (such as the neurotransmitter noradrenaline), and produce an appropriate change in the activity or function of the cell. Many receptors are located within the cell membrane and act to recognize an extracellular signal (such as noradrenaline release) and convert it into an intracellular event (a transmembrane receptor — see below).

The binding of the signal (or ligand) to the receptor is normally *reversible* so that the intensity and duration of the intracellular changes are dependent on the continuing presence of the signal. Thus the interaction between the ligand and its receptor does not involve covalent bonds but weaker, reversible forces such as:

- Ionic bonding — between ionizable groups in the ligand (e.g. $-NH_3^+$) and in the receptor (e.g. $-COO^-$).
- Hydrogen bonding — between amino-, hydroxyl-, keto- functions, etc.

- Hydrophobic interactions — between lipid soluble sites in the ligand and receptor.
- Van der Waals forces — very weak interatomic attraction.

There are numerous possible extracellular signals and therefore a fundamental property of a receptor is its *specificity*, that is, its ability to

respond to only one signal. The ability of receptors to recognize and bind the correct signal depends on an interaction between the receptor molecule and certain specific characteristics of the chemical structure of the signal. The formulae of representative signals or ligands are shown in Fig. 1.1 and it is clear that the differences between them are subtle and occur over a

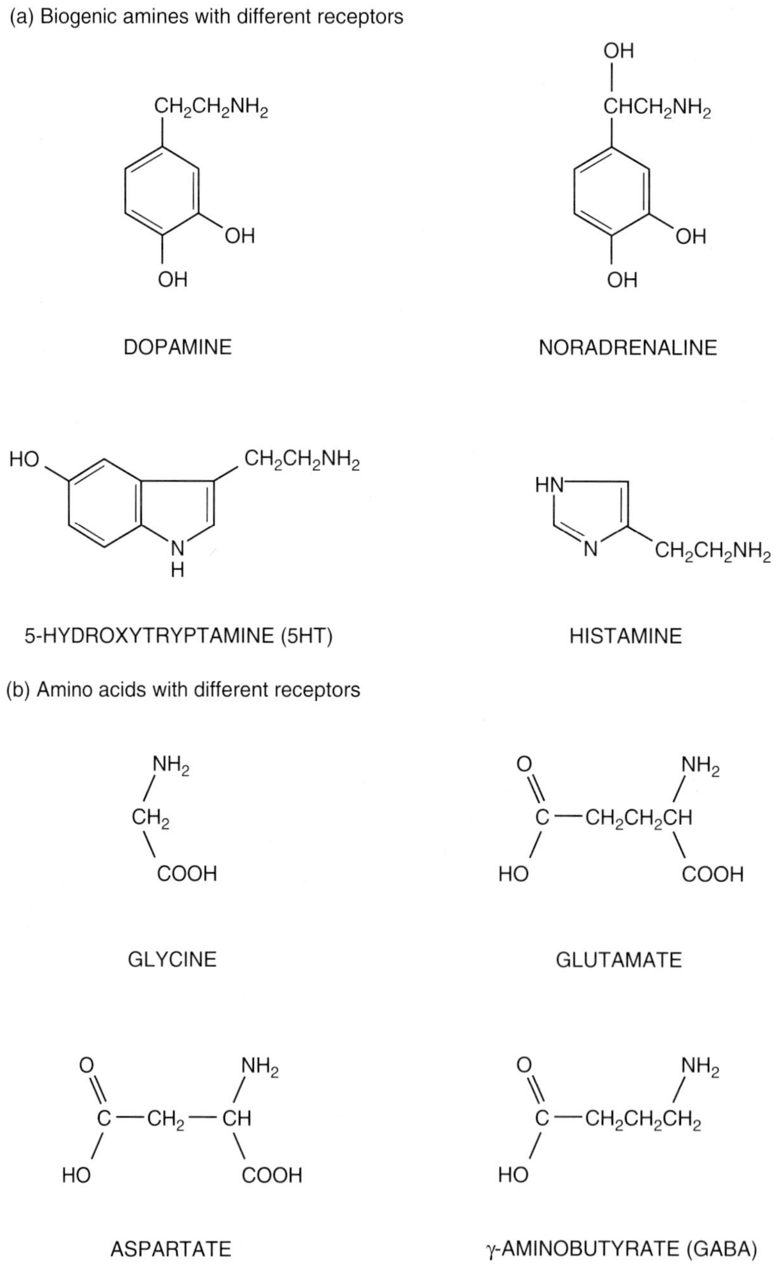

(a) Biogenic amines with different receptors

DOPAMINE

NORADRENALINE

5-HYDROXYTRYPTAMINE (5HT)

HISTAMINE

(b) Amino acids with different receptors

GLYCINE

GLUTAMATE

ASPARTATE

γ-AMINOBUTYRATE (GABA)

Figure 1.1   (a) Biogenic amines with different receptors. (b) Amino acids with different receptors.

small number of interatomic bond lengths. The necessary receptor specificity can only be provided by a structure which has a wide range of different chemical groups for potential inter-actions, such as anion and cation sites, lipid centres, and hydrogen bonding sites. Receptors are proteins, that is polypeptide chains which fold into a tertiary structure and therefore can bring together the necessary specific arrange-ment of bonding types within a small volume — the receptor site (Fig. 1.2).

It should be noted that receptors have a three-dimensional organization in space and therefore require the different aspects of a ligand to be presented in the correct 3-D configuration (rather like fitting a hand into the correct glove). Therefore it is not surprising that different stereo-isomers of the same ligand (whether a normal ligand or a drug) may show very different binding characteristics. Indeed, the different stereo-isomers of some drugs, for example labetalol, may bind to different types of receptor. Thus a racemic drug may be 50% active compound plus 50% inactive or in some cases a mixture of 50% therapeutic and 50% toxic. In addition, the different stereoisomers may undergo different rates of metabolism and elimination. In conse-quence, there has been a trend in recent years for the development of single isomers for therapeutic uses; one of the earliest examples was the use of levodopa in Parkinson's disease.

Although different receptors recognize different ligands, for example noradrenaline receptors bind noradrenaline but not acetylcho-line, there may be a number of receptors which each specifically recognize or bind one parti-cular ligand (e.g. noradrenaline receptors may be α_1, α_2, β_1, β_2 or β_3). This gives rise to subtypes of receptors which may show a tissue or organ specific distribution within the body (see below). Until recently, receptor subtypes were recognized when agonists or antagonists were developed which affected some but not all of the effects of the main receptor class. Thus, acetylcholine acts via different receptors on ganglia (nicotinic N_1), neuromuscular junction (nicotinic N_2) and smooth muscle (muscarinic). This aspect is discussed later under autonomic nervous system (Chapter 4). Recent develop-ments in molecular biology have enhanced our abilities to detect receptor subtypes; for example, it is now recognized that there are multiple types of muscarinic receptors. However, such recognition is currently outstrip-ping our ability to exploit this knowledge by the use of selective therapeutic agents.

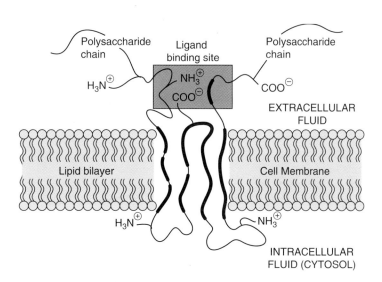

Figure 1.2 Hypothetical transmembrane receptor. The orientation of the receptor within the membrane is achieved by folding of the polypeptide chain plus the presence of hydrophilic centres (such as the extracellular polysaccharide chain) and the hydrophobic regions (shown as thick segments) which orientate the peptide within the cell membrane. The receptor is stabilized across the membrane by the presence of polar amino groups where the chains leave the lipid bilayer and which can interact with the phospholipid end of the bilayer. The ligand binding site represents a small volume in space in which two or more parts of the polypeptide are orientated in such a way as to bind specific ligands only. Other possible ligands may be too large for the site or may show much weaker binding characteristics.

The structure of a hypothetical transmembrane receptor is shown in Fig. 1.2. The binding of an appropriate chemical messenger to the ligand binding site on the extracellular side of the membrane alters the conformation or three-dimensional organization of the receptor protein. The consequence of the conformation change depends on the nature of the receptor.

The numbers of receptors within the cell membrane may be altered during chronic drug treatment, with either an increase in receptor numbers (*up-regulation*) or a decrease (*down-regulation*). The therapeutic effects of tricyclic antidepressants or β-adrenoceptor antagonists develop slowly during regular therapy. This is probably related to adaptive regulation of receptor numbers rather than the recognized acute effects of these drugs, such as the blockade of 5-HT or noradrenaline uptake (tricyclic antidepressants) or of β-adrenoceptors (β-adrenoceptor antagonists). Similarly tolerance to the effects of some drugs (e.g. opiates) may arise from changes in receptor numbers (e.g. opioid receptors), and results in the need for increased doses to produce the same activity.

Ion-channels

The intracellular concentrations of ions such as Na^+, K^+, Ca^{2+}, Cl^- are controlled by ion pumps which move specific ions from one side of the membrane to the other and by ion channels, which may open to allow the selective transfer of ions down their concentration gradients.

Some ion channels show voltage-dependent opening (e.g. the sodium channel which opens in response to a nerve impulse) while others open in response to the presence of a ligand (e.g. chloride channels linked to GABA).

Ligand-gated channels are often complex in nature and may consist of a number of subunits each similar in character to that shown in Fig. 1.2. Subunits may combine to produce a cluster of receptors around a central channel with each orientated so that hydrophilic chains face toward the channel and hydrophobic chains toward the membrane lipid bilayer. The acetylcholine receptor is a good example of this type of structure which comprises five subunits and requires the binding of two molecules of acetylcholine for channel opening. Channel opening is a very rapid process lasting only milliseconds and is usually short lived because the ligand is rapidly inacti-

vated (Chapter 4). Prolonged occupancy of the ligand binding site by acetylcholine leads to a loss of activity possibly due to a further conformational change in the receptor protein which is associated with both receptor occupancy and a closed channel (see muscle relaxants; Chapter 28).

Second messenger systems

In these systems the conformational change in the transmembrane receptor protein, caused by binding of the extracellular ligand, is linked to an intracellular enzyme system. This produces an intracellular message, or second message, which alters the functioning of the cell. There are two complementary second messenger systems, one based on cyclic nucleotides such as cyclic AMP (cAMP) and the other on inositol-1,4,5-triphosphate (IP_3) and diacyl glycerol (DAG). In each case the intracellular enzyme system is linked to the receptor by a guanosine-binding protein (or G-protein) (Fig. 1.3).

The G-protein system consists of subunits; some subunits are lipid soluble and localize and orientate the system within the membrane, whereas other subunits are functional and affect the second messenger system. The functional subunit has three active sites: one for recognition and binding of the transmembrane receptor, one linked to the second messenger enzyme system and a third site which can bind GTP (guanosine triphosphate) or GDP (guanosine diphosphate). This last aspect is of critical importance since it provides a "switch" between the receptor and the second messenger. The G-protein is active when GTP is bound and inactive when GDP is bound. When the extracellular receptor is initially occupied, this third site binds GTP and the second messenger enzyme is "switched on" (see below). However, the G-protein system has GTP-ase activity so that the bound GTP is hydrolysed to GDP and the second messenger enzyme is then "switched off". The strength of binding of the GDP then depends on the presence or absence of a ligand on the extracellular receptor; receptor occupancy lowers the GDP-binding affinity and GTP can replace the GDP and "switch on" the G-protein. However, in the absence of extracellular receptor occupancy the GDP is bound strongly and the second messenger system is "switched off".

Activation (switching on) of the G-protein system may either:

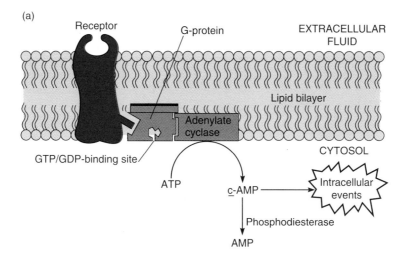

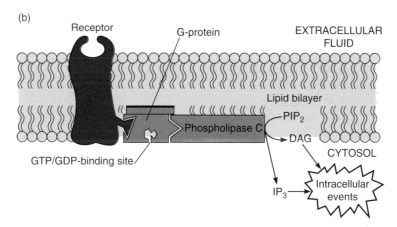

Figure 1.3 Role of G-proteins and second messengers in transmembrane signal transduction. cAMP, Cyclic AMP; IP_3, inositol-1,4,5-triphosphate; DAG, diacylglycerol; PIP_2, phosphatidyl-inositol-4,5-bisphosphate (IP_3 linked to the free glycerol hydroxyl group of DAG via a phosphate diester linkage).

- Activate adenylate cyclase, which increases intracellular cAMP; for example G-proteins linked to β-adrenoceptors or histamine H_2 receptors.

- Inhibit adenylate cyclase, which lowers intracellular cAMP; for example, G-proteins linked to α_2-adrenoceptors and muscarinic (M_2) receptors.

- Activate phospholipase C, which produces second messengers in both the cytoplasm (IP_3) and cell membrane (diacyl glycerol DAG); for example, G-proteins linked to α_1-adrenoceptors and muscarinic (M_1 and M_3) receptors.

The translation of the second messenger into further intracellular responses is complex and may involve changes in enzyme activity or ionic composition either directly or via changes in local intracellular Ca^{2+} concentration.

Tolerance to drug effects may occur without either up-regulation or down-regulation of the numbers of receptors. This phenomenon is termed *desensitization* (a decrease in response with repeated doses) and is seen with various systems. Desensitization may arise from:

- Changes in the functional coupling of the receptor to the G-protein.

- Changes in the G-protein linked enzymes such as adenylate cyclase or phosphodiesterase.

- Depletion of an activation process; for example, chronic administration of organic nitrates may deplete the SH groups necessary for the generation of NO (see angina, Chapter 6); high doses of indirectly acting sympathomimetic amines may cause depletion of neuronal noradrenaline which is necessary for their activity (see Chapter 4).

OTHER SITES OF DRUG ACTION

In addition to actions at ion channels and second messenger systems discussed above, drugs may also bind to and either activate or inhibit other specific sites such as:

- *Cytosolic receptor proteins*; for example, steroids cross the cell membrane and bind to a cytosolic protein. This complex enters the nucleus where cellular protein synthesis is altered.
- *Specific cell membrane ion-pumps*; for example, Na^+/K^+-ATPase in the brain is activated by the anticonvulsant phenytoin and in cardiac tissue is inhibited by digoxin; K^+/H^+-ATPase in gastric parietal cells is inhibited by omeprazole.
- *Specific enzymes*; for example, a number of anticancer drugs inhibit enzymes involved in purine, pyrimidine or DNA synthesis (e.g. methotrexate).
- *Specific organelles*; for example, some antibiotics interfere with the functioning of the bacterial ribosome.
- *Specific transport proteins*; for example, probenecid inhibits renal tubular secretion of anions.

MECHANISMS OF DRUG ACTION

Specific mechanisms of drug action will be introduced throughout this book. In broad terms these compounds can be classified as:

(a) *Agonists* — where the compound binds to the receptor or site of action, produces a conformational change in the receptor and mimics the action of the normal ligand. The action of the compound will be additive with the natural ligand at low concentrations. Drugs may differ in both the affinity or strength of binding and in the rate of binding/dissociation. The affinity of the drug for the receptor determines the concentration necessary to produce a response and therefore is directly related to the *potency* of the drug. In the examples in Fig. 1.4, drug A_1 is more potent than drug A_2 but both are capable of giving a maximal response. For some

compounds a maximal response may require all of the receptors to be occupied whereas for other drugs the maximal response may be produced while some receptors remain unoccupied, that is, there may be spare receptors. The presence of spare receptors becomes important when considering changes in receptor numbers due to adaptive responses during chronic treatment (tolerance) or due to irreversible binding of an antagonist (see later). The rate of binding/dissociation is of negligible importance in determining the rates of onset or termination of effect *in vivo* because these depend mainly on the rates of delivery to and removal from the target organ, that is, on the overall absorption or elimination rate of the drug from the body (Chapter 2).

(b) *Antagonists* — where the compound binds to the receptor but does not cause the necessary conformational change. The compound will block access of the normal ligand. Thus the drug effect may only be detectable when the natural agonist is present (e.g. β-adrenoceptor antagonists lower heart rate particularly when heart rate is increased by stimulation of the sympathetic nervous system). The binding of most clinically useful antagonists is reversible and competitive so that the receptor blockade can be overcome by an increase in the concentration of the natural receptor ligand, or by the administration of an agonist drug. Thus most antagonist drugs move the dose–response graph for an agonist to the right but do not alter the maximum possible response (Fig. 1.4).

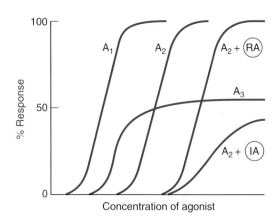

Figure 1.4 Dose–response curves for agonists in the absence or presence of an antagonist. A_1, A_2, two different agonists (A_1 more potent than A_2); A_3, partial agonist; RA, reversible antagonist; IA, irreversible antagonist.

Irreversible antagonists such as phenoxybenzamine bind covalently to their site of action.

(c) *Partial agonists* — where the drug shows both agonist and antagonist properties and the activity expressed at any time is dependent on the concentration of the natural agonist. Stimulation of the receptor produces a submaximal response, possibly due to incomplete amplification of the receptor signal via the G-proteins. A partial agonist will show agonist activity at low concentrations of the natural ligand but the dose–response will not reach the maximal activity even when all receptors are occupied (see Fig. 1.4 — drug A_3). At high concentrations of the natural ligand it will behave as an antagonist by preventing access of the ligand to the receptor, and thereby resulting in a submaximal response.

The *efficacy* of a drug is its ability to produce the maximal response, and therefore agonists may vary in both potency and efficacy. The effect of changes in the numbers of receptors on the dose–response curve for agonists depends on their potency, receptor occupancy and efficacy. This can be illustrated by a consideration of the theoretical situation illustrated in Table 1.1, for a membrane which contains 100 receptors. Drug A is the most potent and there are spare receptors at maximal response. Drug B gives 100% response when 100% of receptors are occupied and drug C is a partial agonist. With downregulation of receptors the response obtained depends upon the extent of downregulation in relation to the extent of occupancy necessary to produce a maximal response (see Table

1.1). [In practice drug effects will be produced at concentrations that do not produce 100% receptor occupancy. Under such circumstances the extent of any effect will depend also on the slope of the dose–response curve, but the concept illustrated in the table will still apply.]

Agonists and antagonists also display a further important property, *selectivity*, that is the extent to which they act preferentially on particular receptor types. Many drugs are specific in that they act only on one class of receptor, for example noradrenergic, but they may affect receptor subtypes, for example β_1 and β_2, to different extents. For such drugs it would be possible to determine dose–response relationships for both receptor subtypes and the selectivity of the drug is the measure of the separation of the dose–response for different receptor subtypes. For example, the β-adrenoceptor antagonist, propranolol, is a non-selective antagonist acting equally on β_1- and β_2-receptors, whereas atenolol shows selectivity towards β_1-receptors, and has less effect on β_2 receptors. The expression of selectivity is dependent on the dose or concentration used since high concentrations will give a maximal blockade at both receptor subtypes (Fig. 1.5).

(d) *Allosteric modulators* — where the drug does not act directly on the ligand/receptor site but may bind elsewhere on the receptor to enhance or decrease the binding of the natural ligand to its receptor. An example is the benzodiazepine class of drugs which alter the affinity of chloride channels for the neurotransmitter GABA.

Table 1.1 Responses for a hypothetical tissue which contains 100 receptors

	Condition	Drug A	B	C
(a) % maximal response with 100 receptors occupied	N	100	100	50
(b) Concentration giving 100% receptor occupancy (μM)	N	1	2	2
(c) Numbers of receptors occupied to give greatest effect seen (100% maximal for A & B, 50% maximal for C)	N	40	100	100
(d) % response at concentrations giving 100% receptor occupancy in normal tissue (see (b) above)	DR (50%)	100	50	25
(e) % response at concentrations given 100% receptor occupancy in normal tissue (see (b) above)	DR (20%)	50	20	10

N, normal tissue.

DR, downregulated tissue so that preparation contains either 50% or 20% of the normal numbers of receptors.

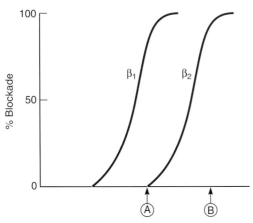

Figure 1.5   Effect of concentration on selectivity. β_1, Dose–response on β_1-adrenoceptor-mediated effects; β_2, dose–response on β_2-adrenoceptor-mediated effects; A, concentration showing maximal selectivity; B, concentration showing no selectivity.

(e) *Enzyme inhibitors/activators* — where the site of action is an enzyme and the drug acts either on the catalytic or allosteric site.

(f) *Non-specific action* — where the presence of the compound has a generalized effect which causes the desired therapeutic outcome. Examples are modulation of neuronal cell membrane fluidity by general anaesthetics and the action of osmotic diuretics on the kidney.

Finally, it must be emphasized that:

- Not all effects seen following drug administration are due to the drug (the placebo effect can be very powerful!).
- Nearly all drugs show multiple effects no matter how receptor selective they are.
- Not all effects produced by a drug will be therapeutically beneficial.

2

Pharmacokinetics

The therapeutic effects seen when a drug is taken by a patient, for example lowering of blood pressure, are determined by the pharmacological properties of the compound. These effects are usually produced by an interaction of the drug with a specific macromolecule, such as a receptor or enzyme (Chapter 1). This aspect is termed the *pharmacodynamics* of the drug and is the subject of subsequent chapters. In contrast, the time to onset of action and the duration and intensity of effect are usually determined by the rate at which the drug is transferred from the site of administration to the site of action and the rate at which it is eliminated from the body by metabolism or excretion. These aspects are called the *pharmacokinetics* of the drug which, as the name implies, is concerned with all processes involved in the movements of the drug within the body.

Pharmacokinetics may be divided into three basic processes:

(1) *Absorption* — The transfer of the drug from the site of administration to the general circulation.
(2) *Distribution* — the transfer of the drug from the general circulation into the different organs of the body.
(3) *Elimination* — the removal of the drug from the body which may involve either *excretion* or *metabolism.*

Each of these processes will be described in terms of their chemical, biochemical and physiological basis and in mathematical terms. For many students the mathematics remain abstract concepts that seem to relate poorly to the more readily understood biology of the processes. To help to relate the biology to the mathematics, those clinical variables which can affect drug handling, such as drug interactions, age and disease, are discussed at the end of the chapter in both biological and mathematical terms.

THE BIOLOGICAL BASIS OF PHARMACOKINETICS

It will be readily apparent to the student familiar with the intermediary metabolism of carbohydrates, fats, proteins, etc. that most of the drug structures given in this book bear little resemblance to such endogenous molecules. Although drugs may bind to particular macromolecular sites, such as the receptor for a specific neurotransmitter, they are only rarely substrates for the carrier processes or metabolizing enzymes which handle the natural ligand. Thus the movement of drugs around the body is usually by simple passive diffusion, whilst metabolism is usually by "drug metabolizing enzymes" of low substrate specificity. However, students should be aware that there are exceptions to each of the generalizations in this chapter but that these generalizations provide an essential framework.

GENERAL CONSIDERATIONS

With the exception of direct intravenous or intra-arterial injections a drug must cross at least one membrane in its movement from the site of administration into the general circulation. The main mechanisms by which drugs can cross membranes are illustrated in Fig. 2.1.

Passage through membrane pores or ion channels down a concentration gradient can only occur for extremely small (mol.wt <100 Da) water soluble molecules, and therefore is applicable only to therapeutic ions such as lithium and radioactive iodide.

Carrier mediated processes include *facilitated diffusion* in which energy is not consumed and the drug cannot be transported against a concentration gradient and *active transport*, an energy-dependent mechanism resulting in accumulation of the drug on one side of the membrane. In each case the drug substrate resembles the natural ligand sufficiently to bind to the carrier macromolecule, but the strength of binding is such that it is also readily released. Examples include levodopa (Chapter 25) which crosses the blood–brain barrier by facilitated diffusion and base analogues such as 5-fluorouracil (Chapter 55) which undergoes active uptake. Drugs that bind to carrier proteins but are only slowly released act as inhibitors of the carrier, for example probenecid inhibits the secretion of anions such as penicillins by the renal tubule.

Pinocytosis could be regarded as a form of "carrier" mediated entry into the cell cytoplasm. This process is normally concerned with the uptake of macromolecules, but attempts are currently underway to utilize it for targeted drug uptake by incorporating the drug into a lipid vesicle or liposome.

Passive diffusion down a concentration gradient applies to all drugs. The drug must pass into the phospholipid bilayer (see Fig. 2.1), and therefore has to have a degree of lipid solubility. Eventually a state of equilibrium will be reached in which equal concentrations of the diffusible form of the drug are present in solution on each side of the membrane.

A number of reversible and irreversible processes can influence the total concentration of drug present on each side of the membrane (Fig. 2.2). Ionization of the drug is a fundamental property of most drugs and will occur whenever the drug is in solution. Drug receptors are formed by the three-dimensional arrangement of a specific section of a protein, and drug binding requires both lipid and water solubility sites within the drug molecule; the latter are usually produced by an ionizable functional group, for example:

$$DCOOH \rightleftharpoons DCOO^- + H^+$$
$$H^+ + D\text{–}NH_2 \rightleftharpoons D\text{–}NH_3^+$$

In general terms the ionized form of the molecule is of negligible lipid solubility compared with the unionized form. Thus the ease with which a drug can enter and therefore cross a lipid bilayer is determined by the lipid solubility of its unionized form. Drugs which are fixed in their ionized form such as quaternary amines,

$$-\overset{\displaystyle |}{\underset{\displaystyle |}{C}}-\overset{\displaystyle |}{\underset{\displaystyle |}{N}}{}^{\oplus}-\overset{\displaystyle |}{\underset{\displaystyle |}{C}}-$$

cross membranes extremely slowly or not at all.

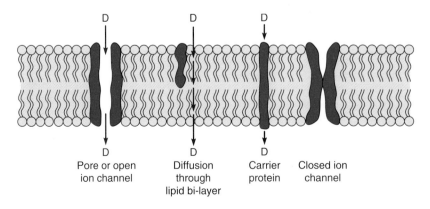

Pore or open ion channel   Diffusion through lipid bi-layer   Carrier protein   Closed ion channel

Figure 2.1 The passage of drugs across membrane bilayers. D, drug molecule.

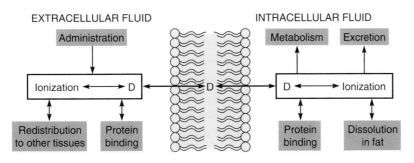

EXTRACELLULAR FLUID   INTRACELLULAR FLUID

Figure 2.2 Passive diffusion and factors which can affect the concentration of drug freely available in solution (as an equilibrium between unionized and ionized forms).

For ionizable groups which exist as an equilibrium, the extent of ionization in pure water is given by the acid dissociation constant K_a. For the equation

$$\text{conjugate acid} \rightleftharpoons \text{conjugate base} + H^+$$

$$K_a = \frac{[\text{conjugate base}]\,[H^+]}{[\text{conjugate acid}]}$$

The value of K_a is normally low (e.g. 10^{-5}) and therefore it is easier to compare compounds using the negative logarithm of the K_a, that is the pK_a (e.g. 5). For *acidic functional groups* such as –COOH, the ionized form is the conjugate base (–COO$^-$) and therefore the stronger the acid, the greater the value of K_a and the smaller the value of pK_a. Thus strongly acidic groups (such as –SO$_3$H) have a pK_a of 1–2 whilst weakly acid groups (such as the phenolic –OH) have a pK_a of 9–10. In contrast, for *basic functional groups* such as –NH$_2$ the ionized form is the conjugate acid (–NH$_3^+$) and therefore the stronger the base the lower will be the K_a and the higher the pK_a. Thus strongly basic groups (such as –NH$_2$) have a pK_a of around 10–11 while weakly basic groups (such as R$_3$N, where R is an alkyl group) have a pK_a of about 2–3.

The pH of body fluids is controlled by the buffering capacity of the ionic groups present in endogenous molecules. Therefore the extent of ionization of a drug in the body is determined by both pK_a of the drug and the pH of the fluid in which it is dissolved. The relationship is given by the Henderson–Hasselbach equation:

$$pH = pK_a + \log \frac{[\text{conjugate base}]}{[\text{conjugate acid}]}$$

or

$$pH - pK_a = \log \frac{[\text{conjugate base}]}{[\text{conjugate acid}]}$$

When the drug is 50% ionized then

$$[\text{conjugate base}] = [\text{conjugate acid}]$$

and

$$\frac{[\text{conjugate base}]}{[\text{conjugate acid}]} = 1$$

and

$$\log \frac{[\text{conjugate base}]}{[\text{conjugate acid}]} = 0$$

$$pH = pK_a$$

When the pH exceeds the pK_a then $(pH - pK_a)$ is greater than zero and [conjugate base] exceeds [conjugate acid]. For an acid group this means that there is greater than 50% ionization, while for a basic group there is less than 50% ionization. Conversely when the pH is less than the pK_a then $(pH - pK_a)$ is less than zero and [conjugate acid] exceeds [conjugate base]. Under these conditions the ionization of bases is increased while that of acids is decreased (Fig. 2.3). Some drugs have more than one ionizable functional group and therefore the relationship between pH and ionization is more complex.

Such basic physicochemical properties are important where the fluids on each side of a membrane (see Fig. 2.2) are at different pH values, for example in the stomach and renal tubule where the pH of the extracellular fluid is significantly less than that of the cell

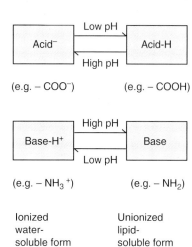

Figure 2.3 The effect of pH on drug ionization.

cytoplasm. At equilibrium there will be equal concentrations of diffusible (unionized) drug on each side of the membrane, but the concentration of ionized drug (see Fig. 2.2) will be determined by the pH of the solution and the pK_a of the drug (see Fig. 2.3). Therefore, the total concentration of drug will be higher on the side of the membrane where it is most ionized, a concept known as pH partitioning (Fig. 2.4). This has implications for drug absorption from the stomach and the renal elimination of drugs, the clinical importance of which will become apparent when considering treatment of drug overdose by altering the urine pH (Chapter 57).

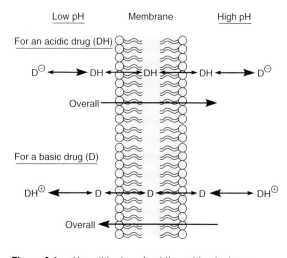

Figure 2.4 pH partitioning of acidic and basic drugs.

ABSORPTION

Absorption from the gut

The most common route of administration of medicines is orally by tablets, capsules or syrups, for reasons of ease and convenience; however, this route is the most complex and presents the greatest number of barriers prior to reaching the systemic circulation. A number of factors can affect the rate and extent to which a drug can pass from the gut lumen into the general circulation.

(i) *Drug structure*
As described above a drug needs to be lipid soluble to cross membranes. Therefore highly polar acids and bases, for example tubocurarine, tend to be absorbed only slowly and much of the dose is voided in the faeces without undergoing absorption. An additional problem is that the drug structure may make it unstable either at the low pH of the stomach, for example penicillin G, or in the presence of digestive enzymes, for example insulin and cocaine. Such compounds have to be given by injection.

Drugs that are weak acids or bases may undergo pH partitioning between the gut lumen and mucosal cells. Thus acidic drugs will be least ionized in the stomach lumen and most absorption would be expected at this site. However, the potential for absorption in the stomach is decreased by a low surface area and the presence of a zone at neutral pH on the immediate surface of the gastric mucosal cells. In consequence even weak acids such as aspirin tend to be absorbed mainly from the small intestine. Basic drugs are most ionized in the stomach so that absorption does not occur until the drug has passed from the stomach to the small intestine.

(ii) *Formulation*
Most tablets disintegrate and dissolve rapidly and completely so that all the dose becomes available for absorption. However, some formulations disintegrate slowly so that the rate at which the drug is absorbed is limited by the formulation rather than the transfer of the dissolved drug across the gut wall. This is the basis for *modified-release formulations* (e.g. slow-release) in which the drug either is incorporated into a complex matrix from which it diffuses or is administered in a crystallized form which dissolves only slowly. Dissolution of a tablet in the stomach can be prevented by coating it in an acid-insoluble layer, producing an *enteric-coated formulation*.

(iii) *Gastric emptying*

The rate of gastric emptying determines the rate at which a drug is delivered to the major site of absorption, the small intestine. A delay between dose administration and the detection of the drug in the circulation is seen frequently after oral dosing and is usually due to delayed gastric emptying. The co-administration of drugs which slow gastric emptying, for example anticholinergics, can alter the rate of drug absorption.

Food has a complex effect on drug absorption since it reduces the rate of gastric emptying and can alter the total amount of drug absorbed.

(iv) *Metabolism*

Drugs taken orally have to pass four major metabolic barriers before they reach the general circulation for distribution to the body tissues:

(1) *Intestinal lumen* — which contains digestive enzymes secreted by the mucosal cells and pancreas. These enzymes are able to split amide, ester and glycosidic bonds. In addition, the lower bowel contains large numbers of aerobic and anaerobic bacteria capable of performing a range of metabolic reactions, especially hydrolysis and reduction.
(2) *Intestinal wall* — which is rich in enzymes such as monoamine oxidase (MAO), L-aromatic amino acid decarboxylase and those responsible for the phase 2 conjugation reactions (see below).
(3) *Liver* — which is the major site of drug metabolism in the body (see below).
(4) *Lung* — which has a high affinity for the uptake of many basic drugs and is the main site of metabolism for many local hormones via MAO or peptidase activity.

The effect of metabolism at these sites is that only a fraction of the administered oral dose may reach the general circulation. This process is known as *first-pass metabolism* because it occurs at the first passage through these organs. The liver is generally the most important site of first-pass metabolism, and this can be avoided by administration of the drug to a region of the gut from which the blood does not drain into the hepatic portal vein, for example the buccal cavity and rectum. A good example is the buccal administration of glyceryl trinitrate (Chapter 6).

Absorption from other routes

Percutaneous administration

The human epidermis and especially the stratum corneum represents an effective permeability barrier to water loss and to the transfer of water-soluble compounds. Although lipid-soluble drugs are able to cross this barrier the rate and extent of entry are very limited. In consequence this route is only really effective for use with potent non-irritant drugs, such as glyceryl trinitrate, or to produce a local effect.

Intradermal and subcutaneous injection

This avoids the barrier presented by the stratum corneum and entry into the general circulation is limited largely by the blood flow to the site of injection. However, these sites only allow the administration of small volumes of drug and tend to be used for local effects such as local anaesthesia, or to limit the rate of drug absorption, for example insulin.

Intramuscular injection

The rate of absorption from the site of injection depends on two variables: the local blood flow and the water solubility of the drug. Absorption of drugs can be prolonged either by incorporation of the drug into a lipid vehicle or by formation of a sparingly soluble salt, such as procaine penicillin, thereby creating a depot formulation.

Inhalation

Although the lungs possess the characteristics of a good site for drug absorption, that is, they have a large surface area and extensive blood flow, inhalation is rarely used to produce systemic effects. The principal reason for this is the difficulty of delivering drugs to the alveoli. Thus inhalation is largely restricted to:

(1) Volatile compounds — such as general anaesthetics.
(2) Potent agents — such as ergotamine for migraine since this route avoids the gastric stasis which is a common feature of a migraine attack.
(3) Locally acting drugs — such as bronchodilators used in asthma.

The last two groups present technical problems for administration since the drugs are not volatile and have to be given either as aerosols containing the drug or as fine particles of the solid drug. Particles greater than 10 μm in diameter settle out in the upper airways which are poor sites for absorption, and the drug then passes back up the airways via ciliary motion and is eventually swallowed. Even when the administration technique generates mostly small particles (i.e. $5 \mu m$ or less) it has been estimated that only 5–10% of the dose may be absorbed across the airways. If the particles are less than $1 \mu m$ in diameter then they are not deposited in the airways and are exhaled.

Minor routes

Although drugs may be applied to all body surfaces and orifices this is usually to produce a local and not a systemic effect. However, absorption with subsequent metabolism and excretion may be important in removing the compound from the body, or producing unwanted systemic actions.

DISTRIBUTION

Distribution is the process by which the drug is transferred from the general circulation into the tissues. For most drugs this occurs by simple diffusion of the unionized form across cell membranes until equilibrium is reached (see Fig. 2.2 and above). Once an equilibrium has been established any process which removes the drug from one side of the membrane will result

in a movement of drug across the membrane to re-establish the equilibrium. Considering the processes shown in Fig. 2.2:

(a) *Administration* — immediately after drug administration the concentration in extracellular fluid is high and therefore there is a net transfer of drug into tissues and the tissue-to-plasma concentration ratio will rise.

(b) *Ionization* — is a simple pH-dependent equilibrium (see above).

(c) *Redistribution to other tissues* — can occur during input, when plasma concentrations are increasing and during elimination, when plasma concentrations fall. When drugs are given by intravenous administration there is an extremely high initial plasma concentration and the drug may rapidly enter and equilibrate with well-perfused tissues such as the brain, liver and lung (Table 2.1). However, poorly perfused tissues will not have reached equilibrium and so the drug will continue to enter these tissues and thereby lower the plasma concentration. Since the rapidly perfused tissues remain in equilibrium with plasma during this phase, the lowering of plasma concentrations will result in a transfer of drug back from those tissues into the plasma (Fig. 2.5). In reality the uptake into well-perfused tissues is so rapid that they may be assumed to equilibrate instantaneously with plasma and, therefore, represent part of the "central" compartment (see later).

Table 2.1 Relative organ perfusion rates in humans*

Organ	% Cardiac output	Blood flow ($ml\ min^{-1}\ 100\ g^{-1}$)
Well perfused		
Lung	100	1000
Adrenals	1	550
Kidneys	23	450
Thyroid	2	400
Liver	25	75
Heart	5	70
Intestines	20	60
Brain	15	55
Placenta (full term)	—	10–15
Poorly perfused		
Skin	9	5
Skeletal muscle	16	3
Connective tissue	—	1
Fat	2	1

*Except for the placenta the data are for an adult male under resting conditions.

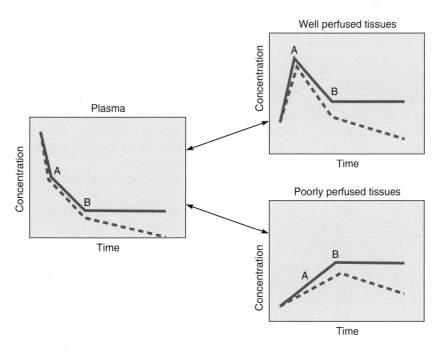

Figure 2.5 A simplified scheme for the redistribution of drugs between tissues. In this diagram the initial decrease in plasma concentrations is due to uptake into well-perfused tissues, which essentially reaches equilibrium at point A. Between points A and B the drug continues to enter poorly perfused tissues which results in a decrease in the concentrations in both plasma and well-perfused tissues. At point B all tissues are in equilibrium. NB — the scheme has been simplified by representing the phases as discreet linear steps and also by the omission of any removal process. The presence of a removal process would produce a parallel decrease in all tissues from point B (shown as - - - - -).

(d) *Elimination processes* — The processes of elimination (i.e. metabolism and excretion) are discussed in detail later. They lower the intracellular drug concentration *in the organ of elimination* so that there is a transfer from plasma to maintain the intracellular concentration. The resultant lowering of the concentration of drug in plasma results in drug transfer from other tissues into plasma in order to maintain their equilibria. Thus there is a net transfer from other tissues to the organ of elimination. Figure 2.5 illustrates how elimination (shown as a dotted line) in well-perfused tissues such as the liver can produce a parallel decrease in drug concentrations in both plasma and poorly perfused tissues.

(e) *Protein binding* — many drugs show an affinity for specific sites on proteins which results in a reversible association or binding:

Drug + protein ⇌ Drug–protein complex

Binding sites occur on circulating proteins such as albumin and α_1-acid glycoprotein and on intracellular proteins. The drug–protein binding interaction resembles drug–receptor interaction in some ways; for example, it is a reversible, saturable process and different ligands can compete for the same site. However, it differs in two extremely important respects:

(1) Drug–protein binding is of low specificity and does not result in any pharmacological effect, but serves simply to lower the concentration of free drug in solution. Thus the "non-receptor" protein binding actually lowers the concentration of drug available to act at the receptor.

(2) Because of the large amounts of "non-receptor" protein in the body the "protein-bound drug" can represent a major part of the total drug present in the body. In contrast the amount of drug bound to receptors usually represents only a minute fraction of the total body load.

The rapidly *reversible* nature of protein binding is important since protein-bound drug can act as a depot. If the intracellular concentration of unbound drug decreases, for example due to metabolism, then this will affect all the equilibria shown in Fig. 2.2. Drug will dissociate from intracellular protein-binding sites, and some will transfer across the membrane from plasma, until the intracellular equilibria are re-established. As a result the extracellular (plasma) concentration of unbound drug will decrease and therefore drug will dissociate from plasma protein-binding sites and also enter the plasma from other tissues until a transmembrane equilibrium is re-established. At equilibrium the ratio of the total amount of drug in the extracellular and intracellular compartments is determined by the ratio of the intra- and extracellular binding affinity constants.

The *competitive* nature of the binding process is shown by competition between different drugs and also between drugs and natural, endogenous ligands. Administration of a second highly protein-bound drug to a patient receiving maintenance therapy with a drug showing reversible plasma protein binding will result in displacement of the initial drug and thereby an increase in its unbound or free concentration. This unbound drug will then be able to cross membranes and to act at either extra- or intracellular receptors. Thus there is the potential for a therapeutically important drug interaction, with a potentiation of the response to the initial drug (Table 2.2). In practice such protein-binding interactions are frequently of limited duration since the extra free drug is available for metabolism and excretion. The most important interaction involving the displacement of an endogenous ligand is the potentially dangerous increase in free unconjugated bilirubin (which binds to albumin) that can occur if jaundiced neonates are given drugs such as sulphonamides which bind to the same sites.

The saturable nature of the binding process is rarely of importance for acidic drugs because of the large excess of albumin compared with the dose usually prescribed. Saturation of binding to α_1-acid glycoprotein may occur for basic drugs because of the low protein concentrations normally present.

Certain drugs, because of their chemical reactivity, undergo covalent binding to plasma or tissue components such as proteins or nucleic acids. When the binding is essentially irreversible, as for example the interaction of some cytotoxic agents with DNA, then this should be considered as an *elimination process*. In contrast the covalent binding of thiol-containing drugs such as the hypotensive drug captopril to proteins via the formation of a disulphide bridge may be slowly reversible. In such cases the covalently bound drug will not dissociate in response to a rapid decrease in the concentration of unbound drug (as happens when the blood passes through a major organ of elimination such as the kidney) and therefore represents a slowly equilibrating reservoir of drug.

Distribution to specific organs

Although the distribution of drugs to all organs is covered by the general considerations discussed above, two systems require more detailed description: the brain, because of the difficulty of drug entry and the fetus, because of the potential for toxicity.

Brain

Lipid-soluble drugs, such as the anaesthetic thiopentone, readily pass from the blood into the brain, and for such drugs the brain represents a typical well-perfused tissue (see Fig. 2.5; Table 2.1). In contrast the entry of water-soluble drugs into the brain is much slower than into other well-perfused tissues and this has given rise to the concept of a "blood–brain barrier". The functional basis of the barrier is reduced capillary permeability due to three components: (i) "tight junctions" between adjacent endothelial cells; (ii) a decrease in the size and number of pores in the cell membranes; and (iii) the presence of a surrounding layer of astrocytes. Since drug molecules have to pass through membranes and cannot diffuse through pores or between cells,

Table 2.2 Examples of drugs which undergo extensive plasma protein binding and which may show therapeutically important interactions

Bound to albumin	Bound to α_1-acid glycoprotein
Clofibrate	Chlorpromazine
Digitoxin	Propranolol
Frusemide	Quinidine
Ibuprofen	Tricyclics
Indomethacin	Lignocaine
Phenytoin	
Salicylates	
Sulphonamides	
Thiazides	
Tolbutamide	
Warfarin	

only lipid-soluble compounds can readily enter the brain. Water-soluble endogenous compounds such as carbohydrates and amino acids are needed for normal brain functioning and there are specific transport processes for these. Some drugs, for example levodopa, may enter the brain via these transport processes and in such cases the rate of transport of the drug will be influenced by the concentrations of competitive endogenous substrates. There is limited drug-metabolizing ability in the brain and drugs leave by diffusion back into plasma, by active transport processes in the choroid plexus, or by elimination in the cerebrospinal fluid.

Fetus

Lipid-soluble drugs can readily cross the placenta and enter the fetus. The placental blood flow is slow compared with that in the liver, lung and spleen (Table 2.1) and thus the fetus may equilibrate slowly with the maternal circulation. Highly polar and large molecules (such as heparin) do not readily cross the placenta. Since the fetal liver has only low levels of drug-metabolizing enzymes, the fetus relies on maternal elimination processes to lower the concentration in the maternal circulation so that the drug can diffuse back across the placenta. After delivery the baby may show effects from drugs received *in utero* via the placenta, and such effects may be prolonged because the infant now has to rely on its own immature elimination processes.

ELIMINATION

Elimination is the removal of drug from the body, and may involve *metabolism*, in which the drug molecule is transformed into a different molecule, and/or *excretion*, in which the drug molecule is expelled in the body's liquid, solid or gaseous "waste".

Metabolism

Lipid solubility is an essential property of most drugs since it allows the compound to cross lipid barriers and hence to be given via the oral route. Metabolism is the principal step for the elimination of lipid-soluble chemicals from the body, since it converts a lipid-soluble molecule, which would be reabsorbed from the kidney tubule, into a water-soluble species which is capable of rapid elimination in the urine. Strictly speaking the drug itself is eliminated as soon as it is transformed into a metabolite because this is a different compound; however, metabolism considers the elimination of the unwanted carbon skeleton of the drug and this may involve a complex series of biotransformation reactions (see later). It is important to realize that metabolism produces a new chemical entity which may show different pharmacological properties. In most cases the increase in polarity which accompanies metabolism results in a decrease in activity although there are numerous examples of altered or enhanced activity due to biotransformation. Some drugs are inactive in the form administered and require a process of metabolic activation to exert their therapeutic effect (these are called *prodrugs*). It should be remembered that for some compounds, first-pass metabolism may limit the amount that enters the general circulation following oral administration.

The various steps of drug metabolism can be divided into two phases (Fig. 2.6). Although many compounds undergo both phases of metabolism it is possible for a chemical to undergo only a Phase 1 or a Phase 2 reaction.

Phase 1 metabolism includes a number of reactions which may modify the drug molecule, and produce a suitable site for a Phase 2 or *conjugation* reaction. Thus Phase 1 reactions are often described as *preconjugation* reactions. The enzymes involved in these reactions are of low substrate specificity and can metabolize a vast range of drug substrates. In this section drug

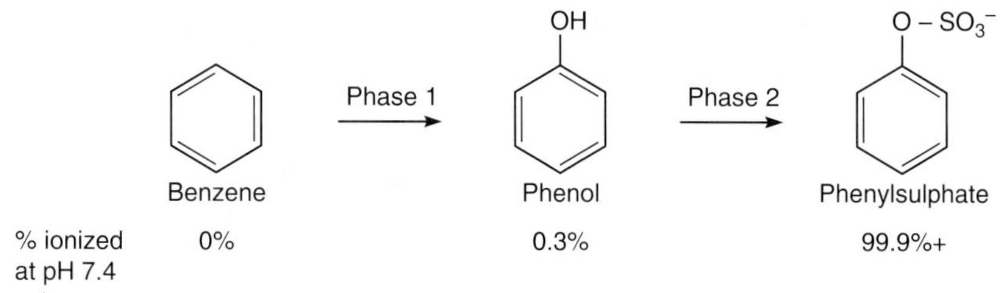

	Benzene	Phenol	Phenylsulphate
		OH	$O-SO_3^-$
% ionized at pH 7.4	0%	0.3%	99.9%+

Benzene →(Phase 1)→ Phenol →(Phase 2)→ Phenylsulphate

Figure 2.6 The two phases of drug metabolism.

metabolism is discussed in terms of the functional groups which may be found in different drugs, rather than individual specific compounds. (In the following tables Ar refers specifically to an aromatic group and R to an alkyl or in some cases an aromatic group.)

Phase 1

Oxidation is by far the most important of these reactions and can involve attack at carbon, nitrogen or sulphur atoms (Table 2.3a). In most cases an oxygen atom is retained in the metabo- lite although some reactions, such as dealkylations, result in loss of the oxygen atom in a small fragment of the original molecule. Oxidation reactions are catalysed by a diverse group of enzymes of which the cytochrome P450 system is the most important. *Cytochrome P450* is a family of membrane-bound enzymes (Table 2.3b) which are present in the smooth endoplasmic reticulum of the cell (Fig. 2.7a). The amounts of cytochrome P450 in extrahepatic tissues are low compared with those in liver and thus the liver is the major site of drug oxidation.

Table 2.3a Oxidation reactions

Oxidation at carbon atoms

Aromatic	$ArH \longrightarrow ArOH$
Alkyl	$RCH_3 \longrightarrow RCH_2OH \longrightarrow RCHO \longrightarrow RCOOH$
Dealkylation	$ROCH_3 \longrightarrow ROH + HCHO$
	$RNHCH_3 \longrightarrow RNH_2 + HCHO$
Deamination	$RCH_2NH_2 \longrightarrow RCHO + NH_3$
	$RCH(CH_3)NH_2 \longrightarrow RCO(CH_3) + NH_3$

Oxidation at nitrogen atoms

Secondary amines

$$\overset{H}{\underset{|}{R-N-R}} \longrightarrow \overset{OH}{\underset{|}{R-N-R}}$$

Tertiary amines $R_3N \longrightarrow R_3N{\rightarrow}O$

Oxidation at sulphur atoms

Thioethers $R-S-R \longrightarrow \overset{O}{\underset{\uparrow}{R-S-R}}$

Table 2.3b The cytochrome P450 superfamily

Isoenzyme	Typical substrate	Comments
CYP1A	Theophylline	Induced by smoking
CYP2A	Testosterone	Induced by polycyclic hydrocarbons (e.g. smoking)
CYP2B	Numerous	Induced by phenobarbitone
CYP2C	Numerous	Constitutive 2C18 shows genetic polymorphism
CYP2D	Debrisoquine/sparteine	Constitutive 2D6 shows genetic polymorphism
CYP2E	Nitrosamines	Induced by alcohol
CYP3A	Nifedipine/cyclosporine	Main constitutive enzyme induced by carbamazepine
CYP4	Fatty acids	Induced by clofibrate

Notes:
Human liver contains at least 20 isoenzymes of cytochrome P450.
Families 1–4 are related to drugs and their metabolism.
Families 17, 19, 21 and 22 are related to steroid biosynthesis.

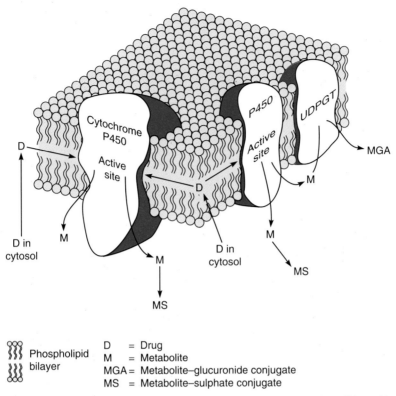

Phospholipid bilayer

D = Drug
M = Metabolite
MGA = Metabolite–glucuronide conjugate
MS = Metabolite–sulphate conjugate

Figure 2.7a Drug metabolism in the smooth endoplasmic reticulum. The lipid-soluble drug (D) partitions into the lipid bilayer of the endoplasmic reticulum. The cytochrome P450 oxidizes the drug to a metabolite (M) which is more water soluble and diffuses out of the lipid layer. The metabolite may undergo a phase 2 (conjugation reaction) with UDP-glucuronyl transferase (UDPGT) in the endoplasmic reticulum or sulphate conjugation in the cytosol.

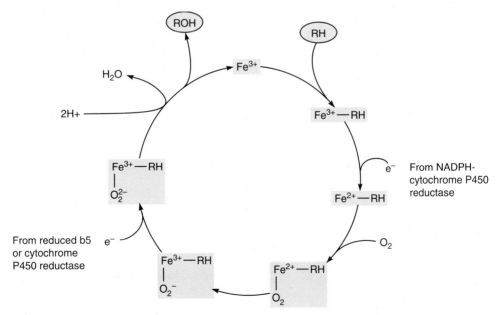

Figure 2.7b The oxidation of substrate (RH) by cytochrome P450. Fe^{3+}, the active site of cytochrome P450 in its ferric state; RH, drug substrate; ROH, oxidized metabolite. Cytochrome b5 is present in the endoplasmic reticulum and can transfer an electron to cytochrome P450 as part of its redox reactions.

Table 2.4 Reduction reactions

Reduction at carbon atoms
  Aldehydes $RCHO \longrightarrow RCH_2OH$
  Ketones $RCOR \longrightarrow RCHOHR$

Reduction at nitrogen atoms
  Nitro groups $ArNO_2 \longrightarrow ArNO \longrightarrow ArNHOH \longrightarrow ArNH_2$
  Azo group $ArN{=}NAr' \longrightarrow ArNH_2 + H_2NAr'$

Reduction at sulphur atoms

$$\qquad\qquad\qquad\quad O$$
$$\qquad\qquad\qquad\quad \uparrow$$
  Sulphoxides $R{-}S{-}R \longrightarrow R{-}S{-}R$
  Disulphides $R{-}S{-}S{-}R' \longrightarrow RSH + HSR'$

Cytochrome P450 is a haemoprotein which can bind both the drug and molecular oxygen and catalyses the transfer of one oxygen atom to the substrate while the other oxygen atom is reduced to water:

$$RH + O_2 + NADPH \longrightarrow ROH + H_2O$$
$$+ H^+ \qquad\qquad\qquad + NADP^+$$

The reaction involves initial binding of the substrate to the ferric (Fe^{3+}) form of cytochrome P450 (Fig. 2.7b) followed by a reduction (via a specific cytochrome P450 reductase) and binding of molecular oxygen. The cytochrome P450 drug/oxygen complex is further reduced following which molecular rearrangement occurs with splitting off of the reaction products and regeneration of ferric cytochrome P450.

Although cytochrome P450 can effect oxidations at nitrogen and sulphur atoms these are frequently performed by a second enzyme of the endoplasmic reticulum, the *flavin-containing mono-oxygenase*, which also requires molecular oxygen and NADPH. Although these two microsomal enzyme systems are responsible for the majority of oxidation reactions on foreign compounds, a number of other enzymes such as alcohol dehydrogenase, aldehyde oxidase and monoamine oxidase may be involved in the oxidation of specific functional groups.

Reduction can occur at unsaturated carbon atoms, and at nitrogen and sulphur centres (Table 2.4), although such reactions are less common than oxidations. Reduction reactions can be performed both by the body tissues and also by the intestinal microflora. The tissue enzymes include cytochrome P450 and cytochrome P450 reductase, both of which can perform reduction reactions under anaerobic conditions. In addition, appropriate functional groups may be reduced by cytosolic aldehyde reductase and ketone reductase. Also, xanthine oxidase and aldehyde oxidase can reduce drugs at the same time as they oxidize their normal substrates (e.g. xanthine or an aldehyde).

Hydrolysis and *hydration* reactions (Table 2.5) both involve addition of water to the drug molecule. In the case of hydrolysis the drug molecule is split by the addition of water in a reaction comparable to that in the intermediary metabolism of polysaccharides and polypeptides. A number of enzymes present in many tissues are able to hydrolyse ester and amide bonds in drugs. The intestinal flora are also an important site of hydrolysis for esters and amides such as drug conjugates eliminated in the bile (see later). In hydration reactions the water molecule is retained in the drug metabolite. The hydration of the epoxide ring to produce a dihydrodiol (Table 2.5) is performed by a microsomal enzyme epoxide hydrolase. This is an important reaction in the metabolism and toxicity of a number of aromatic compounds.

Table 2.5 Hydrolysis and hydration reactions

Hydrolysis reactions
  Esters
  $RCO.OR' \longrightarrow RCOOH + HOR'$
  Amides
  $RCO.NHR' \longrightarrow RCOOH + H_2NR'$

Hydration reactions
  Epoxides

Table 2.6 Major conjugation reactions

Reaction	Functional group	Activated species	Product
Glucuronidation	–OH –COOH –NH$_2$	UDPGA (uridine diphosphate glucuronic acid)	
Sulphation	–OH –NH$_2$	PAPS (3′-phosphoadenosine 5′-phosphosulphate)	–O–SO$_3$H –NH–SO$_3$H
Acetylation	–NH$_2$ –NHNH$_2$	Acetyl-CoA	–NH–COCH$_3$ –NHNH–COCH$_3$
Methylation	–OH –NH$_2$ –SH	*S*-Adenosyl methionine	–OCH$_3$ –NHCH$_3$ –SCH$_3$
Amino acid	–COOH	Drug – CoA	CO–NHCHRCOOH
Glutathione	Various	—	Glutathione conjugate

Phase 2

Phase 2 or conjugation reactions involve the biosynthesis of a covalent chemical bond between the drug and a normal tissue constituent or endogenous substrate. Energy to synthesize the bond is supplied by activation of either the drug or the endogenous substrate. The types of Phase 2 reactions are listed in Table 2.6 and it is clear that in most cases the reaction involves an activated endogenous substrate. The products of conjugations are usually of greater water solubility and lower toxicity than the substrate, although there are exceptions to both of these generalizations.

Glucuronide synthesis utilizes uridine-diphosphate glucuronic acid (UDPGA) as the activated endogenous substrate, which is synthesized from UDP-glucose. The enzymes which transfer the glucuronic acid moiety to the drug (UDP-glucuronyl transferases) are in the endoplasmic reticulum, close to the cytochrome P450 system the products of which frequently undergo glucuronidation (Figure 2.7a). Glucuronide synthesis occurs in many tissues, especially the gut wall and liver, where it may contribute significantly to the first-pass metabolism of substrates such as simple phenols. In contrast *sulphate* conjugation is performed by a cytosolic enzyme which utilizes high energy sulphate (3′-phosphoadenosine-5′-phosphosulphate or PAPS) as the endogenous substrate. The capacity for sulphate conjugation is limited

by the availability of the endogenous substrate (PAPS) rather than the transferase enzyme, and sulphate conjugation is highly dose dependent. Saturation of sulphate conjugation contributes to the metabolic events involved in the liver toxicity seen in paracetamol overdose.

The reactions of *acetylation* and *methylation* frequently produce a decrease in the polarity of the product since they block an ionizable functional group. These reactions mask potentially active functional groups such as amino- and catechol moieties and it is likely that the enzymes are primarily involved in the detoxication of neurotransmitters, such as noradrenaline or local hormones such as histamine.

The conjugation of drug carboxylic acid groups with *amino acids* is of interest since the drug is converted to a high energy form, a CoA derivative, prior to the formation of the conjugate bond. The reaction occurs largely with simple aryl (aromatic) and arylacetic acid compounds (Table 2.6). The enzymes involved in formation of the drug–acyl-CoA derivative are the mitochondrial intermediate chain length fatty acyl CoA synthetases; conjugation with the amino acid is effected by acyl-CoA : amino acid N-acyltransferases.

An important conjugation reaction related to drug toxicity is that with the tripeptide *glutathione* (L-α-glutamyl-L-cysteinylglycine). This reaction is catalysed by a family of transferase enzymes and the drug metabolite is covalently bound to the thiol group in the cysteine

(Fig. 2.8). The substrates are often reactive drugs or activated metabolites, which are inherently unstable (see Chapter 56). Thus glutathione conjugation may be regarded as a true detoxication reaction and acts as a scavenging agent to protect the cell from toxic damage. The initial glutathione conjugate can undergo a series of reactions, either in the tissues or the gut lumen which illustrate well the complexity of drug metabolism, since the molecule undergoes hydrolysis, conjugation and oxidation (Fig. 2.8).

Another good example of a drug which undergoes a complex array of biotransformation reactions is sulphinpyrazone (Fig. 2.9). These involve oxidation by the tissues at various sites in the molecule including the sulphoxide group, reduction by the gut microflora at the sulphoxide group and conjugation with glucuronic acid of phenolic metabolites, as well as at the carbon in position 4 of the heterocyclic ring (which is a very rare reaction only found in man). This drug also illustrates how metabolism can alter pharmacological properties since sulphinpyrazone is a potent uricosuric, while its sulphide metabolite has potent anti-aggregatory activity against platelets.

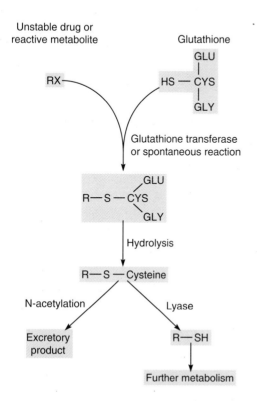

Figure 2.8 The formation and further metabolism of glutathione conjugates.

Excretion

Drugs and their metabolites may be eliminated from the circulation by various routes, dependent on the physicochemical properties of the molecule.

Fluids — urine, sweat, tears, milk, etc. These routes are most important for low molecular weight polar compounds and the urine is the major route. Milk is of importance because of the potential for exposure of the suckling infant.

Solids — faeces, hair, etc. Drugs enter the gastrointestinal tract by various mechanisms (see below) and this route is most important for high molecular weight compounds. The detection of foreign compounds sequestered into hair is not of quantitative importance but due to the slow growth of hair, the distribution of a drug along the hair can be used to indicate drug intake during the preceding weeks.

Gases — expired air. This route is only of importance for volatile compounds.

Excretion via the urine

There are three processes involved in the handling of drugs and their metabolites in the kidney.

(a) *Glomerular filtration* — all molecules less than about 20 000 Da undergo filtration through the 70–80 Å pores in the glomerular membrane, due to the positive hydrostatic pressure. Approximately 20% of the non-protein bound drug enters the filtrate together with a similar amount of plasma water. Thus the unbound drug concentration remaining in plasma is not altered. Plasma proteins and protein-bound drug are not filtered and remain in the blood leaving the glomerulus. Thus the efficiency of glomerular filtration of the drug is influenced by the extent of its binding to plasma protein.

(b) *Reabsorption* — the glomerular filtrate contains a number of constituents which the body cannot afford to lose. Thus there are specific tubular uptake processes for carbohydrates, amino acids, vitamins etc., while most of the water is also reabsorbed. Drugs may pass from the tubule into the plasma if they are substrates for the uptake processes (very rare) or if they are lipid soluble. The urine is concentrated on its passage down the renal tubule and the tubule-to-plasma concentration gradient increases so that only the most polar and least diffusible molecules will remain in the urine. The pH of urine is usually less than that of

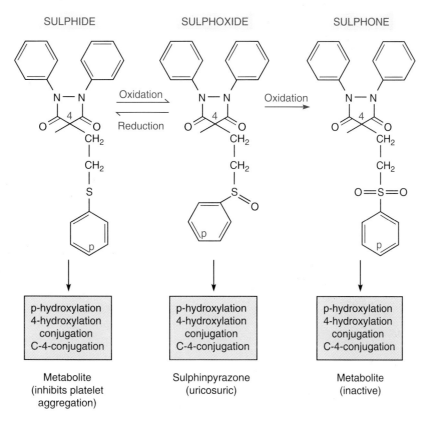

Figure 2.9 The pathways of metabolism of sulphinpyrazone in man and animals. This figure illustrates that a single drug may generate a large number of metabolites, which may possess different pharmacological properties.

plasma, so that pH partitioning may either increase or decrease the tendency of the compound to be reabsorbed (see earlier).

(c) *Tubular secretion* — the renal tubule has secretory mechanisms for both acidic and basic compounds, and drugs and their metabolites may undergo an active carrier-mediated elimination. Because secretion lowers the plasma concentration of unbound drug by an active process, there will be a rapid dissociation of any drug–protein complex so that even highly protein-bound drugs may be cleared almost completely from the blood in a single passage through the kidney.

The total urinary excretion of drug results from the balance of these three processes, that is:

$$\text{Total excretion} = \text{Glomerular filtration} \\ + \text{Tubular secretion} \\ - \text{Reabsorption}$$

Excretion via the faeces

The most important mechanism by which drugs enter the gut lumen is via uptake into hepato-cytes and subsequent elimination in the bile. The bile is the principal route of elimination of larger molecules, which in man is those with a molecular weight greater than about 500 Da. Conjugation with glucuronic acid increases the molecular weight of the substrate by almost 200 Da and therefore the bile is an important site of elimination of glucuronide conjugates.

Once the drug, or its conjugate, has entered the intestinal lumen via the bile, it passes down the gut and eventually may be eliminated in the faeces. However, some drugs may be reabsorbed from the lumen of the gut and re-enter the hepatic portal vein. Thus the drug recirculates between the liver, bile, gut lumen and hepatic portal vein. This is described as an *entero-hepatic circulation*, and it can maintain the drug concentrations in the general circulation because some will not be taken up from the hepatic portal vein by the liver and thereby escape into the systemic circulation. Highly polar glucuronide conjugates excreted into the bile undergo little reabsorption in the upper intestine, but the bacterial flora of

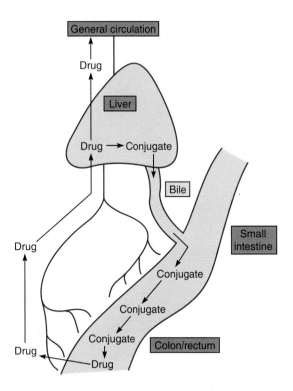

Figure 2.10   The enterohepatic circulation of drugs.

the lower intestine may hydrolyse the conjugate back to the original substrate and glucuronic acid. The original substrate will have a greater lipid solubility and therefore be absorbed from the gut lumen and enter the hepatic portal vein (see Fig. 2.10).

THE MATHEMATICAL BASIS OF PHARMACOKINETICS

The use of mathematics to describe the fate of a drug in the body can be complex and rather daunting for undergraduates. Nevertheless, a basic understanding is invaluable for an appreciation of many aspects of drug handling and for the rational prescribing of drugs. The following account describes the fate of a single dose of a drug and the mathematics of absorption, distribution and elimination, before brief considerations of chronic administration and factors which can affect pharmacokinetic processes.

GENERAL CONSIDERATIONS

Two different but complimentary approaches are used:

(1) *Compartmental analysis* — in which the plasma concentration–time curve is described by an equation containing one or more exponential functions. This approach gives a precise description of concentration–time relationships and allows the prediction of the concentration of the drug in plasma at any time after dosing. This approach requires an appropriate model to be defined and fitted to the data. However, it provides little information on the physiological disposition of the compound.

(2) *Model independent analysis* — may be related more closely to the physiological processes governing the disposition of the chemical and therefore is more useful in predicting and assessing the influence of variables such as disease, age and the administration of other compounds. However, this approach cannot be used to predict the concentration at any time after dosing (unless the compound fits the simplest model possible).

The model independent methods are of greater potential value to medical undergraduates and are the basis of the following account.

Each of the three basic processes of absorption, distribution and elimination will be described in terms of *rate*, that is the speed at which a process occurs, and *extent*, that is the proportion of the dose which is handled by the process.

Before each process is considered in detail it is necessary to define the different types or orders of reaction which commonly occur. If we consider a simple decrease in concentration (e.g. during drug elimination) there are two important types of reaction possible:

(a) *Zero order reactions* — in which the change in concentration $\dfrac{\mathrm{d}C}{\mathrm{d}t}$ occurs at a fixed amount per time, that is:

$$\frac{\mathrm{d}C}{\mathrm{d}t} = -k$$

The units of k (the reaction rate constant) will be an amount per unit time (e.g. $\mu\mathrm{g}\ \mathrm{ml}^{-1}\ \mathrm{min}^{-1}$ or $\mu\mathrm{g}\ \mathrm{min}^{-1}$). A graph of concentration against time will produce a straight line with a slope of $-k$ (Fig. 2.11); examples are ethanol (see Chapter 58) and phenytoin (see Chapter 24).

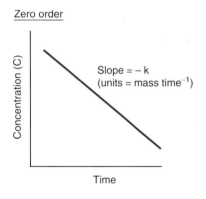

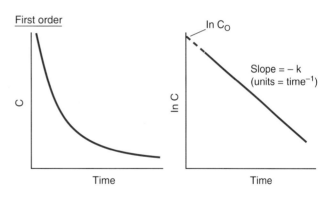

Figure 2.11   Zero and first-order reactions.

(b) *First order reactions* — in which the change in concentration is proportional to the concentration available for the process, that is:

$$\frac{dC}{dt} = -kC$$

The units of k are time^{-1} (e.g. min^{-1}) and k may be regarded as the proportional change in unit time. A graph of concentration against time will produce an exponential decrease since the rate of change will be high at high concentrations, but low at low concentrations (Fig. 2.11). Such a curve can be described by an exponential equation:

$$C = C_0 \, e^{-kt}$$

where C is the concentration at time t and C_0 is the initial concentration (when time $= 0$).

This equation may be written more simply by taking natural logs:

$$\ln C = \ln C_0 - kt$$

and therefore a graph of $\ln C$ (the natural log of the concentration) against time will produce a straight line with a slope of $-k$ and an intercept of $\ln C_0$ (Fig. 2.11).

Most physiological processes are first order reactions with respect to the substrate, that is the rate of reaction is proportional to the amount of substrate available. Examples are diffusion down a concentration gradient and glomerular filtration. Protein-mediated reactions, that is metabolism and active transport, are first order at low concentrations. However, as the substrate concentration increases the protein can become saturated with substrate and the rate of reaction cannot increase in response to a further increase in concentration.

The process then occurs at a fixed maximum rate and the reaction is therefore zero order. If the substrate concentration subsequently decreases so that protein sites become available again, then the change in concentration will proceed at a rate proportional to the concentration available, that is the reaction will revert to first order.

ABSORPTION

The mathematics of absorption apply to all "non-intravenous" routes, for example oral, inhalation, percutaneous, etc., and are illustrated by absorption from the gut lumen.

Rate of Absorption

The rate of absorption after oral administration is determined by the rate at which the drug is able to pass from the gut lumen into the circulation. For lipid-soluble drugs the rate of absorption is greater than the rate of elimination and therefore the plasma concentration–time curve after an oral dose (Fig. 2.12) may be divided into two phases as shown in Fig. 2.12a; the initial steep increase from which the absorption rate constant (k_a) can be calculated and the terminal slope which gives the elimination rate constant (k). In Fig. 2.12a the absorption is essentially complete by point B since the subsequent data are fitted by a single exponential rate constant (the elimination rate). The absorption rate constant (k_a) cannot be calculated directly from the initial slope because elimination occurs as soon as any drug reaches the general circulation. If all the drug entered the circulation instantaneously (at $t = 0$) then the initial

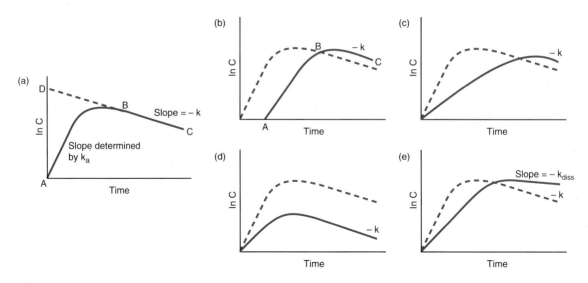

Figure 2.12 Plasma concentration–time curves following oral administration.
(a) General profile (A, start of absorption; B, end of absorption; B–C, elimination (rate = k); D, initial concentration if instantaneous absorption). (This "normal" profile is given as a dotted line in b–e.)
(b) Influence of gastric emptying — delay between $t = 0$ and A.
(c) Influence of food — slower absorption $\therefore$ a reduction in k_a.
(d) Decrease in bioavailability (due to incomplete dissolution of formulation, decomposition, increased first pass metabolism).
(e) Slow release formulation — the rate at which the drug can be eliminated is limited by the rate at which the formulation disintegrates (k_{diss}).

concentrations would be given by point D and the value of k_a would be infinity. In practice k_a is calculated from the difference between the line D–B for each time point and the actual concentration measured (given by the line A–B in Fig. 2.12a).

A number of factors can affect this apparently simple pattern:

(1) *Gastric emptying* — basic drugs undergo negligible absorption from the stomach. Therefore there can be a delay of up to an hour between drug administration and the detection of drug in the general circulation (Fig. 2.12b).

(2) *Food* — can affect the pattern by altering gastric emptying and by affecting the value of k_a (Fig. 2.12c).

(3) *Decomposition or metabolism prior to or during absorption* — the amount of drug which will be able to reach the general circulation will be reduced but the absorption rate will not be affected. Therefore the curve is parallel but at lower concentrations (Fig. 2.12d).

(4) *Modified-release formulation* — if a drug is eliminated rapidly then during regular dosing the plasma concentrations will show rapid swings and patients may have to take the drug at very frequent intervals, for example every 2–3 h (see later). This can be avoided by giving a tablet which releases drug at a slow and usually predictable rate, known as a "modified-release" formulation. These act almost like an intravenous infusion (see later) and the terminal slope is determined by the dissolution rate of the formulation not the elimination rate of the drug (Fig. 2.12e). This results in prolonged plasma concentrations.

Extent of Absorption
The parameter which describes the extent of absorption is the *bioavailability* (F), which is the fraction of the dose which reaches the systemic circulation. For oral administration some of the dose may never reach the general circulation due to two reasons:

(1) *Incomplete absorption* — loss in the faeces either because the molecule is too polar to be absorbed or the tablet did not release all of its contents.

(2) *First-pass metabolism* — in the gut lumen, during passage across the gut wall, or by the liver.

The bioavailability of a drug is determined by comparison of data obtained after oral administration (when the fraction F enters the general circulation as the parent drug) with those following intravenous administration (when 100% enters the general circulation as the parent drug). The amount in the circulation cannot be compared at only one time point since intravenous and oral dosing will show different concentration–time profiles. This is avoided by using the total area under the curve (AUC) from $t = 0$ to $t = $ infinity:

$$F = \frac{\text{AUC}_{\text{oral}}}{\text{AUC}_{\text{iv}}}$$

if the oral and intravenous doses are equal,

or $\qquad F = \dfrac{\text{AUC}_{\text{oral}}}{\text{AUC}_{\text{iv}}} \times \dfrac{\text{dose}_{\text{iv}}}{\text{dose}_{\text{oral}}}$

for different doses.

This calculation assumes that the metabolism is first order. The concept of AUC is discussed later under *clearance*.

An alternative method is to measure the total urinary excretion *of the parent drug* (Aex) following oral and intravenous doses. Even though the urine may be a minor route of elimination the ratio of excretion unchanged after oral to excretion unchanged after intravenous dosing will give the bioavailability:

$$F = \frac{\text{Aex}_{\text{oral}}}{\text{Aex}_{\text{iv}}}$$

for two equal doses,

or $\qquad F = \dfrac{\%\ \text{Dose in urine as parent drug after oral dosing}}{\%\ \text{Dose in urine as parent drug after iv dosing}}$

DISTRIBUTION

This applies to the *reversible* movement of drug from the blood into the tissues such as occurs immediately following an intravenous bolus dose (single rapid injection) and its re-entry into blood as the parent drug during elimination.

Rate of Distribution

The rate of distribution usually can only be measured following an intravenous bolus dose. Some drugs reach equilibrium between blood/plasma and tissues very rapidly and a distinct distribution phase is not seen; only the terminal elimination phase is seen (Fig. 2.13a). Most drugs take some time to distribute into and equilibrate with the tissues. This is shown as a rapid decrease, prior to the terminal elimination phase (which is given the symbol β) (slope B–C in Fig. 2.13b). In Fig. 2.13b the processes of distribution are complete by point B. The distribution rate constant cannot be derived from the slope A–B because elimination starts as soon as the drug enters the body. If distribution had been instantaneous then the initial concentration would be given by the point D and the distribution rate would be infinity. In practice the distribution rate (α) is calculated for the difference between the line D–B for each time point and the actual concentration measured (given by the line A–B in Fig. 2.13b). Clearly situations a and b in Fig. 2.13 have to be described by different models. Figure 2.13a is described as a one-compartment model and all tissues are in equilibrium instantaneously. Figure 2.13b is described as a two-compartment model in which the drug initially enters and reaches instantaneous equilibrium with one compartment (blood and possibly well-perfused tissues) prior to entering more slowly and equilibrating with a second compartment (possibly poorly perfused tissues — refer back to Fig. 2.5). This is shown schematically in Fig. 2.14.

The rate of distribution is dependent on two main variables:

(1) For *water-soluble drugs*, the rate of distribution depends on the rate of passage across membranes, that is the permeability characteristics of the drug.

(2) For *lipid-soluble drugs*, the rate of distribution depends on the rate of delivery to those tissues, such as adipose, which accumulate the drug.

For some drugs the natural logarithm of the plasma concentration–time curve shows three distinct phases and such curves require three exponential rates and represent a three-compartment model. Although two- or three-compartment models may be necessary to give a mathematical description of the data they are of limited practical value since we rarely know which tissues belong to

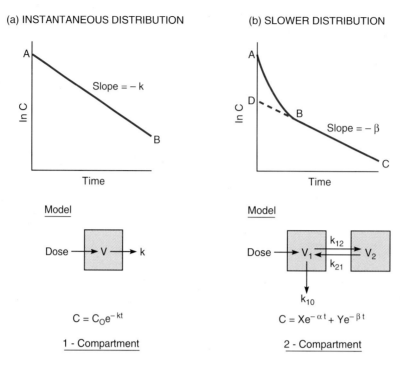

Figure 2.13 Plasma concentration–time curves for the distribution of drugs into one- and two-compartment models. k, α, β, k_{10}, k_{12}, k_{21} are rate constants. α and β are composite rate constants determined by k_{10}, k_{12} and k_{21}. V are volumes. X and Y are constants. (Note: the equation for a 2–compartment system is usually written as $C = Ae^{-\alpha t} + Be^{-\beta t}$ where A and B are constants equivalent to X and Y; X and Y were used to avoid confusion with points A and B on the graph.)

which compartment and more importantly which compartment contains the receptor or site of action of the drug. Thus compartmental analysis has been replaced in recent years by simpler and more physiologically based methods.

Extent of Distribution

The extent of distribution of a drug from blood or plasma into tissues can be determined in animals by measuring concentrations in both blood and all the tissues of the body. However, in man only the blood concentration can be measured and therefore the measurement of distribution has to be made from the amount remaining in blood, or more usually plasma, after completion of distribution. The parameter which describes the extent of distribution is the apparent volume of distribution (V):

$$V = \frac{\text{Total amount of drug in the body}}{\text{Plasma concentration}}$$

In the simple example shown by Fig. 2.13a, if a dose of 20 mg is injected this will mix instantaneously into the volume V. If the initial plasma concentration is $2\,\mu\mathrm{g\,ml}^{-1}$ (equivalent to point

A on Fig. 2.13a) then the apparent volume of distribution will be given by:

$$V = \frac{\text{Total amount (dose)}}{\text{Plasma concentration}} = \frac{20\,000\,\mu\mathrm{g}}{2\,\mu\mathrm{g\,ml}^{-1}}$$

$$= 10\,000\,\mathrm{ml} = 10\,\text{litres}$$

In other words, after giving the dose it *appears* that the drug has been dissolved in 10 litres of plasma. However, plasma volume is only 3 litres and therefore some of the drug must have left the plasma and entered tissues to give the low concentration present ($2\,\mu\mathrm{g\,ml}^{-1}$).

In the more complex example shown in Fig. 2.13b, the dose of 20 mg will distribute instantaneously only into V_1, which is usually termed the *central compartment*. Measurement of the initial concentration (point A in Fig. 2.13b) will not represent distribution into V_2 and the volume calculated will under-represent the true extent of distribution (see Fig. 2.14). Distribution into V_2, which is usually termed the *peripheral compartment*, is not complete until point B in Fig. 2.13b. However, by the time point B is reached there will have been considerable elimi-

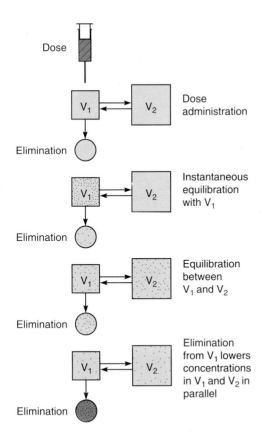

Figure 2.14 Schematic diagram of drug distribution. (Note at equilibrium the total concentrations in V_1 and V_2 may be different due to protein binding, etc.).

Table 2.7 The apparent volume of distribution and plasma-protein binding of selected drugs

Drug	V (litres kg^{-1})	% Binding
Warfarin and frusemide	0.1	99
Aspirin	0.2	49
Gentamycin	0.3	<10
Propranolol	3.9	93
Nortriptyline	18.5	95
Chloroquine	185.7	61

Note:
The apparent volume of distribution (V) is given in litres kg^{-1} body weight and therefore for chloroquine the total volume of distribution will be 13 000 litres per 70 kg patient.

nation and so the total amount of drug in the body is no longer known. This can be overcome by using the elimination phase (B–C in Fig. 2.13b) to back extrapolate to the intercept (point D) which is the concentration which would have been obtained if distribution into V2 had been instantaneous:

$$V = \frac{\text{Total amount}}{\text{Concentration}}$$

$$= \frac{\text{Dose}}{\text{Concentration at point D}}$$

Alternative equations for the calculation of V are presented later.

The apparent volume of distribution is independent of dose or concentration and can be used to calculate either the dose necessary to give a particular concentration or the total body load present at the time a concentration was measured.

The apparent volume of distribution is simply

an indication of the amount of drug remaining in the blood or plasma and provides no information on where the drug has accumulated. Thus a high apparent volume of distribution could result from either reversible accumulation in adipose tissue due to dissolution in fat or reversible accumulation in liver and lung due to high intracellular protein binding. The actual distribution can be determined only by measurement of tissue concentrations.

The apparent volume of distribution is usually calculated using the total concentration in plasma, that is, free (unbound) + protein bound. Therefore a low volume of distribution can result if a drug is highly bound to plasma proteins but not to tissue proteins; but if the drug shows an even higher affinity for tissue (lipid or protein; see Fig. 2.2) then it will have a high volume of distribution. Therefore there is no relationship between plasma protein binding and the apparent volume of distribution (see Table 2.7). The apparent volume of distribution reflects the relative affinity of plasma and tissues.

If the tissues have an extremely high affinity then little drug will remain in the blood; the calculated apparent volume of distribution will be extremely high and may greatly exceed the body weight. Chloroquine is a good example of such a drug (Table 2.7) and the value obtained illustrated clearly the fact that the apparent volume of distribution should be regarded as a mathematical ratio not as an indication of physiological distribution to an actual volume of plasma!

ELIMINATION

Elimination can also be described in terms of both *rate* and *extent*. The extent of elimination will eventually be 100%, that is, all the drug in the circulation will be removed and therefore it is the rate at which the drug is eliminated which is of importance.

Rate of Elimination

The rate of elimination normally determines the duration of drug action and the frequency with which a drug must be taken to maintain therapeutic plasma concentrations during chronic administration.

The decrease in plasma concentration after an intravenous bolus dose is shown in Fig. 2.15 and it is apparent that the terminal elimination phase represents an exponential decline, that is:

$$C = C_0\, e^{-kt}$$

or

$$\ln C = \ln C_0 - kt.$$

A parameter characteristic of an exponential decrease is the *half-life*, that is, the time taken for any concentration to decrease to one-half. The half-life is independent of concentration (Fig. 2.15) and is a characteristic for that particular drug. The half-life can be related to the rate constant k by substituting $C_0 = 2$ and

$C = 1$ into the above equation, when t will be one half-life or $t_{1/2}$, that is:

$$\ln 1 = \ln 2 - k\, t_{1/2}$$
$$0 = 0.693 - kt_{1/2}$$
$$t_{1/2} = \frac{0.693}{k}$$

The half-life is an important variable during repeated drug administration since it determines both the time taken for plasma concentrations to stabilize when the daily dose is modified and also the number of doses necessary each day to prevent large fluctuations in concentration (see later). The half-lives of drugs range from a few minutes to many days (and in rare cases, weeks). Precise knowledge about the half-life of every drug is not necessary and therefore in this book we have used the descriptive terms given in Table 2.8 to indicate the approximate half-life and the influence this would have on clinical use of the drug.

The rate at which a drug can be eliminated from the body and therefore the half-life is dependent on *two* variables:

(a) *The activity of the metabolizing enzymes or excretory mechanisms.* The organs of elimination (usually liver and kidneys) remove drug that is brought to them via the blood. Providing first order kinetics apply, that is the process is not saturated, then a constant *proportion* of the drug carried in the blood will be removed, indepen-

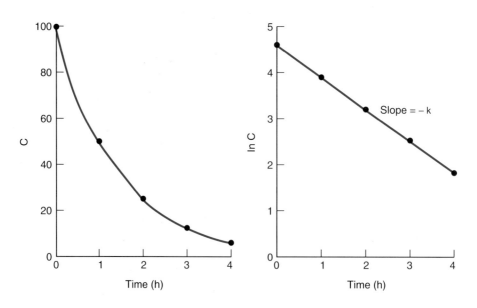

Figure 2.15 The elimination half-life of a drug in plasma. Within each hour the concentration decreases by 50% $\therefore t_{1/2} = 1\,\text{h}$.

Table 2.8 Half-life descriptions

Description	Half-life	Doses per day for chronic treatment	Comment
Very short	<1 h	—	Usually specified in text
Short	1–6 h	3–4	A modified-release formulation may be preferred
Intermediate	6–12 h	1–2	
Long	12–24	1	
Very long	>24 h	1	Usually specified in text due to risk of accumulation

dent of the concentration in the blood. In effect a constant proportion of the blood flow to the organ can be regarded as being cleared of drug. The more active the process (e.g. hepatic metabolism) the greater will be the proportion of the blood flow cleared of drug. The proportion of the blood flow cleared of drug will have units of volume per time (e.g. ml min^{-1}). This is termed the *plasma clearance (CL)* of the drug which may be regarded as the volume of plasma cleared of drug per unit time and is the best indication of the activity of the eliminating processes. The greater the value of plasma clearance, the greater will be the rate at which the drug will be removed from the body, that is:

$$k \propto CL$$

$$CL = \frac{\text{Rate of elimination from the body}}{\text{Plasma concentration}}$$

$$\left(\frac{\text{e.g. } \mu\text{g min}^{-1}}{\text{e.g. } \mu\text{g ml}^{-1}} = \text{ml min}^{-1} \right)$$

(b) *The extent to which the drug has passed from the blood into tissues.* The organs of elimination can only act on drug that is delivered to them via the blood supply. If, after equilibration with tissues, the blood or plasma concentration is very low, that is the apparent volume of distribution is very high, then the rate at which the drug can be eliminated will be limited by the rate of delivery, that is:

$$k \propto \frac{1}{V}$$

Thus the overall rate of elimination is dependent on the two variables CL and V, that is:

$$k = \frac{CL}{V} \quad \text{or} \quad t_{1/2} = \frac{0.693\ V}{CL}$$

This is illustrated in Fig. 2.16 and Table 2.9. The elimination rate constant (or half-life) is the best indication of *changes* in drug concentration and for many drugs this will relate to changes in therapeutic activity following a single dose. Clearance is the best measurement of the ability of the organs of elimination to remove the drug and determines the plasma concentrations (and therefore therapeutic activity) at *steady state* (see later).

Clearance can be calculated from k and V using the equation given above, but it is usually determined using a model-independent method

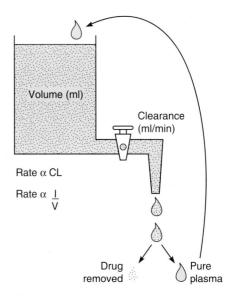

Figure 2.16 The relationship between clearance, volume of distribution and overall elimination rate. The drug is eliminated by the clearance process, which removes a fixed volume of plasma per unit time. The drug is then separated and the pure plasma added back to the tank to maintain a constant volume (the apparent volume of distribution). The fluid therefore continuously recycles via the clearance process and the concentration of drug decreases exponentially. The time taken for one cycle is equal to the volume divided by the clearance (the greater the volume the greater the time needed, but the greater the clearance the shorter the time).

Table 2.9 Pharmacokinetic parameters of selected drugs

	Clearance (ml min^{-1})	Apparent volume of distribution (litres/70 kg)	Half-life (h)
Warfarin	3	8	37
Digitoxin	4	38	161
Diazepam	27	77	43
Valproic acid	76	27	5.6
Digoxin	130	640	39
Ampicillin	270	20	1.3
Lignocaine	640	77	1.8
Propranolol	840	270	3.9
Imipramine	1050	1600	18

Note:
The drugs are arranged in order of increasing plasma clearance. A long half-life may result from a low clearance (e.g. digitoxin), a high apparent volume of distribution (e.g. imipramine) or both.

which is not dependent on accurate determination of the intercept at $t = 0$ (point D on Fig. 2.13b). The method uses the area under the plasma concentration–time curve (AUC) as follows:

$$CL = \frac{\text{Rate of elimination from the body}}{\text{Plasma concentration}}$$

(see above).

The rate of elimination from the body is equivalent to the rate of change of the amount in the body (A_b) with time, that is:

$$CL = \frac{\mathrm{d}A_b}{\mathrm{d}t} \Big/ C \quad \text{where } C \text{ is plasma concentration}$$

rearranging $\qquad CL \times C = \dfrac{\mathrm{d}A_b}{\mathrm{d}t}$

and $\qquad CL \times C\,\mathrm{d}t = \mathrm{d}A_b$

If the equation is integrated between $t = 0$ and $t = $ infinity then the change in body load to infinity ($\mathrm{d}A_b$) will equal the total dose given:

$$CL \times \int_0^\infty C\,\mathrm{d}t = \text{Dose}.$$

The integral between $t = 0$ and $t = $ infinity of $C\,\mathrm{d}t$ is the area under the concentration–time curve to infinity:

$$CL \times \text{AUC} = \text{Dose}$$

or

$$CL = \frac{\text{Dose}}{\text{AUC}}$$

This is an important and useful equation and allows an easy estimate of the ability of the body to remove the drug from the circulation. Factors to be considered in the use of this equation are:

(1) The dose used has to be the dose in the circulation and available to the organs of elimination. For the intravenous route then the dose is that administered; however, for the oral route only a fraction (F; see earlier) may reach the general circulation and therefore the dose used in the calculation should be the administered dose $\times F$. That is:

$$CL = \frac{\text{Dose}_{iv}}{\text{AUC}_{iv}} = \frac{\text{Dose}_{oral} \times F}{\text{AUC}_{oral}}$$

rearranging

$$F = \frac{\text{AUC}_{oral}}{\text{AUC}_{iv}} \times \frac{\text{Dose}_{iv}}{\text{Dose}_{oral}} \quad \text{(see earlier).}$$

(2) The AUC should be the area under the concentration–time curve not the ln concentration–time curve, and should be extrapolated to infinity.

(3) The equation can be used to calculate the apparent volume of distribution and is more reliable than the extrapolation method given above (Fig. 2.13b):

$$CL = \frac{\text{Dose}}{\text{AUC}} = kV$$

$$V = \frac{\text{Dose}}{\text{AUC} \times k} \quad \text{or} \quad \frac{\text{Dose}}{\text{AUC} \times \beta}$$

(for a two-compartment system).

(4) The equation is valid for *constant intravenous infusion* (Fig. 2.17). During infusions the drug concentration in plasma increases until a steady state is reached. At steady state the rate of infusion is exactly balanced by the rate of elimination from the body. The rate of elimination equals clearance times plasma concentration at steady state (C_{ss}):

$$CL = \frac{\text{Rate of elimination from body}}{\text{Plasma concentration } (C_{ss})}$$

$$\text{Rate of elimination} = CL \times C_{ss}$$

$$\therefore \quad \text{Rate of infusion} = CL \times C_{ss}$$

$$CL = \frac{\text{Rate of infusion}}{C_{ss}}$$

Clearance and volume of distribution can also be calculated using the AUC between zero and infinity and the terminal slope (see Fig. 2.17).

The plasma clearance is the sum of all clearance processes, for example metabolic, renal, biliary, airways, etc., and therefore is the best measure of functional status of the elimination

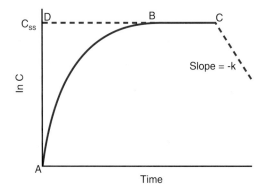

Figure 2.17 Constant intravenous infusion (between points A and C). Steady state is reached at point B and the steady-state concentration (C_{ss}; given by D) can be used to calculate clearance: $CL = $ rate of infusion$/C_{ss}$ (see text). Clearance can also be calculated from the area under the total curve (AUC) and the total dose infused between A and C. The slope on cessation of infusion is the terminal elimination phase (k or β). The distribution phase is not usually detected since distribution is occurring throughout the period A to C. The apparent volume of distribution can be calculated as: $V = $ Dose$/($AUC $\times k)$. The *increase* to steady state is determined by the *elimination* rate constant and it takes approximately four to five half-lives to reach steady state.

processes. Measurement of specific processes such as metabolic clearance or renal clearance would require specific measurement of the rate of elimination by that process. In practice this is only really possible for *renal clearance* (CL_r). The renal clearance can be calculated from the rate of excretion in urine (*as the parent drug*) during a urine collection and the mid-point plasma concentration, that is:

$$CL_r = \frac{\text{Rate of excretion in urine}}{\text{Plasma concentration (mid-point)}}$$

$$\left(\text{e.g.} \ \frac{\mu\text{g min}^{-1}}{\mu\text{g ml}^{-1}} = \text{ml min}^{-1} \right)$$

Alternatively if the urine is collected until no more parent drug can be measured then:

$$CL_r = \frac{\text{Total amount in urine}}{\text{AUC}}$$

Measurement of renal clearance can be useful in a number of ways:

(1) Comparison of renal clearance with plasma clearance will show the importance of the kidney in the overall elimination of the compound. This can be of value in predicting the potential impact of renal disease.
(2) [Plasma clearance – renal clearance] is equivalent to metabolic clearance for most drugs and this can be of value in predicting the potential impact of liver disease.
(3) Comparison of renal clearance (CL_r) with GFR allows an estimate of the extent of reabsorption after allowance for protein binding (if $CL_r <$ GFR) or active secretion (if $CL_r >$ GFR).
(4) Renal clearance can be affected by altering kidney function — for example by changing the urine pH (see later).

The biliary clearance of a drug can be measured using the above approach, but in practice is seldom done due to the difficulty of collecting bile samples.

Extent of Elimination

The extent of elimination is of limited value since eventually all the drug will be removed from the body. Measurement of total elimination in urine, faeces and expired air as parent drug and metabolites can give useful insights into the extent of absorption, metabolism and renal and biliary elimination.

CHRONIC ADMINISTRATION

Long-term or chronic drug therapy is designed to maintain a constant concentration of the drug in blood with an equilibrium established between blood and all tissues of the body including the site of action. In practice a constant concentration can only be achieved by an intravenous infusion which has continued long enough to reach steady state (Fig. 2.17). During constant infusion the time to reach steady state is dependent on the elimination half-life and steady state is approached after four or five half-lives. Since the half-life is dependent on both clearance and apparent volume of distribution each of these can contribute to the delay in achieving steady state. A drug with a large volume of distribution will have a long half-life and therefore it will take a longer time to reach steady state. It is easy to envisage the slow filling of such a high volume of distribution during regular administration. However, once steady state has been reached, the plasma and tissues are in equilibrium and the distribution rate constant and apparent volume of distribution will not affect the plasma concentration. The only processes which can alter the steady-state concentration of drug are those of elimination or clearance, that is:

$$C_{ss} = \frac{\text{Rate of infusion}}{CL} \quad \text{(see above)}$$

Most chronic administration is via the *oral route* and therefore the rate and extent of absorption need to be considered. Also oral therapy is by intermittent doses and therefore there will be a series of peaks and troughs between doses (Fig. 2.18). The *rate* of absorption will influence the inter-dose profile since very rapid absorption will exaggerate fluctuations, while slow absorption will dampen down the peak. The *extent* of absorption or bioavailability (*F*) will influence the average steady-state concentration because it affects the dose entering the circulation and therefore the rate of drug input. The rate of input during chronic oral therapy is given by:

$$\frac{D \times F}{T}$$

where *D* is administered dose, *F* is bioavailability, and *T* is interval between doses.

At steady state the input is balanced by the elimination, that is:

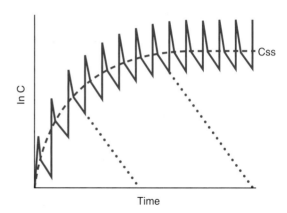

Figure 2.18 Chronic oral therapy (———) compared with intravenous (– – – –) infusion at the same dosage rate. The oral dose shows very rapid absorption and distribution followed by a more slow elimination phase within each dose interval. Cessation of therapy after any dose would produce the line shown as ....

$$\frac{D \times F}{T} = CL \times C_{ss}$$

(C_{ss} is the average steady-state concentration). Therefore:

$$C_{ss} = \frac{D \times F}{T \times CL}$$

Clearly the value of C_{ss} can be increased either by increasing the dose or by decreasing the dose interval. Factors such as concurrent drug therapy or disease will affect the value of C_{ss} by altering clearance and hence could influence the potential for benefit and/or toxicity.

Loading Dose

A therapeutic problem may arise when a rapid effect is required for a drug which has a long or very long half-life, because the steady-state conditions will not be reached until 2–4 days if the half-life is 12–24 h or >4–5 days if the half-life is >24 h. The delay between the initiation of treatment and the attainment of steady state may be avoided by the administration of a *loading dose*. A loading dose is a high initial or first dose which, as the name implies, is designed to "load up" the body. In principle, this is done by giving as the first dose an amount of drug equivalent to the total body load at steady state. This will avoid the slow build up to steady state, and the steady state can then be maintained by giving the dosage regimen which would eventually have resulted in the same steady-state concentration.

The amount of drug equivalent to the steady-state body load is the required or target steady-state plasma concentration (C_{ss}) multiplied by the apparent volume of distribution (V). That is:

$$\text{Loading dose} = C_{ss} V$$

In cases where C_{ss} or V are not known, then the loading dose can be calculated based on the proposed maintenance regimen. This is done by replacing C_{ss} in the above equation by

$$\frac{\text{D} \times F}{T \times CL} \quad \text{(see above)}$$

(where Dose and T refer to the maintenance regimen) and by replacing V in the above equation by $\dfrac{CL}{k}$ (see earlier). Then:

$$\begin{aligned} \text{Loading dose} &= \frac{\text{D} \times F}{T \times CL} \times \frac{CL}{k} \\ &= \frac{\text{D} \times F}{T \times k} \\ &= \frac{\text{D} \times F \times 1.44 \times t_{1/2}}{T} \end{aligned}$$

It is clear from this last equation that the magnitude of any loading dose compared with the maintenance dose is proportional to the half-life. Good examples of this are the cardiac glycosides digoxin and digitoxin, which are compared in Table 2.10.

The values given in Table 2.10 are to illustrate the concept of a loading dose: the doses used clinically should take into account body weight, age and the presence of severe renal or liver impairment. The loading dose may need to be given in two or three fractions over a period of about 24–36 h. The reason for this is that during distribution of the loading dose there are higher (non-steady-state) concentrations in the blood and rapidly equilibrating tissues and lower (non-steady-state) concentrations in the slowly equilibrating tissues (see Fig. 2.5). The excessive concentrations in rapidly equilibrating tissues may give rise to toxicity. This can be minimized by giving the loading dose in fractions which would allow distribution of one fraction before the next was given. The fractional loading doses should be given within the period of the normal dose interval.

FACTORS AFFECTING PHARMACOKINETICS

The following account considers a number of factors which could influence drug handling, based on the likely effect on the physiological processes of absorption, distribution and elimination. The impact of these effects on the pharmacokinetic profile is then considered based largely on the possible changes in bioavailability, apparent volume of distribution and clearance.

Drug interactions

Drugs can have a number of effects on pharmacokinetic processes (see Fig. 2.19):

(1) *Gastrointestinal transit* — drugs such as metoclopramide, which increase gastrointestinal motility, can reduce the lag time prior to absorption following an oral dose. If the drug is poorly absorbed the total time available for absorption may decrease so that bioavailability could decrease. Drugs such as

Table 2.10 Pharmacokinetics and dosage for digoxin and digitoxin

	Digoxin	Digitoxin
Elimination half-life (days)	1.6	7
Time to steady state (days; $4 \times t_{1/2}$)	6	28
"Therapeutic" plasma concentrations (ng ml^{-1} or μg l^{-1})	0.5–2.0	10–35
Volume of distribution (litres per 70 kg)	600	40
Typical loading dose ($C_{ss} \times V$)	up to 1.2 mg	up to 1.4 mg
Bioavailability (F)	0.75	>0.9
Normal oral maintenance dose $\left(\dfrac{\text{Dose} \times F}{T}; \text{ mg day}^{-1} \right)$	0.125–0.5	0.05–0.2
Typical loading dose (maintenance dose $\times$ 1.44 $\times$ $t_{1/2}$)	0.3–1.2 mg	0.5–2.0 mg

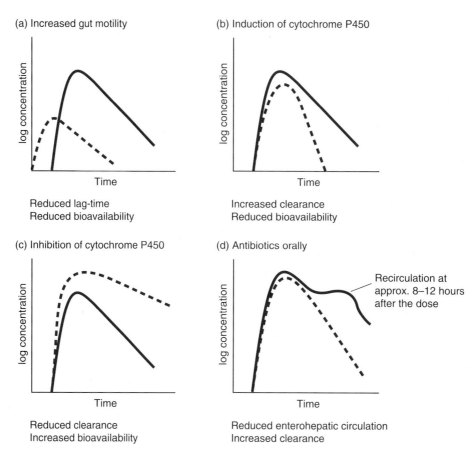

Figure 2.19   The possible effects of drug interactions on the pharmacokinetics of a single oral dose. The drug given alone is shown by (————) and when in the presence of the interacting drug by (– – – –). In example (d) the drug normally shows an enterohepatic circulation which is indicated by the secondary peak which is abolished by the antibiotic.

propantheline which decrease gastrointestinal motility would have the opposite effect.

(2) *Antibiotics* — can affect the gut flora and thereby reduce enterohepatic recirculation, especially of drug conjugates. This can result in an increase in clearance, because the drug would not re-enter the blood, and therefore a reduction in the AUC of a single dose and C_{ss} during chronic dosing. The clinical significance of this is illustrated by possible failure of the oral contraceptive in patients given large oral doses of poorly absorbed, broad-spectrum antibiotics.

(3) *Chelating agents* — such as cholestyramine, could sequester either the drug, which would decrease bioavailability, or its biliary metabolites, which could increase clearance by interrupting the enterohepatic circulation (e.g. warfarin).

(4) *Enzyme induction* — drugs such as phenobarbitone and phenytoin increase the amount of cytochrome P450 in the liver (Table 2.11). This increases hepatic metabolism of P450 substrates both during absorption, which may result in an increased first pass metabolism and decreased bioavailability, and during systemic metabolism, which may result in an increased clearance. The increase in clearance would result in decrease in the terminal half-life.

(5) *Enzyme inhibition* — drugs such as cimetidine (Table 2.11) inhibit cytochrome P450 and therefore the effects seen with P450 substrates are the opposite of those produced by inducing agents, that is, an increase in bioavailability, a decrease in clearance and an increase in terminal half-life.

(6) *Protein binding* — competition for plasma protein binding can produce a complex series of changes. The decreased binding in the plasma may result in an increase in the apparent volume of distribution, which

Table 2.11 Common inducers and inhibitors of cytochrome P450

Inducers	Inhibitors
Barbiturates	Cimetidine
(esp. phenobarbitone)	Allopurinol
Phenytoin	Isoniazid
Carbamazepine	Chloramphenicol
Griseofulvin	Disulfiram
Rifampicin	Quinine
Glutethimide	Erythromycin

would result in an increase in terminal half-life. However, the increase in free drug may facilitate an increase in extraction by the organs of elimination, that is, an increase in clearance would result in a decrease in terminal half-life. Overall the effect of such interactions on pharmacokinetics is of limited importance compared with the increase in free drug and increase in pharmacological effect. The clinically important interactions are those in which the initial drug is highly protein bound and shows a narrow therapeutic range, (e.g. tolbutamide and warfarin) while the displacing drug is given in large doses (e.g. salicylate and sulphonamides) and can displace significant amounts of the initial drug. If the protein binding of a drug is decreased from 99 to 98% this minor change results in a doubling of the free drug concentration from 1 to 2%. Since it is the free drug that interacts with receptors this could result in a greatly increased therapeutic and/or toxic effect (see Chapter 56).

(7) *Renal secretion* — the renal tubular secretion of acidic drugs can be blocked by compounds such as probenecid and aspirin. This results in a decrease in renal clearance. If this is the major route of elimination there will also be a decrease in plasma clearance and hence the half-life will be increased.

(8) *Renal pH* — the renal clearance of weakly acidic and basic drugs is dependent on the pH of the urine. Urine pH affects the ionization of the drug in the renal tubule and hence its tendency to be reabsorbed. The renal clearance of acidic drugs can be increased by increasing urine pH (e.g. with $NaHCO_3$) to increase ionization while the renal clearance of basic drugs is increased by reducing the urine pH (e.g. with NH_4Cl).

Age

Age affects the body composition with respect to fat, muscle and water content and could alter the distribution characteristics of a drug. However, of far greater importance is the fact that the extremes of age — neonates and the elderly — show a reduced renal function and a decreased drug metabolizing ability due to lower enzyme activity (neonates) or reduced liver size and perfusion (elderly). Thus the extremes of age tend to show a decrease in plasma clearance, whether the drug is handled primarily by the liver or the kidneys. The decrease in clearance means that lower and less frequent doses may need to be given to these age groups.

Disease

Diseases can affect absorption, distribution and elimination. Conditions, such as achlorhydria and coeliac disease can influence both the rate and extent of absorption of an oral dose. Distribution can be affected by the changes in plasma proteins which can accompany disease states, for example there is an increase in plasma α_1-acid glycoprotein in arthritis while cirrhosis is associated with a decrease in plasma albumin concentration. These changes could affect the apparent volume of distribution of drugs and hence their half-lives. Hepatic and renal diseases can decrease the ability of the organ of elimination to remove the drug from the blood, and hence there is a decrease in plasma clearance. This results in an increase in terminal half-life and an increase in steady-state plasma concentration.

Pharmacogenetics

There are wide interindividual differences in drug-metabolizing ability in normal healthy subjects. These arise from genetically determined differences in the basal level of expression of the enzyme and can give rise to about two- to three-fold differences in bioavailability, systemic clearance and half-life.

In most cases there is a normal (Gaussian) distribution of enzyme activity in the population. However, for some enzymes there is poly-

Table 2.12 Pharmacogenetic differences in drug-metabolizing enzymes

Enzyme	Incidence of deficiency* or slow metabolizers	Typical substrates
Plasma pseudocholinesterase[†]	1 in 3000	Suxamethonium (succinylcholine)
Alcohol dehydrogenase	5–10% (about 90% in Asians)	Ethanol
Cytochrome P4502C18	5% (about 20% in Asians)	S-Mephenytoin
Cytochrome P4502D6	5–10%	Debrisoquine, sparteine, metoprolol, dextromethorphan
Cytochrome P4502C?	Very rare	Phenytoin
N-Acetyltransferase	Approx 60% (about 5% in Japanese)	Isoniazid, hydralazine, procainamide
Methyltransferase	0.5%	6-Mercaptopurine

*For Caucasians.
[†]A number of variants are known.

morphic expression of the enzyme activity and it is possible to divide the population into two groups — "fast metabolizers" and "slow metabolizers". This metabolizing status is genetically determined and therefore is an underlying characteristic of the individual. Slow metabolizers have high plasma concentrations of the parent drug but lower concentrations of the metabolite(s). In some cases the polymorphism arises from altered transcription of the normal enzyme protein, but frequently the "slow metabolizer" DNA codes for a modified enzyme protein with an altered binding site and which has a decreased substrate affinity. Drug-metabolizing enzymes showing polymorphism or enzyme deficiencies are given in Table 2.12.

Genetically determined expression of enzyme activity can be affected also by ethnic origins. Ethnic origins can affect the proportion of the population showing a genetic deficiency or polymorphism (see Table 2.12). In addition, the extent of metabolism in the general population may be different, for example subjects from the Indian subcontinent show a two- to three-fold slower elimination of cytochrome P4503A substrates than Caucasians.

3

Drug Discovery, Evaluation and Safety

"One of the features which is thought to distinguish man from other animals is his desire to take medicines" (Sir William Osler, 1849–1919). Initially, most of these were of botanical or zoological origin. However, the past 50 years have seen first an increase in the use of organic chemicals, and secondly the recent introduction of "natural molecules" based on recombinant DNA technology; examples include erythropoietin and human insulins. Thirdly, major improvements have occurred in antimicrobial chemotherapy. These have revolutionized the chances of patients surviving severe infections such as lobar pneumonia, the mortality of which was 27% in the pre-antibiotic era but fell to 8% (and subsequently less) following the introduction of sulphonamides and later penicillins.

The introduction of new drugs has been bought at a price of significant toxicity. One of the most dramatic episodes occurred in the United States in 1937 when in a period of 2 months, 76 people died of renal failure after taking an elixir of sulphanilamide which contained diethylene glycol. This tragedy led to the establishment of the Food and Drugs Administration and to the development of the science of preclinical toxicity testing. The need for stringent testing was emphasized further by the occurrence of phocomelia and cardiac defects in infants born to mothers who consumed thalidomide in the first trimester of pregnancy. The thalidomide disaster led to the establishment of the precursor of the UK Committee on Safety of Medicines. It is this committee which is responsible for advising the Secretary of State for Health on the quality, safety and efficacy of all products for which an application is made for licencing. The committee also advises on the safety of medicines that have already been marketed. Another body, the Committee on the Review of Medicines, recently undertook a systematic review of all 39 000 products which were licensed for use in the United Kingdom. As a result many thousands of products had been discontinued by the time the review was completed in 1991.

DRUG DISCOVERY

The discovery of a new drug can be achieved in several different ways. First, new chemical entities are subjected to a battery of screening tests that are designed to detect particular types of biological activity. These include studies of animal behaviour, as well as work on isolated tissues. In general, this is not an efficient type of research since at best only one compound out of several thousand screened is eventually marketed as a medicine. A second approach involves the synthesis and testing of chemical analogues of existing medicines. In general, the products of this research lead to minor advances in absorption, potency or a more selective action. But, unexpected additional properties may become evident when the compound is tried in man. For example, the thiazide diuretics and sulphonylurea type of oral hypoglycaemics represent minor modifications of the sulphanilamide antibiotic molecule.

More recently, attempts have been made to design substances to fulfil a particular biological role. This may entail the synthesis of a naturally occurring substance, its precursor or antagonist. A good example is that of levodopa, used in the treatment of Parkinson's disease. Others include the histamine H_2 receptor antagonists and omeprazole, the first proton pump inhibitor. Logical drug development of this type depends, however, on a detailed understanding of human physiology both in health and disease.

PRECLINICAL DRUG TESTING

Before a new product can be tried in man, several months, even years, are spent on toxicological studies including:

- Acute (single dose) studies in two or more animal species by two or more routes of administration.
- Repeated dose studies in two animal species by all routes of administration intended for use in man.
- Reproduction studies (fertility, teratogenicity and developmental).
- Mutagenicity and lifetime carcinogenicity studies.

Preclinical toxicity testing in animals is discussed further in Chapter 56.

PREMARKETING CLINICAL STUDIES

The purposes of premarketing clinical studies are first to establish that the drug has a useful action in man; secondly, to confirm that it is non-toxic and thirdly, to establish the nature of common (type A) unwanted effects (see Chapter 56). Traditionally, premarketing clinical studies have been subdivided into three phases but the distinction between these is blurred and there are differences of opinion about the classification system which follows.

PHASE I STUDIES

This term is used to describe the first few administrations of a new drug to man. These may be carried out either by pharmaceutical companies or in volunteer units associated with major hospitals. Subjects taking part in phase I studies can be either healthy volunteers recruited by open advertisement or they may be patients suffering from the condition in which the drug will be used.

The first few administrations are usually by mouth in a dose which (after scaling for weight) may be as low as one-fiftieth of the minimum calculated to produce an effect seen in animals. Depending upon what is found, the dose may be then built up either in small increments or by doubling until a pharmacological effect is observed or an unwanted action occurs. During these studies toxic effects are looked for by means of routine haematology and biochemical investigations of liver and renal function and other tests including an ECG will be performed as appropriate. It is also usual to study the disposition, metabolism and main pathways of elimination of the new drug at this stage. Such studies help to identify not only the most suitable dose and route of administration in future studies but also the choice of appropriate animal species for further toxicity studies. Investigations of drug metabolism and pharmacokinetics often necessitate the use of isotopically labelled β-emitting compounds containing ^{14}C or ^{3}H.

PHASE II STUDIES

During phase II, detailed studies of the clinical pharmacology of the new compound are performed by skilled investigators. An important aspect of these studies is an attempt to define the relationship between dose and response. In addition, further studies are undertaken in special groups: for example, elderly people if it is intended that the drug will be used in that population. Other studies which may be undertaken include a dissection of the mechanism of a drug's action and studies of the potential interaction with other agents. During phase II studies, some evidence of a beneficial effect may emerge. However, the large subjective element in human illness may make it difficult to distinguish between pharmacological and placebo effects. In order to prove that it is a drug itself which has efficacy, it is necessary to undertake formal clinical trials.

PHASE III STUDIES

Clinical trials seek to establish that a drug works in comparison with a placebo that looks (and tastes) similar to the active compound. Alternatively, and additionally, they seek to establish the advantages and disadvantages of the new compound in comparison with the best available treatment. For example, new antihypertensive drugs might be compared with a diuretic, a β-adrenoceptor blocker, a calcium channel blocker or an angiotensin converting enzyme inhibitor.

Clinical trials are of two main types, either within-patient or between-patient comparisons (Fig. 3.1). In the former, a patient is randomized to commence treatment with either the new compound or its comparator before "crossing-over" to the alternative therapy. By contrast, between-patient comparisons involve randomization to receive one or other of two (or more) treatments. Within-patient comparisons can usually be performed on a smaller number of patients (about half that required in between-patient studies). A further advantage is that the patient acts as his or her own control and that most other variables are therefore eliminated. However, such studies often take longer for the individual patient and there may be carry-over effects from one treatment that affect the apparent efficacy of the alternative therapy. Studies of this type may be difficult to

WITHIN PATIENT TRIAL

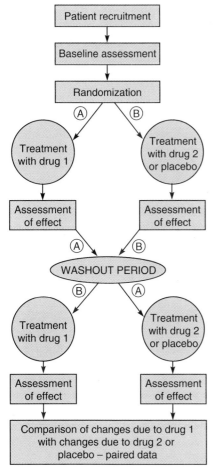

BETWEEN PATIENT TRIAL

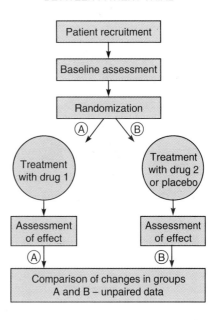

Figure 3.1 The design of clinical trials.

interpret when there is a pronounced seasonal variation in the severity of a condition such as Raynaud's disease or hay fever.

The advantages and disadvantages of between-patient comparisons follow in large part from what has been outlined above. They require roughly twice as many participants, each of whom will usually be studied for lesser periods of time. Carry-over effects are avoided but it is not possible to provide a perfect match between patients entering the two or more treatment groups. Nevertheless, this approach to the evaluation of new drugs is preferred by many drug regulatory authorities.

Whichever form of comparison is made, measurements of benefit (and adverse effects) are made at regular intervals using a combination of objective and subjective techniques. Examples of objective measurements include those of blood pressure, heart rate and exercise tolerance in the case of an antianginal agent or size of finger joints, grip strength and the number of additional paracetamol tablets consumed in the case of an antiarthritic drug. Subjective measurements could include keeping a diary of the number of anginal attacks experienced and the duration of morning stiffness and intensity of pain (using visual analogue scales) respectively. Throughout these studies careful attention is paid to the detection and reporting of both unwanted effects (type A reactions) and other unpredictable type B reactions (Chapter 56). However, the majority of the latter are not seen prior to the marketing of a new drug because they occur only once in every 10 000 or so patients treated with the drug. It is salutory to note that by the time that a drug is marketed only 2000–3000 people may have taken the drug, usually for short periods. Only a few hundred people may have 6 months or more of exposure to the new compound and the total experience may amount to no more than 500 patient years (500 patients taking the drug for 6 months = 250 patient years).

PHASE IV STUDIES: POSTMARKETING SURVEILLANCE (PHARMACOVIGILANCE) AND FURTHER STUDIES OF EFFICACY

As a consequence of the low frequency of occurrence of certain adverse drug reactions and the tendency to avoid the inclusion of children, the old and women of childbearing age in premarketing clinical studies, the full spectrum of bene-

fits and risks of medicines do not become clear until after marketing. Another factor is the widespread use of other medicines with which serious interactions have not previously been anticipated or studied.

Two main systems of postmarketing surveillance (pharmacovigilance) are in use in the UK. The first and most important is known as the "yellow card system": it depends upon doctors reporting suspected serious adverse reactions directly to the Medicines Control Agency using postage prepaid cards (or slips available in the *British National Formulary* (BNF), GP prescribing pads and the *Monthly Index of Medical Specialties* (MIMS)). In some health regions (Mersey, West Midlands, Northern and Wales) yellow cards are sent to centres located in Liverpool, Birmingham, Newcastle-upon-Tyne and Cardiff. In addition to reporting suspected serious adverse effects of established drugs, doctors are asked to supply information about *all* unwanted effects of medicines that have been marketed recently. These products are identified by the use of inverted black triangles in the *BNF*, *MIMS* and drug Data Sheets. Each year the Medicines Control Agency receives some 20 000 yellow cards/slips. In return for their efforts, doctors are supplied at regular intervals with an information circular about current drug-related problems.

The second form of pharmacovigilance involves systematic postmarketing surveillance of recently marketed medicines. This may be organized by the pharmaceutical company responsible for the manufacture of the new drug (companies also receive information via their representatives). Alternatively, the drug may be the subject of Prescription Event Monitoring (PEM). This involves the supply of information on prescribing for individual patients by the Prescription Pricing Authority to a unit in Southampton and the subsequent distribution of "green cards" to the patients' general practitioners with a request that they complete all details about the patient and events which occurred and then return the cards to Southampton where the data are analysed.

PEM has the advantage that it does not require doctors to make a value judgement concerning the cause of an event such as a broken leg. An event of this type may be coincidental or it could be due to drug-related hypotension, ataxia or metabolic bone disease. In a recent PEM study, broken limbs were found to be common amongst patients receiving terodiline for urinary incontinence. Subsequent analysis has suggested that these fractures were due to syncope associated with a rare form of ventricular tachycardia known as torsade de pointes.

Finally, detailed monitoring of adverse reactions to drug therapy takes place in certain hospitals. These data contribute further to our overall knowledge.

4

The Autonomic Nervous System

The autonomic nervous system (ANS) is an important site for drug action because:

- The ANS either controls or contributes to the control of the functioning of all of the major organ systems of the body (apart from the brain).
- The ANS utilizes two different neurotransmitters and a number of receptor subtypes which allow specific pharmacological and therapeutic manipulation.

The ANS is subdivided into two main branches:

- *Parasympathetic nervous system* (PNS) — utilizes acetylcholine as the final transmitter at the effector organs which acts via muscarinic receptors.
- *Sympathetic nervous system* (SNS) — utilizes noradrenaline as the final transmitter at most effector organs which acts via adrenoceptors.

The basic arrangement for both branches of the ANS is similar in that the neurone innervating the effector organ is linked to the central nervous system via a ganglion. The distribution and neuronal interconnections differ between the two branches. The PNS is responsible for controlling single organs and the ganglion is close to the organ; there are few or no interconnections between ganglia. The SNS is involved in the "flight or fight" response and many of

the ganglia are close to the spinal column (the paravertebral sympathetic ganglion chain) and are interconnected. Because the nerve fibres leaving the spinal column may interconnect with more than one ganglion, the whole system can be fired simultaneously. Where the sympathetic nerves are involved in specific control of organ function (e.g. the emptying of the bladder or rectum) the preganglionic sympathetic fibres are longer and the postganglionic cell bodies are grouped together in ganglia (see Fig. 4.1). This chapter will deal with the ANS in relation to its potential for allowing specific therapeutic effects via the different neurotransmitters and receptor subtypes present.

Many organ systems are innervated by both the PNS and SNS and these may have opposite effects giving rise to the concept of physiological antagonism between the two branches of the ANS. Table 4.1 shows the principal organ systems, their ANS innervation, their response to PNS and SNS stimulation and the principal neurotransmitter released at postganglionic fibre/effector organ junctions.

GANGLION BLOCKADE

Some drugs are able to block the acetylcholine receptors in the postsynaptic membrane of the ganglia of both PNS and SNS (see later).

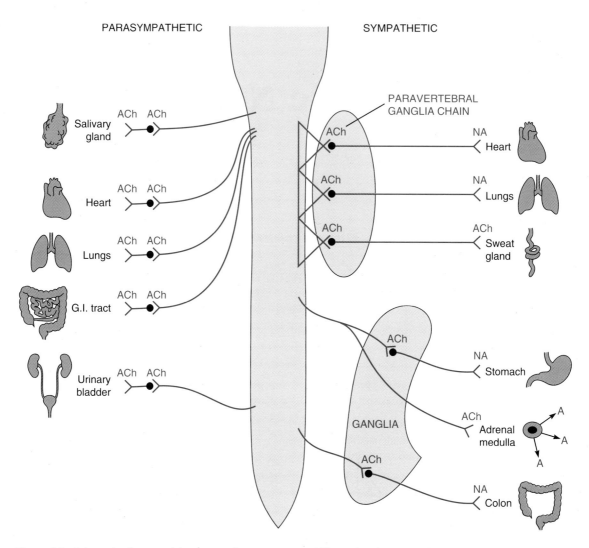

Figure 4.1 Schematic diagram of the autonomic nervous system illustrating the types of organization — with the sympathetic shown on the right and the parasympathetic shown on the left. ACh, acetylcholine; NA, noradrenaline; A, adrenaline. The ganglia innervating some organs are not part of the paravertebral chain but are grouped together to form the coeliac, superior mesenteric and inferior mesenteric ganglia.

Because of their generalized non-specific actions they have very restricted clinical use (Chapter 7). However, their effects in a resting individual indicate the balance between PNS and SNS drives to different organ systems under such circumstances (Table 4.2).

This balance between PNS and SNS drives is affected by activities which may either produce a slight increase in SNS drive, for example exercise, or a massive SNS drive combined with release of adrenaline from the adrenal medulla (flight or fight response). Antagonists at autonomic ganglia nicotinic N_1 receptors may produce either competitive blockade

(mecamylamine) or depolarizing blockade (hexamethonium; not used clinically); these different mechanisms of action are explained in Chapter 28 which describes the effects of competitive and depolarizing blockers on the acetylcholine receptors of the neuromuscular junction.

RECEPTOR TYPES AND SUBTYPES

There are two neurotransmitters involved in the autonomic nervous system — acetylcholine (ACh) and noradrenaline (NA) (Fig. 4.1); these

Table 4.1 Autonomic nervous system innervation of the major organ systems

Organ system	Parasympathetic NS		Sympathetic NS	
	Effect	Receptor type	Effect	Receptor type
Heart				
Rate	↓	M	↑	β_1, β_2
Contractility	↓ in atria	M	↑	β_1
Vascular smooth muscle				
In skin/gut	(Dilate)	(M)	Constrict	α_1
In skeletal muscle	(Dilate)	(M)	Dilate	$\beta_2{}^*$
Bronchial smooth muscle	Constrict	M	Dilate	β_2
Gastrointestinal tract:				
Motility	↑	M	↓	α_1, β_2
Sphincter tone	↓	M	↑	α_1
Secretions	↑	M	(↓)	?
Uterine smooth muscle	—	—	↑	α_1
tone in pregnancy	—	—	↓	β_2
Urinary bladder				
Detrusor	↑	M	(↓)	β_2
Sphincter	↓	M	↑	α_1
Penis	Erection	M	Ejaculation	α_1
Skin				
Pilomotor muscles	—	—	↑	α_1
Sweat glands	—	—	Secretion	M
			Local secretion	α_1
Eye				
Radial muscle	—	—	↑	α_1
Sphincter muscle	↑	M	—	—
Ciliary muscle	↑ - near vision	M	(↓ - far vision)	β_2
Metabolic functions				
Hepatic glycogenolysis	—	—	↑	$\beta_2; \alpha$
Skeletal muscle				
Glycogenolysis	—	—	↑	$\beta_2{}^*$
Fat cell lipolysis	—	—	↑	$\beta_1; \alpha; \beta_3{}^*$
Pancreas insulin secretion	↑	M	↓	α

Note: only the principal receptor types are shown.
↑ *or* ↓ increase *or* decrease: contraction *or* relaxation.
Functions in brackets are of doubtful physiological significance.
*Respond to circulating adrenaline; no noradrenergic innervation.
M = Muscarinic receptor; α and β = noradrenergic receptors.

act via different receptors. Adrenaline, released from the adrenal medulla, acts on NA receptors. However, there are a number of different receptor subtypes for each neurotransmitter.

ACETYLCHOLINE RECEPTORS

There are three main types of receptors which were named after a plant (nicotine) or fungal (muscarine) alkaloid shown to have a specific agonist action:

- *Nicotinic* (N_1) — occur on all ganglia of both the sympathetic and parasympathetic branches of the ANS.
- *Nicotinic* (N_2) — occur on the somatic motor nerves, that is the neuromuscular junction (see Chapter 27) and therefore are not a part of the ANS. N_2 receptors differ from N_1

Table 4.2   The effects of ganglion blockade in a resting subject

Organ	Effect of ganglion blockade	Predominant system
Heart	Increased rate	PNS
Vascular smooth muscle	Decreased tone/dilation	SNS
Bronchial smooth muscle	Little effect/slight dilation	PNS
Gastrointestinal tract	Decreased motility	PNS
Urinary bladder	Urinary retention	PNS
Penis	Blocked erection and ejaculation	PNS/SNS
Sweat glands	Blocked secretion	SNS
Eye	Dilation of pupil	PNS
	Loss of accommodation	PNS

receptors in their agonist/antagonist ligand-binding characteristics.

- *Muscarinic* (M) — occur at the PNS postganglionic fibre/effector organ junction. These receptors are also present on most sweat glands (but not on the palms of the hands) which are innervated by the SNS. Recently, application of molecular biology has recognized the presence of five subtypes of muscarinic receptor; experimental studies have demonstrated that at least three of these show different antagonist specificities: M_1 (in the CNS and excitatory at autonomic ganglia), M_2 (in the heart) and M_3 (in smooth muscle/secretory glands). (Although selective therapeutic agents are not currently available, students should be aware of future possibilities in the area.)

NORADRENALINE RECEPTORS

There are five known noradrenergic receptor (adrenoceptor) subtypes, 4 of which are of current therapeutic importance:

α_1 — postsynaptic receptors of the SNS (see Table 4.1); activate phospholipase C

α_2 — presynaptic receptors on the postganglionic fibres of SNS; inhibit NA release via inhibition of adenylate cyclase. Also postsynaptic in some tissues

β_1 — postsynaptic receptors of the SNS (Table 4.1); activate adenylate cyclase

β_2 — postsynaptic receptors of SNS (Table 4.1); also presynaptic where they enhance NA release; activate adenylate cyclase

β_3 — present on adipocytes and enhance lipolysis via activation of adenylate cyclase; not

blocked by most β-adrenoceptor antagonists; physiological importance is unclear.

Examples of drugs acting on these different adrenoceptor subtypes are shown in Table 4.3. The clinical uses of drugs which act on these receptors are discussed in later chapters.

DRUGS ACTING ON THE BIOSYNTHESIS, RELEASE AND CATABOLISM OF NEUROTRANSMITTERS

ACETYLCHOLINE

A scheme for the synthesis and release of acetylcholine is given in Fig. 4.2. Acetylcholine is synthesized in the cytosol and stored in membrane-bound vesicles as a complex with ATP and proteoglycans. Acetylcholine is a quaternary amino derivative:

$$CH_3-\overset{\overset{\displaystyle CH_3}{\displaystyle |}}{\underset{\underset{\displaystyle CH_3}{\displaystyle |}}{N^{\oplus}}}-CH_2 . CH_2 . O . COCH_3 \quad \text{acetylcholine}$$

The quaternary amino group is shared by many drugs which affect acetylcholine receptors or metabolism. Drugs may act on many of the processes in Fig. 4.2:

(1) *Synthesis* — no therapeutic example.

(2) *Storage* — carbachol can displace ACh from vesicles.

(3) *Release* — release is caused by black widow spider poison and blocked by botulinum toxin which is derived from the bacterium *Clostridium botulinum* and which is used therapeutically by local injection for muscle dyskinesia, for example torticollis.

Table 4.3 Drugs acting on the autonomic nervous system

Receptor	Agonists	Antagonists
Acetylcholine		
N_1	Carbachol	Trimetaphan
	Bethanechol	Mecamylamine
M	Pilocarpine	Atropine
		Hyoscine
		Propantheline
Noradrenaline		
α_1	Phenylephrine	Prazosin
		Phenoxybenzamine $(+\alpha_2)$
		Phentolamine $(+\alpha_2)$
α_2	Clonidine	Phentolamine $(+\alpha_1)$
		Yohimbine
		Phenoxybenzamine $(+\alpha_1)$
β_1	Dobutamine	Propranolol $(+\beta_2)$
	Isoprenaline $(+\beta_2)$	Atenolol
β_2	Salbutamol	Propranolol $(+\beta_1)$
	Isoprenaline $(+\beta_1)$	

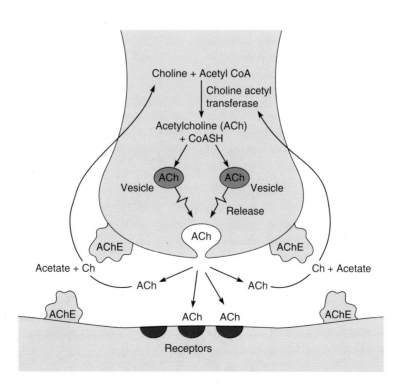

Figure 4.2 The synthesis and release of acetylcholine (ACh). The receptor may be N_1, N_2 or M. The release is in response to the nerve impulse opening voltage-sensitive Ca^{2+} channels and the influx of Ca^{2+} causes fusion of the vesicle and cell membranes. The released ACh is very rapidly hydrolysed by acetylcholine esterase (AChE) into choline and acetate. This represents the only inactivation process. The choline is taken back into the neurone and reutilized.

(4) *Metabolism* — acetylcholine esterase (AChE) is an important site of drug action. The enzyme is located on pre- and postsynaptic membranes adjacent to the synapse so that little intact acetylcholine escapes. The active site of the enzyme has two critical features: an *anionic site*, which forms an ionic bond to the quaternary nitrogen of the choline part, and a *hydrolytic site*, which contains a serine moiety the OH group of which accepts the acetyl group from acetylcholine and transfers it to water to complete the hydrolysis reaction. Drugs acting at this site may:

- Inhibit the enzyme by simple reversible binding to the anionic site, for example edrophonium (Chapter 29).

- Bind to the anionic site and transfer a carbamoyl group $[(CH_3)_2–N–C=O]$ from the drug to the serine OH group. The carbamoyl group is hydrolysed slowly from the serine so that prolonged and profound (but reversible) inhibition of the enzyme occurs, for example neostigmine, pyridostigmine (Chapter 29).

- React with the serine OH group (with or without binding to the anionic site) to produce a phosphorylated enzyme. This product is stable to hydrolysis and causes *irreversible* inhibition of the enzyme. Such permanent changes in enzyme activity are not of great clinical value but compounds in this group may be encountered clinically as a result of accidental and intentional poisoning; they form an important group of environmental chemicals — the organophosphate pesticides (which have a limited clinical use in ophthalmology, for example ecothiopate, and have been used as nerve gases for chemical warfare). The active serine OH group may be regenerated by administration of pralidoxime, which is an antidote to organophosphate poisoning.

It should be appreciated that AChE inhibitors produce diverse effects since they increase acetylcholine concentrations at all nicotinic and muscarinic receptor sites. For example, when an acetylcholine esterase inhibitor is used to overcome reversible neuromuscular blockade (Chapter 28) it produces effects on the gastrointestinal tract and heart which can be blocked by co-administration of an antimuscarinic agent.

(5) *Reuptake* — the choline produced from acetylcholine hydrolysis is an essential nutrient which is in limited supply in the body and therefore there is an active process for reuptake of choline into the neurone to prevent loss. This transport is blocked by the quaternary nitrogen compound hemicholinium, which thereby indirectly prevents acetylcholine synthesis, storage and release. This compound has no clinical use.

(6) *Presynaptic receptors* — the release of acetylcholine may be modulated (fine tuned) by presynaptic receptors (not shown in Fig. 4.2). There is evidence that the presynaptic membrane of postganglionic parasympathetic fibres may have a variety of receptors, for example muscarinic (inhibit transmitter release), nicotinic (enhance release) and α_2-adrenergic (inhibit release). The importance of these receptors in the clinical effects of drugs is unclear at present and may be limited by the low receptor selectivity of currently available agents.

NORADRENALINE

A scheme for the synthesis and release of noradrenaline is given in Fig. 4.3. As the name suggests, the structures of catecholamine neurotransmitters contain two important binding characteristics recognized by the receptors:

Dopamine and noradrenaline differ only in the nature of X (which is either **H** or **OH** respectively) and yet they bind to completely different receptors; noradrenaline and adrenaline differ only in Y (which is either **H** or **CH₃** respectively) and they bind to similar receptors, but with different selectivity.

Catecholamine neurotransmitters are synthesized from inactive precursors, starting with tyrosine which provides the basic backbone and requires metabolism at the aromatic ring (to produce a catechol) and at the amino acid end

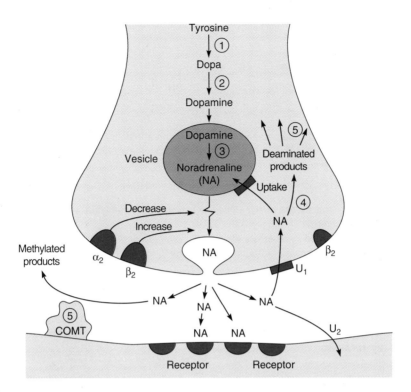

Figure 4.3 The synthesis and release of noradrenaline. The post-synaptic receptors may be α_1, β_1 or β_2. The release mechanism via exocytosis is similar to that of acetylcholine (see Fig. 4.2). The released NA is inactivated mostly by rapid reuptake into the neurone via an active transport process — uptake 1 (U_1); some is also removed by uptake into the post-synaptic effector organ (U_2) and by metabolism (enzyme 5). The NA in the cytoplasm is taken back into the vesicle by a second transport system. The synthesis and metabolism of NA utilizes a number of different enzymes:

(1) *tyrosine hydroxylase* — cytosolic enzyme converts tyrosine to *levodopa*:

This is the rate-limiting step in catecholamine synthesis.

(2) *L-amino acid decarboxylase* — cytosolic enzyme converts levodopa to *dopamine*:

Dopamine is a neurotransmitter in its own right acting on specific dopamine (D_1 and D_2) receptors.

(3) *dopamine-β-hydroxylase* — present within the vesicles of noradrenergic neurones converts dopamine to *noradrenaline*:

(4) *monoamine oxidase* (MAO) — a mitochondrial enzyme which converts noradrenaline into an *inactive hydroxyaldehyde*:

The product undergoes further metabolism by oxidation (to an hydroxy acid), reduction· (to a glycol) and methylation (via enzyme 5).

(5) *catechol-O-methyltransferase* (COMT) — adds a methyl group to the 3-hydroxy of the catechol group to produce an *inactive* product *normetanephrine*:

$$HO\!-\!\underset{HO}{\diagdown}\!\!\!\diagup\!\!\!-\!\underset{\underset{OH}{|}}{CH}\!-\!\underset{\underset{NH_2}{|}}{CH_2} \longrightarrow HO\!-\!\underset{CH_3O}{\diagdown}\!\!\!\diagup\!\!\!-\!\underset{\underset{OH}{|}}{CH}\!-\!\underset{\underset{NH_2}{|}}{CH_2}$$

O-methylation also occurs with the products of enzyme 4 (MAO).

The adrenal medulla contains an additional enzyme which converts noradrenaline into *adrenaline*:

$$HO\!-\!\underset{HO}{\diagdown}\!\!\!\diagup\!\!\!-\!\underset{\underset{OH}{|}}{CH}\!-\!\underset{\underset{NH_2}{|}}{CH_2} \longrightarrow HO\!-\!\underset{HO}{\diagdown}\!\!\!\diagup\!\!\!-\!\underset{\underset{OH}{|}}{CH}\!-\!\underset{\underset{NHCH_3}{|}}{CH_2}$$

The enzyme is a specific methyltransferase enzyme phenylethanolamine-*N*-methyltransferase (*not* COMT which adds the methyl to the other end of the molecule).
The presynaptic membrane has α_2-and β_2-receptors which may inhibit (α_2) or enhance (β_2) transmitter release.
Noradrenaline storage granules also contain ATP and neuropeptide Y, the function of which is unclear.

to produce an amine (Fig. 4.3). Inactivation processes also act on these critical receptor-binding regions by methylating the catechol group (COMT) or removing the amino function (MAO).

Drugs can act on these processes at several steps:

(1) *Synthesis* — the hypotensive drug α-methyl-dopa (Chapter 7) was "designed" to block noradrenaline synthesis (but actually acts via its metabolite α-methylnoradrenaline which is an α_2-agonist). Levodopa is administered to provide a substrate for dopamine synthesis within the CNS (Chapter 25).

(2) *Storage* — the carrier-mediated reuptake of noradrenaline from the cytoplasm into the vesicles is blocked by reserpine, which depletes stored noradrenaline and reduces SNS output.

(3) *Release* — indirectly acting sympathomimetic agents, such as tyramine, do not stimulate postsynaptic receptors but are taken up into the neurone (often by uptake 1) and act via the release of noradrenaline from cytoplasm and storage vesicles. Also adrenergic neurone-blocking drugs such as guanethidine and debrisoquine (Chapter 7) enter the neurone and act presynaptically to prevent the release of noradrenaline vesicles, thereby reducing SNS output.

(4) *Reuptake into the neurone* — is via a specific transport process which is different in neurones releasing different neurotransmitters, for example noradrenaline, dopamine

and 5-hydroxytryptamine. (Newer therapeutic agents are beginning to exploit these differences). Blockade of noradrenaline reuptake by drugs such as tricyclic antidepressants (Chapter 23) and cocaine (Chapter 58) increases the synaptic concentration of noradrenaline, and increases the activity of the SNS. Some polar drugs which act presynaptically, for example guanethidine (Chapter 7), enter the neurone via this active uptake process (uptake 1).

(5) *Metabolism* — MAO inhibitors (MAOIs) block the major pathway of metabolism of noradrenaline and other aminergic neurotransmitters containing a primary amino group [–CH_2NH_2]. MAOIs are used mainly for their effects on aminergic transmitters within the CNS rather than the SNS and are discussed in the section on antidepressants (Chapter 23) and Parkinson's disease (Chapter 25) — COMT inhibitors are currently under investigation as an adjunct to levodopa therapy for Parkinson's disease.

(6) *Presynaptic receptors* — the clinical importance of specific presynaptic receptors was first recognized during the development of an α-agonist for use as a nasal decongestant. Unexpectedly the drug produced severe hypotension, an effect incompatible with a postsynaptic α-agonist. The receptor responsible was subsequently shown to be the presynaptic α_2-receptor which acts to inhibit noradrenaline release. This reduces the activity of the SNS and

thereby lowers blood pressure; after this discovery a whole new class of drugs was developed. Therapeutic drugs which act via a specific α_2-agonist effect include clonidine and α-methylnoradrenaline (the metabolite of α-methyldopa) (Chapter 7).

Students should familiarize themselves with the autonomic nervous system and the sites of drug action presented above. Such knowledge is fundamental to understanding both the principal mechanisms of action for some drugs and the source of unwanted effects for others.

Cardiovascular System

Introduction to the Cardiovascular System

MAINTENANCE OF CARDIAC OUTPUT

There are four major determinants of cardiac output:

- Preload: this reflects ventricular end-diastolic volume, which in turn is related to ventricular filling pressure and to venous return.
- Heart rate.
- Myocardial contractility.
- Afterload: the systolic wall tension, which reflects the resistance to ventricular emptying.

In the healthy heart, changes in cardiac output are achieved mainly by changes in heart rate and preload. The influence of afterload assumes a greater importance when myocardial contractility is impaired.

The relationship between preload and stroke volume (the amount of blood ejected from the ventricle during systole) is shown in Fig. 5.1. The degree of stretch of the ventricular muscle (preload) determines the force of cardiac contraction (the Frank–Starling phenomenon). The curve describing this relationship is governed by intrinsic myocardial contractility: thus the curve is shifted downwards in the failing ventricle and upwards when contractility is augmented, for example by sympathetic nervous stimulation. The normal range of ventricular filling pressures falls on the steep part of the curve for a heart with normal contractility, making stroke volume sensitive to changes

in preload. In the failing ventricle, the curve is flatter indicating that the cardiac output is less dependent on changes in preload.

A similar family of curves describes the relationship between afterload and stroke volume (Fig. 5.2). Afterload is determined largely by peripheral resistance but also by the size of the ventricle. Enlargement of this chamber increases wall tension and the heart must generate greater pressure both to initiate and to maintain contraction. Preload and afterload are therefore interrelated. In the healthy ventricle, a

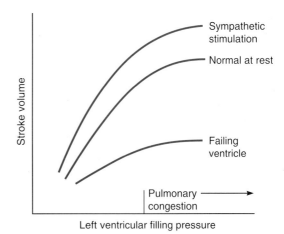

Figure 5.1 The Frank–Starling phenomenon: the relationship between preload (left ventricular filling pressure) and stroke volume at different states of myocardial contractility.

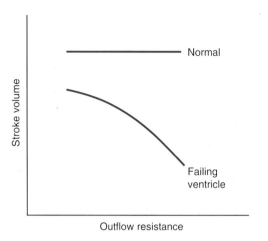

Figure 5.2 The relationship between afterload (outflow resistance) and stroke volume in the presence of normal and reduced myocardial contractility.

rise in afterload is met by an increase in myocardial contractility to maintain stroke volume. In the failing ventricle, inability to augment contraction leads to a progressive fall in stroke volume as afterload rises.

CIRCULATORY REFLEXES AND THE CONTROL OF BLOOD PRESSURE

Systemic blood pressure is determined by the cardiac output and by peripheral resistance. It is maintained within fairly narrow limits by a series of physiological reflexes that respond to both acute and chronic changes in blood pressure. The two most important regulatory systems are:

- The sympathetic nervous system.
- The renin–angiotensin–aldosterone system.

An acute reduction in systemic blood pressure is detected by baroreceptors in the aorta and carotid arteries and inhibits their rate of firing. Afferent inhibitory impulses from these structures are integrated in the vasomotor centres of the sympathetic nervous system. A reduced input of inhibitory impulses triggers the efferent response of sympathetic nervous stimulation. Sympathetic efferents to the heart act mainly through β-adrenoceptors to increase myocardial contractility and heart rate, generating a greater cardiac output (Chapter 4). Efferents to the blood vessels stimulate postsynaptic α-adrenoceptors. The result is arteriolar vasoconstriction which raises blood pressure by increasing afterload, and redistributes blood to maintain perfusion of vital organs. However, it may reduce cardiac output if ventricular function is impaired (Fig. 5.2). Stimulation of venous α-adrenoceptors decreases venous capacitance, increases venous return to the heart (preload), and improves cardiac output (Fig. 5.1).

A slower compensatory mechanism for a reduction in blood pressure is initiated by release of renin from the juxtaglomerular apparatus of the kidney (Fig. 5.3). The major stimuli leading to renin release are reduced renal blood flow (often due to a decrease in blood pressure), excess sodium in the distal renal tubule and direct sympathetic stimulation via β-adrenoceptors.

Renin is a protease which acts on circulating renin substrate (angiotensinogen) to release the decapeptide angiotensin I. This in turn is cleaved by angiotensin converting enzyme

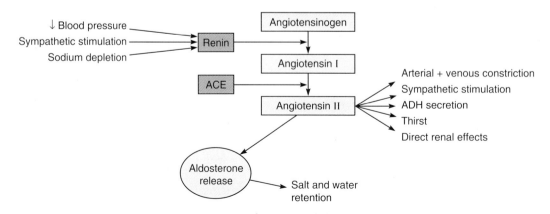

Figure 5.3 The renin–angiotensin–aldosterone system.

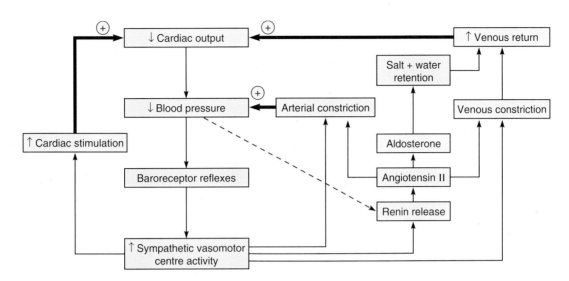

Figure 5.4 Compensatory mechanisms for an acute reduction in blood pressure or cardiac output. ⊕, Compensatory increase in cardiac output or blood pressure.

(ACE) to release the octapeptide angiotensin II. Angiotensin II is a potent vasoconstrictor with a number of additional properties which may alter salt and water balance (Fig. 5.3). It also promotes the release of aldosterone from the adrenal cortex, which acts at the distal renal tubule to conserve salt and water at the expense of potassium loss (Chapter 15). Thus angiotensin II and aldosterone raise blood pressure by vasoconstriction and by increasing circulating blood volume.

The integration of the sympathetic nervous system and renin–angiotensin–aldosterone responses to a fall in blood pressure is shown in Fig. 5.4. These mechanisms prevent hypotension due to peripheral pooling of the blood on standing and on exercise.

Additional control mechanisms involved in the regulation of vascular tone and circulating blood volume include circulating or local hormones and metabolites such as atrial natriuretic peptide, prostaglandins, kinins and adenosine. Their roles may differ in importance between health and disease states.

6

Ischaemic Heart Disease

ANGINA PECTORIS

Angina pectoris is a symptom of reversible myocardial ischaemia and is most frequently experienced as chest pain on exertion, which is relieved by rest. Pain is the consequence of an imbalance between oxygen supply and oxygen demand in the ischaemic area of myocardium (Fig. 6.1). This results from an inability of the coronary blood flow to meet the metabolic demands of the heart, usually due to a fixed atheromatous narrowing of a coronary artery. In some patients, particularly those with long-standing ischaemic heart disease, smaller collateral vessels provide a potential route to by-pass the obstruction. Reversible coronary artery spasm frequently accentuates the reduction in flow produced by fixed obstructions and may occasionally lead to angina in patients with otherwise healthy coronary arteries.

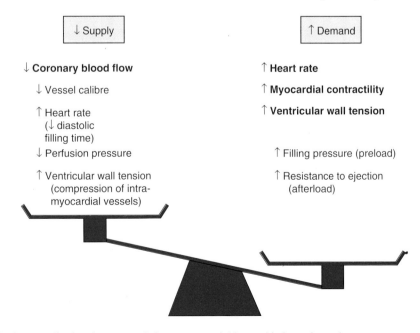

Figure 6.1 The factors affecting the myocardial oxygen supply/demand balance in angina.

Drug treatment for angina is directed to either increasing oxygen supply by improving coronary blood flow or to reducing oxygen demand by decreasing cardiac work. Drugs can be given to relieve rapidly the ischaemia during an acute attack, or as prophylaxis to reduce the risk of subsequent episodes. Three major classes of drug are commonly used to treat angina:

- Organic nitrates.
- β-Adrenoceptor antagonists.
- Calcium antagonists.

ORGANIC NITRATES

Examples: glyceryl trinitrate, isosorbide dinitrate, isosorbide mononitrate.

Mechanism of action and effects

The organic nitrates are vasodilators which relax vascular smooth muscle by mimicking the effects of endogenous endothelium-derived relaxing factor (EDRF). They release nitric oxide free radicals which combine with thiol groups in vascular endothelium to form nitrosothiols. These activate guanylate cyclase which raises the concentration of cyclic GMP (Fig. 6.2) and in turn reduces the availability of intracellular calcium to the contractile mechanism of vascular smooth muscle. Vasodilation is produced in three main vascular beds:

- Venous capacitance vessels which results in peripheral pooling of blood and reduced venous return to the heart. This lowers left ventricular filling pressure ("preload"), which decreases ventricular wall tension and reduces myocardial oxygen demand.
- Arterial resistance vessels, mainly large arteries, which reduce the resistance to ventricular emptying ("afterload"). This is less important than venodilation during long term treatment but it lowers blood pressure, decreases cardiac work and contributes to a reduced myocardial oxygen demand.
- Coronary arteries. Nitrates have little effect on total coronary flow, which may even be reduced due to a decrease in perfusion pressure. However, blood flow through collateral vessels may be improved and nitrates also relieve coronary artery spasm. The net effect is increased blood supply to ischaemic areas of myocardium.

Pharmacokinetics

Glyceryl trinitrate is the most widely used organic nitrate. It is well absorbed orally but undergoes extensive first-pass metabolism in the liver which generates inactive metabolites. This metabolism is saturable and large oral doses of glyceryl trinitrate have useful systemic actions, especially when given as a modified-release formulation to prolong the duration of action. Usually glyceryl trinitrate is given by one of four routes that avoid first-pass metabolism and hence increase bioavailability:

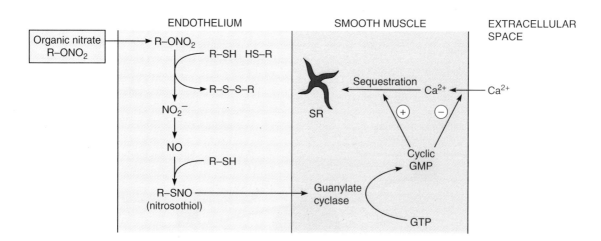

Figure 6.2 Diagram of the cellular action of nitrates. SR, sarcoplasmic reticulum; GTP, guanosine triphosphate; GMP, guanosine monophosphate; $\oplus$, increases; $\ominus$, inhibits.

(1) *Sublingual*: rapid absorption of glyceryl tri-nitrate occurs from the mucosal surface of the mouth but the very short half-life of about 5 min limits the duration of action to approximately 30 min. Tablets lose their potency with prolonged storage; a metered dose aerosol spray is equally effective and more stable.

(2) *Buccal*: the tablet is held between the upper lip and gum and an inert polymer matrix permits slow release of drug to prolong the duration of action.

(3) *Transdermal*: glyceryl trinitrate is absorbed well through the skin and can be delivered from an adhesive patch, via a rate-limiting membrane or matrix. Steady release of the drug maintains a stable blood glyceryl tri-nitrate concentration for at least 24 h.

(4) *Intravenous*: the short duration of action of glyceryl trinitrate is an advantage for intra-venous dose titration.

Isosorbide dinitrate is longer acting than glyceryl trinitrate but still has a short half-life, so that sustained release formulations are often used. It is also given as a chewable tablet for buccal absorption and a rapid onset of action, or by intravenous infusion. Isosorbide dinitrate is well absorbed orally but undergoes extensive first-pass metabolism which produces both active and inactive metabolites. The majority of the sustained clinical effect is due to the forma-tion of isosorbide-5-mononitrate.

Isosorbide-5-mononitrate is not subject to first-pass metabolism, and can be used orally as an alternative to isosorbide dinitrate, when it gives a more predictable clinical response. Since the amount of isosorbide mononitrate absorbed is greater than that generated during first-pass metabolism of the dinitrate, the anti-anginal action with the mononitrate is sustained better than with the dinitrate.

Unwanted effects of nitrates

- Venodilation may lead to postural hypoten-sion, dizziness, syncope and reflex tachycardia.
- Arterial dilation causes throbbing headaches and flushing, but tolerance to these effects is common during treatment with long-acting nitrates.
- Tolerance to the therapeutic effects of nitrates develops rapidly with long-acting formula-tions. This may be due to depletion of

vascular thiol groups or to neurohumoral acti-vation with expansion of blood volume. It can be avoided by a "nitrate-low" period of several hours each day.

β-ADRENOCEPTOR ANTAGONISTS (β-BLOCKERS)

Examples: atenolol, propranolol, pindolol.

Mechanism of action and effects in angina

All β-blockers act as competitive antagonists of catecholamines at β-adrenoceptors. They achieve their therapeutic effect in angina by blockade at the cardiac β_1-adrenoceptor which decreases heart rate, reduces the force of cardiac contraction and lowers blood pressure. These effects are most marked during exercise and reduce myocardial oxygen demand.

Additional properties of β-blockers

Cardioselectivity

Some β-blockers, for example atenolol, are rela-tively selective antagonists at the β_1-adreno-ceptor, a property known as "cardioselectivity" because of their predominant effects on the heart. However, many β-blockers, for example propranolol, have equal or greater antagonist activity at β_2-adrenoceptors; these drugs are referred to as "non-selective" β-blockers. It is important to be aware that even cardioselective β-blockers cause β_2-adrenoceptor blockade at higher doses, that is they are "selective" rather than truly specific for the β_1-adrenoceptor (Chapter 1).

Partial agonist activity

β-Blockers, for example pindolol, can also possess partial agonist activity (Chapter 1) at the β-adrenoceptor. This results in weak stimu-lation of the receptor at rest. When the concen-tration of circulating catecholamines rises, the drug becomes a competitive antagonist while retaining its mild stimulant activity. Exercise heart rate and force of contraction are there-fore reduced less by a partial agonist than by a full antagonist, and myocardial oxygen demand remains higher. For this reason, β-blockers with partial agonist activity may be less effec-tive than full antagonists in patients with severe angina.

Pharmacokinetics

- Lipophilic β-blockers, such as propranolol, are well absorbed from the gut, but undergo extensive first-pass metabolism in the liver, with considerable variability among individuals. Reduction in exercise heart rate is closely related to the plasma concentration of β-blocker. Consequently, dose titration of lipophilic β-blockers is particularly important to achieve the maximum clinical response in angina. Most lipophilic β-blockers have short half-lives.

- Hydrophilic β-blockers, such as atenolol, are less completely absorbed from the gut and are eliminated unchanged by the kidney. The dose range to maintain effective plasma concentrations is narrower than for drugs which undergo metabolism and the clinical response in angina is more predictable The half-lives are usually intermediate.

Unwanted effects

- Blockade of β_1-adrenoceptors: this may precipitate heart failure in patients with poor left ventricular function, who rely on high sympathetic nervous activity to compensate for a reduced cardiac output. The reduction in cardiac output can also impair blood supply to peripheral tissues, which may increase symptoms of intermittent claudication or provoke Raynaud's phenomenon by reducing peripheral blood flow.

  Excessive bradycardia occasionally occurs and β-blockers should be avoided in the presence of an atrioventricular conduction defect ("heart block"). Drugs with partial agonist activity are less likely to cause bradycardia.

- Blockade of β_2-adrenoceptors: bronchospasm may be precipitated in asthmatics and even "cardioselective" drugs are not completely safe.

  Impaired vasodilation in skeletal muscle may exacerbate intermittent claudication, and contribute to the fatigue commonly experienced during β-blocker therapy.

  Insulin-requiring diabetics are prone to prolonged hypoglycaemic episodes while taking non-selective β-blockers. Gluconeogenesis, a component of the metabolic response to hypoglycaemia, is dependent on β_2-adrenoceptor stimulation in the liver. β-Blockers also blunt the autonomic response which alerts the patient to the onset of hypoglycaemia.

Most β-blockers raise the plasma concentration of triglycerides and lower the concentration of high density lipoprotein (Chapter 51). These changes are most marked with non-selective blockers and do not occur if the drug has partial agonist activity.

- Central nervous system effects: these include sleep disturbance, vivid dreams and hallucinations. They are more common with lipophilic drugs, which readily cross the blood–brain barrier. Fatigue and more subtle psychomotor effects, for example lack of concentration, may also reflect "central" actions of β-blockers.

- Sudden withdrawal syndrome: β-adrenoceptor "up-regulation" (Chapter 1) during long-term treatment makes the heart more sensitive to circulating catecholamines. β-Blockers should be stopped gradually in patients with ischaemic heart disease to avoid precipitating unstable angina or myocardial infarction.

- Drug interactions: the calcium antagonist verapamil (see below) has potentially hazardous additive effects with β-blockade, reducing the force of cardiac contraction and slowing heart rate.

CALCIUM CHANNEL ANTAGONISTS (CALCIUM ANTAGONISTS)

Examples: nifedipine, amlodipine, verapamil, diltiazem.

Mechanism of action and effects

Calcium is essential for excitation–contraction coupling in muscle cells. Free calcium must either enter the cell or be released from intracellular stores for contraction to occur. As myofilaments relax, calcium is then either taken up by the sarcoplasmic reticulum or translocated out of the cell. In striated muscle, calcium is readily stored and released by the sarcoplasmic reticulum. However, in smooth muscle (such as that surrounding arteriolar resistance vessels) and to a lesser extent in cardiac muscle, intracellular calcium recycling is poorly developed. Reduced calcium entry into these cells will therefore inhibit muscle contraction.

Calcium antagonists have widely different chemical structures but all act by reducing calcium influx through voltage-operated "L-type" slow calcium channels. They have little effect on receptor-operated channels which respond to endogenous agonists such as nora-drenaline (Fig. 6.3). Despite this, there are important differences among the calcium antagonists.

Actions which may be important in angina include:

- Arteriolar dilation: dihydropyridine derivatives such as nifedipine or amlodipine are the most potent. The reduction in peripheral resistance lowers the blood pressure and therefore the work of the left ventricle which reduces myocardial oxygen demand. The reflex sympathetic nervous system response tends to produce a tachycardia (Fig. 5.4).

- Negative chronotropic effect: verapamil and diltiazem (but not the dihydropyridines such as nifedipine or amlodipine) slow the rate of firing of the sino-atrial node and slow impulse conduction through the atrioventricular node (Chapter 9). This prevents reflex tachycardia from occurring in response to arteriolar dilation.

- Reduced cardiac contractility: many calcium antagonists (particulary verapamil) produce a negative inotropic effect. With nifedipine the reflex tachycardia usually maintains cardiac output. Newer "second generation" dihydro-pyridine derivatives such as amlodipine do not impair myocardial contractility.

- Coronary artery dilation by relief of spasm will improve myocardial blood flow.

Pharmacokinetics

Most calcium antagonists are lipophilic compounds which share many pharmacokinetic properties. They are almost completely absorbed from the gut, undergo extensive and variable first-pass metabolism in the liver, and have short half-lives. Modified-release formulations are widely used to prolong the duration of action. Nifedipine is also available in a liquid-containing capsule formulation; biting the capsule and swallowing the contents leads to a more rapid onset of action. Nifedipine is inacti-vated by metabolism while verapamil and diltiazem have active, although less potent, metabolites. Verapamil can be given intrave-nously, a route that is usually reserved for the treatment of arrhythmias (Chapter 9). If given by this route, first-pass metabolism is avoided and smaller doses must be used.

Amlodipine differs from other calcium antagonists in that it is slowly and incompletely absorbed and does not undergo first-pass meta-bolism. Extensive distribution and slow metabo-lism in the liver give amlodipine a very long half-life of about 1–2 days.

Unwanted effects

- Arterial dilation: headache, flushing and dizzi-ness may be troublesome, although tolerance often occurs with continued use. Ankle oedema, frequently resistant to diuretics, may

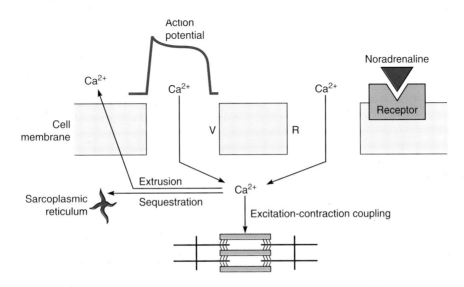

Figure 6.3 Receptor (R) and voltage (V) operated calcium channels in the cell membrane and the intracellular handling of calcium.

be a consequence of increased trans-capillary hydrostatic pressure.

- Reduced cardiac contractility: this may precipitate heart failure in susceptible patients, particularly with verapamil.
- Bradycardia and heart block: verapamil or diltiazem can cause excessive slowing of the heart, particularly if they are used in combination with other drugs that have similar effects on heart rate or atrioventricular nodal conduction, for example digoxin or β-blockers.
- Gastrointestinal: constipation occurs particularly with verapamil, while nifedipine can cause nausea and heartburn. These result from altered gut motility.

MANAGEMENT OF ANGINA

TREATMENT OF AN ACUTE ANGINAL ATTACK

An organic nitrate, most often glyceryl trinitrate, is used sublingually for rapid relief of pain. Swallowing the contents of a nifedipine capsule is also effective.

PROPHYLAXIS OF ANGINA

Regular prophylactic treatment is usually given when angina attacks are frequent. Although sublingual glyceryl trinitrate can be taken before exercise to prevent pain, the protection is short-lived. Many patients will need regular treatment with either a long-acting nitrate, a β-blocker or a calcium antagonist. Monotherapy with a β-blocker or a calcium antagonist that reduces exercise heart rate (verapamil or diltiazem) is usually most effective.

If control of symptoms is incomplete with one drug, combination therapy with two or even three different classes of drugs may be tried. The rationale behind this approach lies in their complementary mechanisms of anti-anginal effect (Fig. 6.4).

UNSTABLE ANGINA

Angina at rest or symptoms which progress rapidly in severity and frequency require intensive treatment both to control symptoms and to reduce the risk of progression to myocardial infarction. β-Blockers are often used in combination with oral or intravenous nitrates. Antiplatelet treatment with aspirin has been shown to improve outcome and is often given with intravenous heparin (Chapter 10). Calcium antagonists have no proven value in this situation but are used in addition to other treatments if these fail to control symptoms.

MANAGEMENT OF ACUTE MYOCARDIAL INFARCTION

Myocardial infarction most commonly arises from thrombosis in a coronary artery. Rupture of an

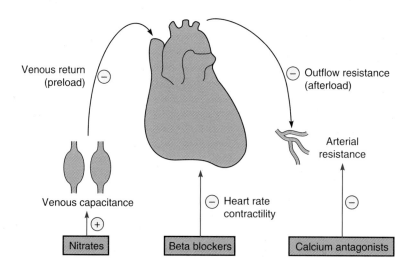

Figure 6.4 Complementary major sites of action for anti-anginal drugs. ⊕, increases; ⊖, decreases – indicate the consequences of drug effects at these sites.

atherosclerotic plaque initiates platelet aggregation with subsequent local thrombosis. Ischaemia rapidly progresses to tissue necrosis which begins subendocardially and extends transmurally over the next few hours, unless reperfusion of the vessel occurs. Natural thrombolysis or the presence of a collateral circulation will in some cases limit the necrosis to a partial thickness infarction. The ischaemia is usually associated with intense, prolonged chest pain and sympathetic nervous stimulation which increases cardiac work.

Drug therapy is directed initially towards two principal goals.

(1) *Pain relief.* An intravenous opiate analgesic such as diamorphine (Chapter 20), is given with an antiemetic. Intramuscular injection should be avoided since a low cardiac output and poor tissue perfusion often delay absorption.

(2) *Thrombolysis.* Natural thrombolysis can be enhanced by intravenous thrombolytic therapy (Chapter 10). The extent of myocardial salvage is determined by the interval between the onset of pain and the start of treatment. Three agents are in wide clinical use: recombinant tissue plasminogen activator (rt-PA), streptokinase and anistreplase. rt-PA produces more rapid reperfusion in a greater percentage of occluded vessels than either streptokinase or anistreplase. The extent of myocardial salvage and consequent reduction in mortality are similar after all three agents, except in patients with anterior infarcts who can be treated within 4 h of the onset of pain. In this subgroup rt-PA, given by an intensive bolus infusion followed by anticoagulation with intravenous heparin, gives the highest survival rate. Streptokinase is used for most patients since it is cheaper and as effective as rt-PA; it does, however, carry a higher risk of producing hypotension. rt-PA is used for patients with severe symptomatic hypotension prior to thrombolytic therapy and for those who have received streptokinase within the previous 12 months, and who are therefore likely to have high titres of neutralizing antibodies (Chapter 10). Thrombolytic therapy significantly reduces mortality if given within 12 h of the onset of pain.

SECONDARY PROPHYLAXIS OF MYOCARDIAL INFARCTION

Secondary prophylaxis to reduce mortality after myocardial infarction has been achieved with several agents:

- Low dose aspirin (Chapter 10) reduces early mortality when started within 24 h after the onset of pain, and may reduce late mortality if continued longterm. Initial benefits may be due to reduced reocclusion of vessels which have undergone natural or therapeutic thrombolysis.

- β-Blockers given intravenously immediately after the infarct and then followed by oral therapy reduce early cardiac rupture after myocardial infarction. Long-term oral use also reduces later deaths, although the mechanism is unknown. Greatest benefit is produced in patients at highest risk, for example those who had serious post-infarct arrhythmias, angina or heart failure. In the latter group, care must be taken not to exacerbate fluid retention.

- Verapamil produces a reduction in late mortality similar to that of β-blockers, but only in patients who have not had signs of heart failure. Diltiazem may reduce early reinfarction in patients with partial thickness (non-Q wave) infarcts. Nifedipine is ineffective in all patient groups.

- Other secondary prevention measures include stopping smoking, regular exercise and the control of abnormal plasma lipids.

- Anticoagulation with subcutaneous heparin (Chapter 10) can prevent deep vein thrombosis, but most patients nowadays are mobilized quickly after a myocardial infarct and the risk is not high. Low dose aspirin has also been shown to reduce the risk of deep vein thrombosis. Heparin will also reduce the formation of an intraventricular clot, which may form especially after large anterior infarcts, and will reduce the chance of cerebral embolism.

Recent evidence suggests that long-term anticoagulation with warfarin (Chapter 10) can also reduce mortality and reinfarction.

7

Hypertension

In most patients, hypertension is characterized by an increased peripheral resistance and a normal or (especially in the elderly) slightly low cardiac output. The cause of hypertension in the majority of patients is unknown (essential hypertension), although genetic factors contribute to its development. A small number of hypertensive patients have secondary hypertension due to recognized underlying disease. This is most often renal, for example glomerulonephritis and renal artery stenosis or endocrine, for example phaeochromocytoma and Conn's syndrome. The most frequent complications of hypertension are coronary artery disease and stroke; heart failure and progressive renal impairment can also occur.

Antihypertensive drugs act either by reducing cardiac output or by lowering peripheral resistance, and can be considered in three groups (Fig. 7.1):

(1) Drugs acting on the sympathetic nervous system:
   β-Adrenoceptor antagonists (β-blockers).
   α-Adrenoceptor antagonists (α-blockers).
   Centrally acting drugs.
   Adrenergic neurone blockers.
   Ganglion blockers.
(2) Diuretics:
(3) Other vasodilators:
   Angiotensin-converting enzyme (ACE) inhibitors.
   Calcium channel antagonists.
   Direct acting vasodilators.

β-ADRENOCEPTOR ANTAGONISTS (β-BLOCKERS)

Examples: atenolol, propranolol, pindolol.

Mechanism of action in hypertension

The hypotensive action of these drugs is believed to have several components. Selective β_1-adrenoceptor blockers are as effective as non-selective drugs indicating that β_2-adrenoceptor blockade makes little contribution. The more important actions are probably:

- Reduction of heart rate and myocardial contractility which decrease cardiac output.
- Blockade of renal juxtaglomerular β-adrenoceptors which reduces renin secretion (Chapter 5).
- Presynaptic β-adrenoceptor blockade in sympathetic nerves supplying arteriolar resistance vessels. These receptors form a positive feedback loop promoting noradrenaline release (Fig. 7.2). Blockade blunts the reflex increase in peripheral resistance which occurs via baroreceptors in response to the fall in cardiac output.
- Compounds with β_2-adrenoceptor partial agonist activity, for example pindolol, produce peripheral vasodilation.

For further details about β-blockers, see Chapter 6.

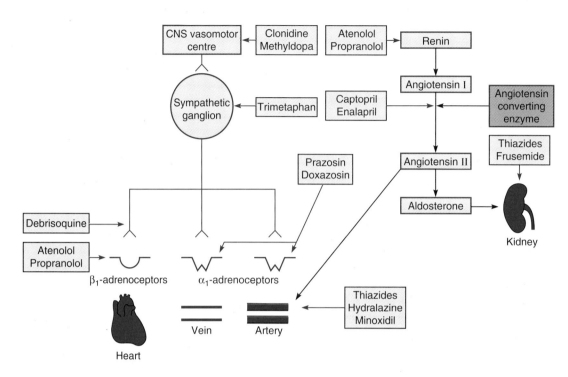

Figure 7.1 Important sites of drug action in hypertension with examples of individual agents.

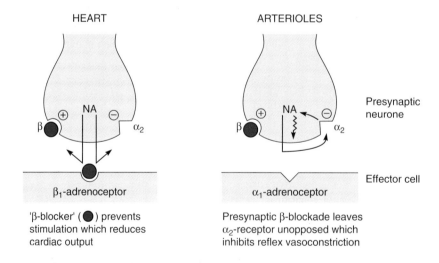

'β-blocker' (●) prevents stimulation which reduces cardiac output

Presynaptic β-blockade leaves α₂-receptor unopposed which inhibits reflex vasoconstriction

Figure 7.2 The action of β-blockers in hypertension.

α-ADRENOCEPTOR ANTAGONISTS (α-BLOCKERS)

Examples — α₁-selective: prazosin, doxazosin;
        — non-selective: phenoxybenzamine.

Mechanisms of action

Blockade of postsynaptic α₁-adrenoceptors lowers blood pressure by:

- Lowering tone in arteriolar resistance vessels.
- Dilating venous capacitance vessels, which reduces venous return and, therefore, cardiac output.
- Selective α₁-adrenoceptor antagonists spare the presynaptic α₂-adrenoceptors. Reflex sympathetic stimulation via baroreceptors to the β₁-adrenoceptors in the heart is, therefore, blunted by a negative feedback

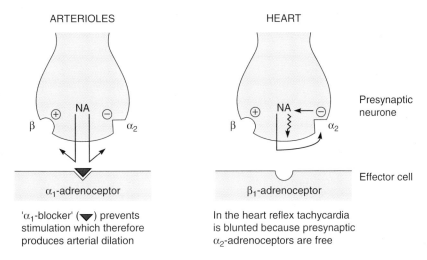

ARTERIOLES

HEART

'α_1-blocker' (▼) prevents stimulation which therefore produces arterial dilation

In the heart reflex tachycardia is blunted because presynaptic α_2-adrenoceptors are free

Figure 7.3 The action of selective α_1-adrenoceptor antagonists in hypertension.

(Fig. 7.3). Non-selective α-blockers do not have this advantage and produce reflex tachycardia; they are now little used in clinical practice except for the perioperative management of phaeochromocytoma.

Pharmacokinetics

Selective α_1-blockers undergo extensive first-pass metabolism in the liver. The compounds differ principally in their plasma half-life and therefore duration of action, for example prazosin has a short half-life, while that of doxazosin is long.

Unwanted effects

- Postural hypotension due to venous pooling. This can be particularly troublesome after the first dose.
- Palpitations due to reflex cardiac stimulation. These occur more commonly with non-selective drugs.
- Lethargy.
- Potentially beneficial effects on plasma lipids with an increase in HDL cholesterol and a reduction in triglycerides (Chapter 51).

CENTRALLY ACTING ANTIHYPERTENSIVES

Examples: methyldopa, clonidine.

Mechanisms of action

These drugs reduce central sympathetic nervous outflow from the vasomotor centre, which reduces both peripheral arterial and venous tone.

Methyldopa and clonidine produce stimulation of central presynaptic α_2-adrenoceptors and inhibit neurotransmitter release. Clonidine is a direct-acting agonist; methyldopa is first metabolized in the nerve terminal as a "false substrate" in the biosynthetic pathway for noradrenaline to produce α-methylnoradrenaline, a potent α_2-adrenoceptor agonist. Clonidine also has some postsynaptic α-adrenoceptor stimulant activity which produces peripheral vasoconstriction.

Pharmacokinetics

Methyldopa is incompletely absorbed from the gut and undergoes dose-dependent first-pass metabolism to an inactive sulphate conjugate. The half-life is short.

Clonidine is completely absorbed from the gut and is eliminated partly by the kidney and partly by liver metabolism. It has a long half-life.

Unwanted effects

- Sympathetic blockade: failure of ejaculation and postural hypotension (unusual with clonidine due to direct peripheral action).
- Unopposed parasympathetic action (unusual with methyldopa): nasal stuffiness (clonidine).
- CNS effects: sedation and drowsiness occur in up to 50% of patients. Depression is occasionally seen.
- Methyldopa induces a reversible positive Coomb's test, due to IgG production, in up

to 20% of patients. Haemolytic anaemia, however, is rare but cross-matching of blood may be difficult.

- Sudden withdrawal of clonidine can produce severe rebound hypertension with anxiety, sweating and tachycardia.

ADRENERGIC NEURONE BLOCKERS

Examples: debrisoquine, guanethidine.

Mechanism of action

These drugs use the active transport mechanism for monoamines (uptake 1) to accumulate in the adrenergic nerve terminal (Chapter 4). Inside the cell they prevent the release of nor-adrenaline from vesicles by interfering with calcium ion responses to the nerve action potential. The inhibition of adrenergic neurone activity produces arterial and venous dilation and a relatively constant heart rate.

Pharmacokinetics

Debrisoquine is fairly well absorbed and undergoes hepatic metabolism by hydroxylation. Most individuals metabolize debrisoquine extensively, but about 8% of the UK population have a genetically determined decreased metabolism of the drug which greatly increases the clinical response. Platelet uptake leads to slow elimination and a long half-life.

Unwanted effects

- Sympathetic blockade: venous pooling produces troublesome postural and exertional hypotension. Inhibition of ejaculation.
- Unopposed parasympathetic actions: increased intestinal secretions with diarrhoea, nasal stuffiness.
- Fluid retention due to renin release (Fig. 5.4).
- Interactions with other drugs acting at the adrenergic neurone. Tricyclic antidepressants compete for uptake into the neurone and reduce the hypotensive response. Neuronal uptake of indirect-acting sympathomimetics (e.g. ephedrine in cold remedies: see Chapter 4) is inhibited, reducing their beneficial action.

GANGLION BLOCKERS

Example: trimetaphan.

Mechanism of action

Competitive blockade of nicotinic (N_1) receptors at autonomic ganglia reduces activity in the sympathetic and parasympathetic nervous systems (Chapter 4). Arterial and venous dilation both contribute to the hypotensive effects.

Pharmacokinetics

Trimetaphan is rapidly metabolized in the liver and has a brief duration of action of only a few minutes. It is given by intravenous infusion or intermittent injection for controlled hypotension during surgery. Since it is highly ionized, oral absorption is very poor. It is eliminated by the kidney.

Unwanted effects

- Sympathetic blockade: postural hypotension, inhibition of ejaculation.
- Parasympathetic blockade: dry mouth, constipation, urinary retention, blurred vision, impotence (see Chapter 4).

DIURETICS

Mechanism of action in hypertension

The sites and mechanisms of action of diuretics on the kidney are considered in Chapter 15. Their initial hypotensive effect is due to intravascular salt and water depletion. However, compensatory mechanisms such as activation of the renin–angiotensin–aldosterone system restore plasma and extracellular fluid volumes (Fig. 5.4) (unless salt and water retention was a major component of the initial hypertension, e.g. in advanced renal failure). Despite this, blood pressure remains lower due to direct arterial dilation. This probably results from reduction of intracellular sodium in the smooth muscle of the arteriolar resistance vessel walls, which decreases responsiveness to circulating vasopressor substances.

WHICH DIURETIC FOR HYPERTENSION?

Three groups of diuretics are used to lower blood pressure.

Thiazide and thiazide-like diuretics

Examples: bendrofluazide, chlorthalidone.

These effectively lower blood pressure in mild to moderate hypertension at doses lower than those required for diuretic effects. This is an advantage since most unwanted effects are dose-related.

Loop diuretics

Example: frusemide.

Loop diuretics are less effective hypotensive agents than thiazides in uncomplicated hypertension. Despite having a more powerful diuretic action, the hypotensive effect is usually shorter than that of a thiazide. However, hypertension with advanced renal impairment, or hypertension resistant to multiple drug treatment is more likely to be associated with fluid retention and will respond better to a loop diuretic than to a thiazide.

Potassium-sparing diuretics

Examples: spironolactone, amiloride, triamterene.

Spironolactone, a specific aldosterone antagonist, is reserved for hypertension due to primary hyperaldosteronism (Conn's syndrome) due to concern about its long-term safety (see Chapter 15). The alternative drugs, amiloride and triamterene, are less effective than thiazides in essential hypertension.

DIRECT-ACTING VASODILATORS

Examples: hydralazine, minoxidil.

Mechanism of action

The direct-acting vasodilators selectively bind to vascular smooth muscle. Hydralazine activates guanylate cyclase leading to the production of cyclic GMP. Activation of the cell membrane potassium pump leading to intracellular potassium accumulation may contribute to the effects of minoxidil.

Pharmacokinetics

Hydralazine is well absorbed from the gut, then undergoes extensive first-pass metabolism in the gut wall and liver, principally by *N*-acetylation.

Some individuals who are genetically determined slow acetylators (Chapter 2) require lower doses of hydralazine and are more susceptible to some of the unwanted effects. The half-life is short.

Minoxidil is well absorbed from the gut, and mainly metabolized in the liver. The half-life is short.

Unwanted effects

- Arterial vasodilation produces flushing and headache. Increased trans-capillary pressure may produce dependent oedema.
- The reflex sympathetic nervous system response to vasodilation causes tachycardia and increased myocardial contractility leading to palpitations. Salt and water retention occurs due to stimulation of the renin–aldosterone system (Fig. 5.4). These compensatory mechanisms, which limit the hypotensive effect of vasodilators, can be blunted by the concurrent use of β-blockers and diuretics.
- Hydralazine may cause a systemic lupus erythematosus-like syndrome. It usually occurs after several months of treatment, is dose-related, and more common in slow acetylators. It resembles the naturally occurring disease but does not produce renal or cerebral damage and is reversible if treatment is stopped. A positive antinuclear antibody is found in many patients who do not develop the syndrome.
- Minoxidil produces hirsutism and therefore is used rarely for women.

ANGIOTENSIN CONVERTING ENZYME (ACE) INHIBITORS

Examples: captopril, enalapril.

Mechanisms of action

Competitive inhibition of angiotensin converting enzyme (ACE), reduces generation of angiotensin II and release of aldosterone (Fig. 7.4). Inhibition of tissue ACE in the vascular wall is believed to be more important for the hypotensive effect of these drugs than an effect on the circulating renin-angiotensin system. Reduced tissue concentrations of angiotensin II lead to arterial and venous dilation. Lack of a reflex tachycardia may be due to stimulation of the vagus nerve or to loss of

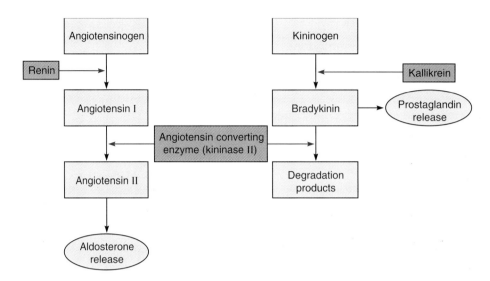

Figure 7.4 The inter-relationship between the renin–angiotensin–aldosterone and the kallikrein–kinin systems.

potentiation of sympathetic nervous activity by angiotensin II (Fig. 5.4).

ACE also degrades vasodilator kinins (Fig. 7.4). Increased kinins or vasodilator prostaglandins may contribute to the hypotensive actions of ACE inhibitors.

Pharmacokinetics

Many ACE inhibitors are water soluble and poorly absorbed from the gut in the active form. These are given as prodrugs which are converted in the liver to the active agent, for example enalapril is converted to enalaprilat. Others, for example captopril, are adequately absorbed as an active molecule. For most compounds, the active drug is excreted unchanged by the kidney. The half-life of captopril is short while that of enalaprilat is long.

Unwanted effects

- Cough: unproductive, not dose-related; may be due to accumulation of kinins in the lung; occurs in up to 10% of patients, and is more common in women.
- Postural hypotension: rare unless there is salt and water depletion, for example due to diuretics. In such patients, profound hypotension can occur, particularly after the first dose.
- Disturbance of taste.
- Rashes.
- Angioneurotic oedema.

CALCIUM CHANNEL ANTAGONISTS

Examples: nifedipine, verapamil, diltiazem.

Mechanism of action

These drugs lower blood pressure principally by arterial vasodilation. For full details see Chapter 6.

NITROPRUSSIDE

Mechanism of action

Nitroprusside is a nitro-vasodilator with a mechanism of action similar to that of organic nitrates (Chapter 6). It produces dilation of arterioles and veins, reducing both peripheral resistance and venous return.

Pharmacokinetics

It is given by intravenous infusion and has a duration of action of less than 5 min. Metabolism to cyanide within red blood cells (by electron transfer from haemoglobin iron) terminates its effect. The cyanide is partly bound in the erythrocyte and partly liberated producing inhibition of cellular cytochrome oxidase. Free cyanide is converted in the liver to less toxic thiocyanate which accumulates with prolonged infusion.

Unwanted effects

- Confusion and psychosis.
- Metabolic acidosis due to inhibition of aerobic metabolism in cells.

TREATMENT OF HYPERTENSION

It is rarely possible to correct the underlying cause of hypertension but the morbidity associated with untreated hypertension is high. Lowering blood pressure produces a substantial reduction in the risk of stroke, heart failure and kidney damage.

Treatment with drugs in young and middle-aged patients with uncomplicated hypertension has not been shown to be beneficial until the phase V diastolic blood pressure is 100 mmHg or greater. In the elderly, the risk of morbid events is much greater, and treatment is desirable if the diastolic blood pressure exceeds 90 mmHg and/or the systolic blood pressure is above 160 mmHg. The treatment of isolated systolic hypertension in the elderly gives similar benefit to treatment of diastolic hypertension.

Treatment prevents coronary artery disease in the elderly, but the evidence is less convincing in the young. This may reflect either the short duration of the trials (up to 5 years) or a failure to reduce other risk factors such as smoking and hypercholesterolaemia. Almost all trials have used treatment regimens based on β-blockers or diuretics. These have shown equal efficacy in younger patients for reducing events, but diuretics are clearly superior to β-blockers in the elderly. Compared with newer agents, these drugs are much slower at reversing left ventricular hypertrophy (which independently predicts the risk of ischaemic heart disease) and they produce potentially atherogenic changes in the plasma lipid profile (Chapter 51).

Although ACE inhibitors, calcium antagonists and α-blockers have theoretical advantages for the prevention of coronary artery disease, these have not been tested in clinical trials. Current opinion is divided between using only β-blockers and diuretics as first-line treatment or giving the newer classes of drug equal prominence. The cost implications of the second option are considerable.

Non-pharmacological treatment with weight loss, alcohol reduction and salt restriction may make drug treatment unnecessary or control with drugs easier to achieve. For mild to moderate hypertension, a single drug will provide good blood pressure control in at least 40% of patients. For more resistant patients, combinations of two or occasionally three drugs from different classes may be necessary, for example a diuretic with a β-blocker, or an ACE inhibitor with a diuretic.

The ganglion blocker, trimetaphan, is used for induction of controlled hypotension during certain surgical procedures. Non-selective α-blockers are given to control hypertension in phaeochromocytoma. Nitroprusside is reserved for severe hypertensive emergencies (such as hypertensive encephalopathy) to produce a rapid but controlled reduction in blood pressure.

8

Positive Inotropic Agents and Heart Failure

Myocardial contractility can be improved by increasing the availability of free calcium in the cell to interact with contractile proteins, or by increasing the sensitivity of the myofibrils to calcium. Only drugs which increase myocardial intracellular calcium are established in clinical use. They affect intracellular calcium by two distinct pathways: an action on the membrane sodium pump, or by increasing in intracellular cyclic AMP.

A major advantage of those positive inotropic drugs that increase myocardial cyclic AMP is an associated enhanced reuptake of calcium by the sarcoplasmic reticulum in diastole. This improves diastolic relaxation in addition to augmenting systolic contractility.

DIGITALIS GLYCOSIDES

Example: digoxin.

Mechanism of action

All digitalis glycosides have a steroid nucleus, and were originally isolated from a species of foxglove (*Digitalis purpura*). The receptor for digitalis is the energy dependent myocyte membrane sodium pump (Na^+/K^+-ATPase). This pump establishes and maintains the Na^+ and K^+ gradients across the cell (Fig. 8.1), producing low intracellular sodium and high intracellular potassium concentrations. Partial inhibition of the pump by digitalis increases the intracellular sodium concentration, and reduces the concentration gradient for sodium across the cell membrane. As a consequence, there is a reduction in the passive transmembrane exchange of Na^+ and Ca^{2+} down their concentration gradients, which increases the intracellular Ca^{2+} concentration. The excess intracellular calcium is stored in the sarcoplasmic reticulum during diastole and released during membrane excitation, leading to enhanced contraction.

Digitalis glycosides also have effects on the cardiac action potential. The direct action of the drug on the myocardium shortens the duration of the action potential (and, therefore, the refractory period of the cell) and produces spontaneous release of calcium from the sarcoplasmic reticulum leading to transient depolarization of the cell immediately following an action potential ("after potentials"). Both effects increase myocardial excitability and automaticity (Chapter 9) which can provoke arrhythmias. By contrast, digitalis glycosides also produce central stimulation of the vagus nerve and enhanced cardiac sensitivity to acetylcholine. These actions decrease automaticity of the sinoatrial node and increase the refractory period of the atrioventricular (AV) node, effects which result in antiarrhythmic activity (Chapter 9).

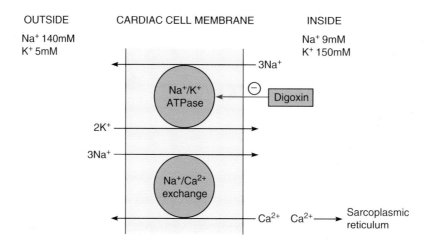

Figure 8.1   The cellular actions of digoxin; $\ominus$, inhibition.

Digitalis glycosides produce distinctive changes on the ECG which include non-specific T wave changes and sagging of the S–T segment ("reverse tick"): these can make identification of myocardial ischaemia difficult.

Pharmacokinetics

Digoxin is the most widely used of the digitalis glycosides in the UK. It is well absorbed from the gut; the kidney is the main route of elimination, partially by active tubular secretion. The half-life of digoxin is very long (about 1.5 days) and considerably longer when renal function is impaired. To achieve an early onset of action, initial loading doses should be given over 24–36 h (Chapter 2). If a rapid response is essential, digoxin can be given by slow intravenous injection.

Other digitalis glycosides are rarely used. Digitoxin is occasionally given in renal failure since it is extensively metabolized and mainly excreted by the gut. However, it has a major disadvantage of a much longer half-life than digoxin (approximately 7 days).

Unwanted effects

Digitalis glycosides have a narrow therapeutic index. Most toxicity is dose-related:

- Consequences of intracellular calcium overload: increased automaticity of AV junctional and Purkinje fibres produces junctional escape beats, junctional tachycardia, ventricular ectopic beats (including bigeminy), or (less commonly) ventricular tachycardia.

- Consequences of increased vagal activity: excessive AV nodal block can occur; when associated with increased atrial automaticity this produces atrial tachycardia with AV nodal block, a rhythm characteristic of digitalis toxicity.

- Gastrointestinal disturbances: anorexia, nausea and vomiting (largely a central effect at the chemoreceptor trigger zone (Chapter 34)), diarrhoea.

- Neurological disturbance: fatigue, malaise, confusion, vertigo, coloured vision (especially yellow halos around lights) possibly due to inhibition of Na^+/K^+-ATPase in the cones of the retina.

- Gynaecomastia or breast enlargement: due to the oestrogen-like steroid structure.

Exacerbating factors for digitalis toxicity

- Hypokalaemia: reduced extracellular potassium increases the effects of digitalis on the Na^+/K^+-ATPase pump. Care must be taken if diuretics are used with digitalis glycosides.

- Renal failure: this is not always obvious in the elderly, who may have a normal plasma creatinine even when renal function is markedly reduced.

- Hypoxaemia: this sensitizes the heart to digitalis induced arrhythmias.

- Hypothyroidism: decreases renal elimination of digoxin.

- Drugs which displace digoxin from tissue binding sites and interfere with its excretion:

these include verapamil (Chapter 6) and quinidine (Chapter 9) which can double the plasma concentration of digoxin. Amiodarone (Chapter 9) produces a less marked effect.

Treatment of digitalis toxicity

- Withhold further drug.
- Potassium supplementation (Chapter 15) for hypokalaemia. This should be given by slow intravenous infusion if there are dangerous arrhythmias, orally otherwise.
- Phenytoin (Chapter 9) is the preferred drug for serious ventricular arrhythmias since it will also reverse AV block.
- Atropine (Chapter 9) for sinus bradycardia or AV block. Temporary transvenous pacing is used for marked bradycardia unresponsive to atropine.
- Digoxin-specific antibody fragments for serious toxicity (Chapter 57).

SYMPATHOMIMETIC INOTROPES

Examples — non-selective β-adrenoceptor agonist: isoprenaline;
— selective β_1-adrenoceptor agonist: dobutamine;
— mixed non-selective β-adrenoceptor- and dopaminergic agonist: dopamine.

Mechanisms of action and effects

These are considered in Chapter 4.

Isoprenaline is a non-selective β-adrenoceptor agonist which increases both myocardial contractility (β_1-adrenoceptors) (Fig. 8.2) and heart rate (β_1- and β_2-adrenoceptors) and produces peripheral arterial vasodilation (β_2-adrenoceptors).

Dobutamine, a synthetic dopamine analogue, is a selective β_1-adrenoceptor agonist which produces a powerful inotropic response with relatively less increase in heart rate and little direct effect on vascular tone.

Dopamine has dose-related actions at several receptors:

- At lowest doses, it selectively stimulates peripheral dopamine (DA) receptors which are structurally distinct from those in the CNS (Chapter 17). This produces renal vasodilation and diuresis (DA_1 receptors) and

peripheral arterial vasodilation (DA_2 receptors which inhibit noradrenaline release from sympathetic nerves).
- At moderate doses, non-selective β-adrenoceptor stimulation produces a positive inotropic response (Fig. 8.2). The tachycardia is greater than with dobutamine, due to direct cardiac β_2-adrenoceptor stimulation and the reflex response to β_2-adrenoceptor mediated peripheral arterial dilation.
- At maximum doses, α-adrenoceptor stimulation produces peripheral vasoconstriction, which also affects the renal arteries and overcomes dopamine-induced renal vasodilation.

Pharmacokinetics

Dobutamine, dopamine and isoprenaline are all administered by intravenous infusion due to their very short half-lives of about 2 min. Inactivation is by the same pathways as noradrenaline (Chapter 4). Downregulation of β-adrenoceptors (Chapter 1) rapidly reduces the response to sustained infusions. Owing to its vasoconstrictor actions, dopamine is usually given into a large central vein.

Unwanted effects

These can be predicted from excessive adrenoceptor stimulation (Chapter 4).

PHOSPHODIESTERASE INHIBITORS

Examples: milrinone, enoximone.

Mechanism of action and effects

Milrinone and enoximone are specific inhibitors of the isoenzyme of phosphodiesterase found in cardiac and smooth muscle (phosphodiesterase III). Their inotropic action is due to increased intracellular cyclic AMP (Fig. 8.2) and is not limited by downregulation of cell surface receptors, unlike that of β-adrenoceptor agonists. However, they produce tachycardia and have the potential to induce serious cardiac rhythm disturbances. Phosphodiesterase inhibition in vascular smooth muscle produces peripheral vasodilation. Because of complementary sites of action, phosphodiesterase inhibitors and β-adrenoceptor agonists will have additive effects on the heart.

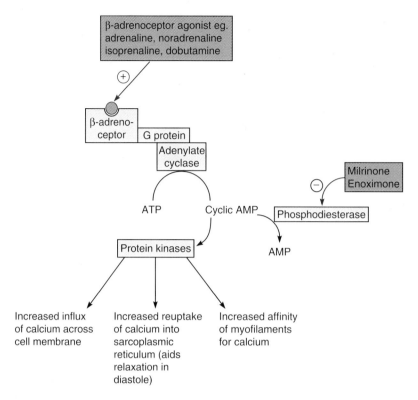

Figure 8.2 Cyclic AMP and myocardial contractility. ⊕, Stimulation; ⊖, inhibition.

Pharmacokinetics

Owing to doubts about their long-term safety these drugs are only available for short-term intravenous infusion. They have short half-lives and are eliminated principally by the kidney.

Unwanted effects

- Mainly those produced by excessive cardiac stimulation, with tachycardia, palpitation and arrhythmia.
- During long-term use, concern has been expressed about excessive myocardial oxygen consumption and metabolic "exhaustion". Serious arrhythmias may also predispose to sudden death.

MANAGEMENT OF HEART FAILURE

ACUTE LEFT VENTRICULAR FAILURE

Left ventricular failure usually results from a sudden inability of the heart to maintain cardiac output and blood pressure. This leads to reflex arterial and venous constriction (Fig 5.4) with a rapid rise in filling pressure of the left ventricle due to increased venous return. The hydrostatic pressure in the pulmonary veins rises until it exceeds the plasma osmotic pressure and produces pulmonary oedema. The principal symptom is breathlessness, particularly orthopnoea or exertional dyspnoea in the early stages, with symptoms present at rest if the condition is severe.

The immediate aim of treatment is to reduce the excessive venous return. Intravenous injection of a loop diuretic (Chapter 15) produces initial venous dilation, increases peripheral venous pooling and relieves symptoms even before the onset of a diuresis. Sublingual glyceryl trinitrate (Chapter 6) also dilates venous capacitance vessels, and is an alternative emergency treatment. An opiate analgesic (Chapter 20) is often given intravenously to relieve distress and breathlessness.

Whenever possible a precipitating or exacerbating cause should be treated, for example arrhythmias, anaemia, thyrotoxicosis. However, many patients will require maintenance treatment with an oral diuretic.

CARDIOGENIC SHOCK

Sudden loss of a large amount of myocardium (e.g. after a large anterior myocardial infarction) can produce a low cardiac output state with pulmonary congestion. In contrast to hypovolaemic shock, the central venous pressure is high in cardiogenic shock. Mortality is high even with intensive treatment but several options are available.

Intravenous dobutamine is usually used as an inotropic agent, often in combination with low-dose dopamine to increase renal blood flow and to encourage a diuresis. An intravenous loop diuretic is also given to augment the diuresis.

Intense venous and arterial constriction can be relieved by intravenous nitroprusside which will improve cardiac output (Fig. 5.2) and relieve pulmonary oedema (Fig. 5.1). Intravenous nitrate is an alternative option to produce predominant venous dilation but is generally less useful than nitroprusside. Because there is a considerable risk of excessive vasodilation and more profound hypotension, facilities for intensive monitoring of cardiac output and central pressures are desirable if a vasodilator is used.

Phosphodiesterase inhibitors combine inotropic and vasodilator properties. They are sometimes used as an alternative to dobutamine and nitroprusside.

CHRONIC HEART FAILURE

Patients with chronic heart failure usually have biventricular failure with pulmonary and peripheral congestion. The compensatory responses of the sympathetic nervous system and renin–angiotensin system to the low cardiac output are often marked. Diuretics (Chapter 15) form the basis of treatment, with a loop diuretic most often used. If fluid retention is resistant to treatment with a loop diuretic the addition of a thiazide or related diuretic should be considered. This will reduce the compensatory distal tubular sodium reabsorption of the excess sodium delivered from the loop of Henle. Most patients should also be given an ACE inhibitor (Chapter 7). These can relieve symptoms of breathlessness and fatigue by their balanced vasodilator action (Figs 5.1, 5.2). Patients with heart failure are at increased risk of sudden death, or death from progressive heart failure. ACE inhibitors reduce mortality in patients with symptomatic heart failure, regardless of its severity, although the mechanism is uncertain. They also reduce mortality in patients who developed heart failure after a myocardial infarction. ACE inhibitors may also slow the progression of asymptomatic left ventricular dysfunction. These actions may be due to prevention of adverse structural remodelling of the infarcted ventricle.

Digoxin is of undoubted benefit for the treatment of fast atrial fibrillation in association with heart failure. Slowing the rate of the ventricular response can improve myocardial performance and relieve symptoms. In sinus rhythm a sustained inotropic effect can be achieved in patients with a dilated poorly contractile ventricle in whom systolic function is markedly impaired. Heart failure with a small heart is less likely to respond. In this situation failure to relax the ventricle in diastole may be a major factor and symptoms arise from reduced ventricular filling and a high filling pressure. Digoxin has no effect on myocardial relaxation. The effect of digoxin on mortality in heart failure is unknown.

Sudden death in heart failure can result from either an arrhythmic or an embolic event. Antiarrhythmic drugs are of uncertain value and most (apart from amiodarone (Chapter 9)) reduce myocardial contractility. Anticoagulation with warfarin (Chapter 10) may prevent the formation of thrombus in a dilated ventricle but the long-term effects on embolic events and mortality are unknown.

9

Cardiac Arrhythmias

PRINCIPLES OF ARRHYTHMOGENESIS

BASIC ELECTROPHYSIOLOGY

Myocardial cells maintain transmembrane ion gradients by movement of the ions through membrane channels. Specific channels exist for sodium and calcium and several for potassium.

The resting potential of a cardiac cell is approximately -80 to $-90\,mV$ compared to the extracellular environment. This is maintained by a transmembrane concentration gradient for potassium. The resting potential comprises phase 4 of the action potential (Fig. 9.1).

Depolarization is initiated by a rapid influx of sodium ions (phase 0) through specific voltage-gated ion channels. Depolarization is triggered when sufficient sodium channels have been opened to allow the cell to reach the threshold potential. In the atrioventricular node this depolarization is due to the slower influx of calcium ions. This results in slower conduction of the impulse through the node than in other parts of

the heart, and is responsible for the conduction delay in the atrioventricular node.

At the end of phase 0 there is an overshoot creating a brief positive intracellular potential, at which point a "gate" in the sodium channel closes and prevents further ion flow. Inactivation of the channel is triggered by the same depolarizing impulse that opens the channel, but occurs far more slowly. Its purpose is to prevent repetitive depolarization. Recovery of the channel to the resting state, when it is closed but no longer refractory to further depolarization, depends on repolarization of the cell.

Repolarization is initiated by the opening of specific potassium ion channels and begins when potassium efflux exceeds sodium influx (phase 1). It is temporarily interrupted by influx of calcium ions which maintains depolarization (phase 2). Finally, potassium efflux increases until it is sufficient to repolarize the cell (phase 3). Sodium and potassium transmembrane concentration gradients are restored by a separate exchange pump.

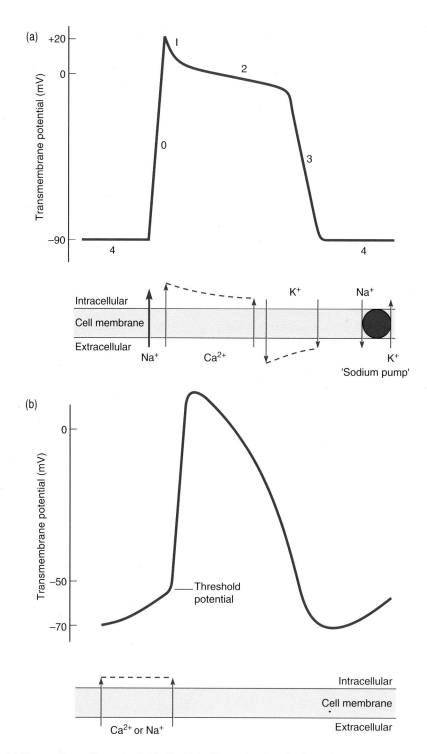

Figure 9.1 (a) The cardiac action potential in Purkinje fibres showing the four phases and transmembrane ion fluxes. (b) The cardiac action potential in a pacemaker cell showing additional ion flux in phase 4.

The heart has several pacemaker cells which differ from non-pacemaker myocardial cells in developing spontaneous depolarization during the resting phase of the action potential. The normal cardiac impulse arises from the sino-atrial node, since these cells have the fastest intrinsic rate of spontaneous depolarization. The specialized electrical conducting tissue of the heart has a cascade of potential pacemakers with progressively slower rates of depolarization. These will only be utilized if higher pacemakers slow or fail. The non-specialized cardiac muscle cells do not show this spontaneous depolarization in the healthy heart, but are linked in a manner that facilitates rapid conduction of an action potential from an adjacent cell. Thus, all cardiac cells have "excitability", or the ability to respond to a stimulus but only specialized conducting tissue has "automaticity" or the ability to initiate a spontaneous discharge.

In phase 4, pacemaker cells have a slow leak of positive ions into the cell. In the sino-atrial and atrioventricular nodes calcium ions are responsible for depolarization until a threshold potential is reached. In other pacemaker cells, sodium ion leakage is the trigger.

During the period between phase 0 and the end of phase 2, the cell is refractory to further depolarization (absolute refractory period) since the sodium channels are inactivated. During phase 3, a sufficiently large stimulus can open enough sodium channels (which have recovered to the resting state) to overcome the potassium efflux. This is the relative refractory period.

MECHANISMS OF ARRHYTHMOGENESIS

Arrhythmias can arise as the result of either abnormal impulse generation or abnormal impulse conduction. Three mechanisms can be identified:

(1) *Re-entry.* This is the cause of most clinically important arrhythmias. If an impulse arrives at an area of tissue when it is refractory to the stimulus, the impulse will be conducted by an alternative route (Fig. 9.2). If this impulse again reaches the "blocked" tissue distally when it has had sufficient time to recover, the impulse will be conducted retrogradely (re-entry). This retrograde conduction is usually slow, because in order to initiate a circuit of electrical activity, the healthy tissue has to be given time to repolarize. Such a mechanism can, therefore, initiate a self-perpetuating "loop" of electrical activity which acts as a pacemaker. The re-entry circuit can be localized within a small area of myocardium. Alternatively it can exist as large circuits, for example between the atria and ventricles.

(2) *Automaticity.* Subsidiary (or ectopic) pacemakers may develop when a site in the myocardium develops a more rapid phase 4 depolarization than the sino-atrial node. This can arise in a site with natural pacemaker activity or if spontaneous depolarization develops in cells which usually have a stable phase 4, for example as a result of ischaemia.

(3) *Triggered activity.* Following a depolarization, a cell may develop oscillating depolarizations ("after potentials") which will initiate an action potential if they depolarize the cell to its threshold. This is a rare

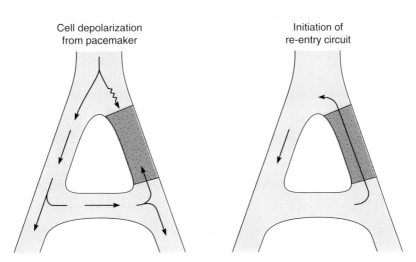

Figure 9.2 Schematic representation of a re-entry circuit. Abnormal conducting tissue initially refractory to stimulation (▨) recovers to permit retrograde depolarization which initiates the circuit.

mechanism of arrhythmogenesis, but may be responsible for the proarrhythmic activity of class I and III antiarrhythmic agents and digitalis glycosides (see below).

EFFECTS OF DRUGS ON THE ACTION POTENTIAL: CLASSIFICATION OF ANTIARRHYTHMIC DRUGS

A widely used classification of antiarrhythmic drugs (the Vaughan Williams Classification) is based on their effects on the action potential (Fig. 9.3).

- *Class I*: These drugs slow the rate of rise of phase 0 by inhibiting fast sodium channels and are known as membrane stabilizers. The class is subdivided according to the effects of the drug on the duration of the action potential:

  IA: increase the duration. Moderate to marked sodium channel blockade is produced. Refractoriness of the cell is prolonged due to multiple potassium channel blockade.

  IB: decrease the duration. Mild to moderate sodium channel blockade is produced, but there is little effect on refractoriness since there is no blockade of potassium channels.

  IC: no effect on the duration. Marked sodium channel blockade is produced, and

refractoriness is increased due to specific blockade of potassium channels responsible for repolarization.

- *Class II*: These are β-adrenoceptor antagonists which reduce the rate of spontaneous depolarization of sinus and atrioventricular nodal tissue and some ectopic foci in phase 4 by indirect blockade of calcium channels, reversing the effects of catecholamines.

- *Class III*: These drugs prolong the duration of the action potential thus increasing the absolute refractory period. This is the result of reduced influx of potassium into the cell.

- *Class IV*: Certain slow calcium channel antagonists have specific actions on the sinoatrial and atrioventricular nodes, stabilizing phase 4 of the action potential.

Three drugs used in the treatment of rhythm disturbances do not fit into this classification: digitalis glycosides, adenosine and atropine.

CLASS IA DRUGS

Indications: supraventricular and ventricular arrhythmias.

DISOPYRAMIDE

Pharmacokinetics

Oral absorption is almost complete, but an intravenous formulation is available for rapid onset of action. Metabolism in the liver generates a less active compound but with greater anticholinergic activity. About half the drug is eliminated unchanged in the urine. Disopyramide has an intermediate half-life.

Unwanted effects

- Powerful negative inotropic effect; disopyramide should be avoided in heart failure.

- Anticholinergic effects (see Chapter 4): especially urinary retention, glaucoma, dry mouth and blurred vision.

PROCAINAMIDE

Pharmacokinetics

Procainamide is well absorbed from the gut, but is also available for intravenous use. Most is

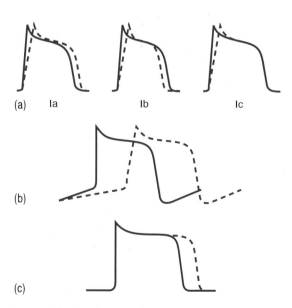

(a) Ia Ib Ic

(b)

(c)

Figure 9.3 (a) Effects of Class I drugs on the cardiac action potential. (b) Effects of Class II and IV drugs on phase 4 of the cardiac action potential. (c) Effect of Class III drugs on the cardiac action potential.

excreted unchanged by the kidney but about 40% is acetylated in the liver. The rate of acetylation is subject to genetic polymorphism and is slow in some individuals (Chapter 2). The plasma half-life is intermediate in fast acetylators.

Unwanted effects

- Gastrointestinal disturbances: nausea, vomiting, anorexia, diarrhoea.
- Negative inotropic effect.
- Systemic lupus erythematosus with fever, arthralgia, rashes, pleurisy. The syndrome is more common in slow acetylators. It usually appears after at least 2 months treatment and is common after 6 months; long-term treatment is therefore usually avoided.

QUINIDINE

Pharmacokinetics

Oral absorption is almost complete and about 30% undergoes first-pass metabolism. Metabolism in the liver is extensive and it has an intermediate half-life. Modified release formulations are frequently used to reduce the peak plasma concentration and minimize unwanted effects. An intramuscular formulation is available.

Unwanted effects

- Gastrointestinal disturbances: nausea, vomiting, abdominal pain, diarrhoea.
- Cinchonism: tinnitus, nausea, visual disturbance.
- Negative inotropic effect.

CLASS IB DRUGS

Indications: ventricular arrhythmias, digitalis toxicity (Chapter 8).

LIGNOCAINE

Pharmacokinetics

Extensive first-pass metabolism to a potentially toxic metabolite prevents oral administration. Intravenous bolus injection (as a loading dose) followed by constant infusion is the usual method of administration. Metabolism in the liver is extensive to less active compounds, one of which also has convulsive activity. The half-life is short.

Unwanted effects

- Nausea and vomiting.
- CNS toxicity: muscle twitching, convulsions, lightheadedness.
- Negative inotropic effect.

MEXILETINE

Pharmacokinetics

Oral absorption is almost complete, but an intravenous formulation is also available. Metabolism in the liver is extensive and the half-life is long.

Unwanted effects

- Nausea and vomiting.
- CNS toxicity: lightheadedness, tremor.
- Hypotension and bradycardia after intravenous use.
- Negative inotropic effect.

PHENYTOIN

This drug is rarely used except for digitalis toxicity (Chapter 8) since it can improve atrioventricular conduction. Further details can be found in Chapter 24.

CLASS IC DRUGS

Indications: supraventricular and ventricular arrhythmias.

FLECAINIDE

Pharmacokinetics

Oral absorption is complete. An intravenous formulation is also available. Most of the drug is eliminated by metabolism; the half-life is long.

Unwanted effects

- Negative inotropic effect.
- CNS toxicity: lightheadedness, anxiety, headache, blurred vision.

PROPAFENONE

Pharmacokinetics

Oral absorption is almost complete but dose-dependent first-pass metabolism can be extensive. Elimination is by hydroxylation which is saturable and shows genetic polymorphism (Chapter 2). The half-life is therefore dose-dependent and much longer in slow metabolizers.

Unwanted effects

- Negative inotropic effect.
- CNS toxicity: as for flecainide.
- Weak β-adrenoceptor antagonist activity can cause bronchoconstriction in susceptible individuals, for example asthmatics.

CLASS II DRUGS: β-ADRENOCEPTOR ANTAGONISTS

Indications: supraventicular and ventricular arrhythmias.

ATENOLOL AND PROPRANOLOL

β_1-Adrenoceptor blocking activity is responsible for the therapeutic effects. The most widely used agents are atenolol and propranolol; these are discussed in Chapter 6. Both can be given intravenously for a rapid onset of action.

ESMOLOL

This is an ultra-short acting cardioselective β-blocker which is used exclusively for the treatment of arrhythmias. Esmolol is most often used when arrhythmias arise during anaesthesia. Esmolol is given by bolus intravenous injection.

Pharmacokinetics

The half-life of esmolol is very short (about 9 min) and its action is terminated by esterase activity in erythrocytes.

BRETYLIUM

Bretylium is now used only for life-threatening ventricular arrhythmias when other agents have failed.

Pharmacokinetics

Oral absorption is poor and bretylium is now only available for parenteral (usually intravenous) use. Selective concentration occurs in the myocardium. Bretylium is excreted unchanged by the kidney and has an intermediate half-life.

Unwanted effects

- Hypotension due to adrenergic neurone blockade.
- Nausea and vomiting after rapid intravenous injection.

CLASS III DRUGS

Indications: supraventricular and ventricular arrhythmias.

AMIODARONE

Pharmacokinetics

Amiodarone has an almost unique profile. It is incompletely absorbed orally, and has a large volume of distribution. Metabolism in the liver produces an active metabolite. Both amiodarone and its metabolite have very long half-lives, averaging 50–60 days. An intravenous formulation is available. The effects seen early after intravenous use are believed to be due to non-competitive β-adrenoceptor blockade, while the class III effect is delayed. A substantial prolonged loading dose regimen is used for both routes of administration.

Unwanted effects

- Gastrointestinal disturbances, for example constipation and nausea, most often occur during the loading period.
- Corneal microdeposits are almost universal but do not produce symptoms.

- Inhibition of peripheral conversion of thyroxine to tri-iodothyroxine (Chapter 44). This produces hypothyroidism.
- Photosensitive skin rashes.
- Progressive pulmonary fibrosis is a rare but serious effect of long-term treatment.
- Drug interactions: the plasma concentrations of warfarin (Chapter 10) and digoxin (Chapter 8) are increased with consequent potentiation of their effects.

Unlike most antiarrhythmic drugs, amiodarone does not have negative inotropic effects and is safe to use in heart failure.

SOTALOL

This is a β-adrenoceptor antagonist with additional class III properties. As with many drugs, sotalol is a racemic mixture; the β-blocking activity resides in the L-isomer and the class III activity in the D-isomer. For details of β-adrenoceptor antagonists see Chapter 6.

Pharmacokinetics

Sotalol is completely absorbed from the gut and excreted unchanged in the urine. The half-life is intermediate.

CLASS IV DRUGS: CALCIUM CHANNEL ANTAGONISTS

Indications: supraventricular arrhythmias.

Verapamil is the main class IV drug. Diltiazem is less potent but occasionally useful. Full details are found in Chapter 6.

OTHER DRUGS FOR RHYTHM DISTURBANCES

DIGOXIN

Digitalis glycosides are not strictly antiarrhythmic. They are, however, useful to control ventricular rate in atrial flutter and atrial fibrillation through their ability to reduce conduction through the atrioventricular node. Digoxin is discussed in Chapter 8.

ADENOSINE

Mechanism of action and effects

Adenosine is a purine nucleotide which has potent effects on the sino-atrial node, producing bradycardia, and also slows impulse conduction through the atrioventricular node. It is therefore only useful in supraventricular arrhythmias. Its action is mediated by specific adenosine receptors.

Pharmacokinetics

Adenosine is given by rapid bolus intravenous injection. The effect is terminated by metabolism in plasma to inosine, and it has a half-life of less than 10 s. The duration of action is less than 1 min.

Unwanted effects

These are common, occurring in about 25% of patients, but are usually transient lasting less than 1 min.

- Bradycardias and atrioventricular block.
- Malaise, flushing, headache, chest pain or tightness, bronchospasm. Adenosine should be avoided in patients with asthma.
- Drug interactions: dipyridamole (Chapter 10) potentiates the effects of adenosine while methylxanthines such as aminophylline (Chapter 11) inhibit its action.

ATROPINE

This is fully discussed in Chapter 4. It is given by intravenous bolus injection and increases conduction through the atrioventricular node via blockade of muscarinic M_2 receptors. Atropine is used specifically for the treatment of sinus bradycardia and atrioventricular block. It is metabolized in the liver and has an intermediate half-life.

PROARRHYTHMIC ACTIVITY OF ANTIARRHYTHMIC DRUGS

All antiarrhythmic drugs have the potential to precipitate serious arrhythmias, particularly ventricular tachycardia or ventricular fibrillation. Several drugs prolong the Q–T interval on the ECG (particularly Class IA agents) which predisposes to a particular polymorphic ventricular tachycardia known as torsade de pointes. This arrhythmia has a characteristic twisting axis on the ECG.

The mechanisms of arrhythmogenesis are variable and include electrophysiological actions (particularly triggered automaticity), haemodynamic changes such as depressed contractility and hypotension, and also local metabolic disturbances. The induced ventricular rhythm disturbances are particularly refractory to treatment.

DRUG TREATMENT OF ARRHYTHMIAS

Arrhythmias producing severe haemodynamic disturbances or which are life-threatening should usually be treated by direct current cardioversion. Drugs can be used for acute treatment of a rhythm disturbance or for prophylaxis. The following is only a guide to choice of drug, which will depend on the specific nature of the arrhythmia, and on an evaluation of co-existing conditions.

SUPRAVENTRICULAR ARRHYTHMIAS

- Atrial or nodal ectopics: drug treatment is rarely required. Avoidance of provoking factors such as caffeine or alcohol may be helpful.
- Atrial flutter or fibrillation: digoxin is usually used to slow the ventricular response. Class II, III or IV drugs are useful alternatives or can be given in combination with digoxin. Class IA or IC agents can be used in atrial fibrillation but may be dangerous in atrial flutter, by slowing the atrial rate but increasing the conduction rate through the atrioventricular node. Class III drugs such as sotalol or amiodarone are particularly effective to maintain sinus rhythm in patients with paroxysmal atrial fibrillation.
- Atrial and junctional tachycardias. Vagotonic manoeuvres (e.g. carotid sinus massage) can terminate an acute episode. Alternatively, adenosine or verapamil can be given intravenously. For prophylactic treatment verapamil, a β-adrenoceptor antagonist or a class IC agent, are usually used. Disopyramide (Class IA) is occasionally useful, or amiodarone (Class III) for resistant arrhythmias.

VENTRICULAR ARRHYTHMIAS

- Ventricular ectopics: drug treatment is rarely needed.
- Ventricular tachycardia: intravenous lignocaine is the treatment of choice for the acute situation. For prophylaxis, mexiletine can be given. A class IC agent, β-adrenoceptor antagonist or amiodarone can also be considered.

BRADYCARDIAS

- Sinus bradycardia: treatment with atropine may be necessary after myocardial infarction or when associated with drug-precipitated hypotension (e.g. streptokinase (Chapter 10) or the first dose of an ACE inhibitor (Chapter 7)).
- Atrioventricular block: atropine is used. If an external or transvenous pacing wire is required, but there is likely to be delay in treatment, then the β-adrenoceptor agonist isoprenaline (Chapter 8) can be used intravenously. However, this usually results in excessive ectopic beats and rarely improves nodal conduction.

10

Haemostasis

BLOOD COAGULATION

The coagulation cascade (Fig. 10.1) involves a series of enzyme reactions which lead to generation of the enzyme thrombin. Once sufficient thrombin has been produced to overcome the effect of circulating antithrombin III, the soluble protein fibrinogen is converted to a fibrin gel. There are two pathways for activation, the intrinsic and extrinsic systems, which amplify the coagulation response and work together to produce the thrombus. The intrinsic system is triggered by contact of blood with a negatively charged surface such as subendothelial collagen. The extrinsic system requires the release of tissue thromboplastin from damaged tissue. The extrinsic pathway is activated rapidly within minutes of endothelial disruption, while activation of the intrinsic system is delayed by more than 10 min. Both processes are substantially slower than platelet aggregation and vasoconstriction which initiate haemostasis.

ANTICOAGULANT AGENTS

Anticoagulation may be achieved with either parenteral or oral drug therapy. A comparison of these classes of drugs is given in Table 10.1.

HEPARIN

Mechanism of action and effects

Heparin is a highly sulphated acidic mucopolysaccharide which has a variable molecular weight. It enhances the action of a circulating protein antithrombin III with which it forms a complex. The major effects of heparin on haemostasis include:

- Inhibition of the activated coagulation factors XIIa, XIa, IXa, Xa and thrombin by enhancing the activity of antithrombin III.
- Inhibition of platelet aggregation.

An additional effect of heparin is activation of lipoprotein lipase which produces lipolysis and also reduces platelet adhesiveness.

Pharmacokinetics

Heparin is inactive orally and is usually given by intravenous infusion or subcutaneous injection. It has a rapid onset of action. Several forms of heparin are available:

- Unfractionated heparin is extracted from porcine intestinal mucosa or bovine lung. The kinetics are dose-dependent: the half-life is very short (about 30 min) at low

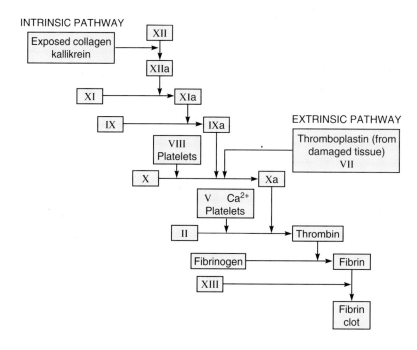

Figure 10.1   The coagulation cascade.

doses, increasing some five-fold at higher doses. Most is metabolized in the liver, with a small amount excreted unchanged by the kidney.

• Low molecular weight heparins are either fractionated heparin or fragments of native heparin. They produce a four times greater inhibition of factor Xa than unfractionated heparin (although their short length reduces inhibition of thrombin). They have about twice the duration of anticoagulant activity and only need to be given once daily. The clinical advantages of these heparins compared to the unfractionated form are uncertain in most situations, but they appear to be more effective for the prevention of perioperative deep venous thrombosis in high risk patients (see below).

Table 10.1   Comparison of heparin and warfarin

	Heparin	Warfarin
Route	Intravenous or subcutaneous	Oral
Onset	Immediate	1–3 days
Duration of action on cessation of treatment	3–6 h	3–5 days
Antagonist	Protamine	Vitamin K_1
Monitoring test	Activated partial thromboplastin time	Prothrombin time
Site of action	Activated clotting factors in plasma	Clotting factor synthesis in liver
Fate in the body	Partially degraded in liver; does not cross placenta	Inactivated in liver; crosses placenta
Individual variability in response	Little	Great: due to genetic differences in kinetics and sensitivity and the effects of other drugs

Heparins do not cross the placenta or enter breast milk.

Control of heparin therapy

The therapeutic index for heparin is low. The degree of anticoagulation with heparin is usually monitored with the activated partial thromboplastin time (APTT, a global test of the intrinsic coagulation pathway) which should be prolonged by 1.5–2.0 times the control value. Monitoring is not required when low-dose subcutaneous heparin is used (see below).

Unwanted effects

- Haemorrhage: this is most common in the elderly, especially if there is a history of heavy alcohol intake. Excessive bleeding can be reversed by administration of fresh frozen plasma or clotting factor concentrate. Alternatively, heparin can be inactivated by intravenous injection of the basic compound protamine which binds strongly to heparin.

- Thrombocytopenia: this is a rare complication due to platelet aggregation. The mechanism is unknown, but arterial thrombosis can occur. Low molecular weight heparin does not affect platelets.

- Osteoporosis is a rare complication which occurs when heparin is given for several weeks.

ORAL ANTICOAGULANTS

Example: warfarin.

Mechanism of action

These drugs are antagonists of vitamin K, which act by inhibiting the hepatic reductase enzyme which converts vitamin K to its active (hydroquinone) form. As a result, the synthesis of vitamin-K dependent clotting factors (II, VII, IX and X) by the liver is impaired. There is a delay in the onset of the anticoagulant effect due to the presence of preformed circulating clotting factors; the delay is principally determined by the decrease in the concentrations of factor VII which is degraded most rapidly.

Pharmacokinetics

Warfarin is the most widely used oral anticoagulant. It is almost completely absorbed from the gut and is highly protein bound to albumin in plasma. It is eliminated by cytochrome P450-mediated hepatic metabolism and has a very long half-life. The plasma concentration does not directly relate to the effect of the drug, which is determined by the balance between the rates of synthesis and degradation of clotting factors. The maximum effect of an individual dose is reflected in the blood coagulation time some 24–36 h later. Warfarin crosses the placenta, and should not be used in the last month of pregnancy. On cessation of treatment the duration of anticoagulant action is determined largely by the time necessary to synthesize new clotting factors.

Control of oral anticoagulant therapy

Since factor VII is the clotting factor that is most sensitive to vitamin K deficiency, a test of the extrinsic coagulation pathway — the prothrombin time — is used as a measure of effectiveness. A prothrombin time about two to four times the control value is usually considered therapeutic.

Unwanted effects

- Haemorrhage. The most effective antidote is phytomenadione (vitamin K_1) which is given intravenously and controls the bleeding within 6 h. However, there will be difficulty in restoring therapeutic anticoagulation for up to 3 weeks unless a very small dose is used. An immediate coagulant effect can be achieved by transfusion of fresh frozen plasma or clotting factor concentrate.

- Rarely, alopecia or allergic reactions.

- Teratogenicity. Avoid in the first trimester of pregnancy.

- Drug interactions are particularly important due to a narrow therapeutic index. Anticoagulant activity may be enhanced by broad spectrum antibiotics which suppress the production of vitamin K by gut bacteria. Some non-steroidal anti-inflammatory drugs (Chapter 31) compete with warfarin for its binding site on plasma proteins. This increases the plasma concentration of free (and therefore active) drug and briefly increases its effects. Amiodarone (Chapter 9) and the H_2 antagonist cimetidine (Chapter 35) inhibit warfarin metabolism. Drugs which induce hepatic microsomal drug-metabolizing enzymes, for example phenytoin, phenobarbitone and alcohol (Chapter 2), reduce the effects of warfarin by increasing its elimination.

CLINICAL USES OF ANTICOAGULANTS

Prevention of venous thromboembolism

Patients at high risk of deep venous thrombosis in hospital (prolonged bed rest, surgery or trauma especially to the pelvis or legs) should receive prophylactic subcutaneous heparin. Low molecular weight heparin may be more effective than unfractionated heparin for patients undergoing orthopaedic surgery. Low doses are used every 8–12 h (or once daily if low molecular weight heparin is given). The risk of bleeding is small but local bruising is common.

Treatment of established venous thrombosis

Intravenous heparin is given for immediate effect for 3–5 days (although some studies suggest that high dose subcutaneous heparin may be equally effective). Warfarin is started simultaneously and continued for at least 6 weeks; the optimal duration is uncertain.

Prevention of arterial thromboembolism

Warfarin is used long-term in patients with prosthetic heart valves to avoid thrombosis of the valve or peripheral emboli. Atrial fibrillation (which can cause atrial thrombus formation) and mural thrombus in the left ventricle following a myocardial infarction are also indications for anticoagulation.

THE FIBRINOLYTIC SYSTEM

Fibrinolysis is the physiological mechanism for dissolving the fibrin meshwork in a thrombus. The process is initiated by activation of plasminogen, a circulating α_2 globulin (Fig. 10.2). Tissue plasminogen activator, released from

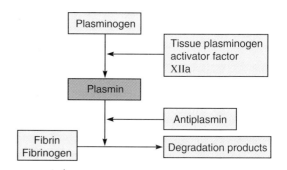

Figure 10.2 The fibrinolytic system.

damaged vessels, cleaves plasminogen to the active enzyme plasmin. Plasmin splits both fibrinogen and fibrin into degradation products; if this occurs at the site of a thrombus, it produces lysis of the clot matrix. The action of plasmin is regulated by circulating antiplasmins which inhibit lysis of a useful thrombus sealing a breach in a vessel wall.

FIBRINOLYTIC OR THROMBOLYTIC AGENTS

Examples: streptokinase, urokinase, anistreplase, recombinant tissue plasminogen activator (rt-PA).

Mechanisms of action

All thrombolytic drugs activate plasminogen and enhance fibrinolysis. Tissue plasminogen activator (rt-PA) is a genetically engineered copy of the naturally occurring substance (Fig. 10.2). Urokinase is also a naturally occurring plasminogen activator which is derived from human urine or kidney cell culture. By contrast, streptokinase is obtained from haemolytic streptococci. Streptokinase is inactive until it forms a complex with circulating plasminogen. The resultant streptokinase–plasminogen complex substitutes for tissue plasminogen activator in the fibrinolytic cascade. Anistreplase is a preformed streptokinase–plasminogen activator complex with a blocking chemical (anisoyl) group at the active site. This group is cleaved by enzymes liberated locally at the site of a thrombus.

The effectiveness of any thrombolytic agent depends on the age of the thrombus and the surface area exposed to the activator.

Pharmacokinetics

All thrombolytic agents are given intravenously or intra-arterially, since oral absorption is negligible. Rt-PA shows a greater affinity for fibrin than for fibrinogen and this potentially produces less systemic thrombolysis. This selectivity is achieved by a preferential action on fibrin-bound plasminogen.

Urokinase and rt-PA are metabolized in the liver. Both streptokinase–plasminogen complex and anistreplase are degraded enzymatically. Streptokinase is partially cleared from the plasma, before it forms an active complex, by combining with circulating neutralizing antibody formed during previous exposure to streptococcal infection. After the use of streptokinase or recent streptococcal infection, neutralizing antibodies are formed which can persist in high titre for at least a year, and substantially reduce the effectiveness of subsequent therapy with streptokinase. The half-life of streptokinase is longer than that of urokinase or rt-PA due to slow combination with plasminogen. That of anistreplase is also longer and determined by the rate of activation at the clot surface.

Both streptokinase and anistreplase have a slower onset of action than urokinase or rt-PA and the re-perfusion of occluded vessels is slower. However, re-occlusion is more common after use of the short-acting drugs. Anistreplase produces prolonged thrombolysis after a single intravenous bolus injection. Streptokinase is usually given as a short (1 h) infusion for the treatment of coronary artery occlusion although longer infusion periods may be required for peripheral arterial occlusions. Infusions of rt-PA and urokinase are often given over longer periods, usually for between 3 and 24 h depending on the condition being treated.

Unwanted effects

- Haemorrhage: this is usually minor, but can occasionally be serious, for example intra-cerebral haemorrhage. Bleeding can be stopped by antifibrinolytic drugs (see below) or by transfusion of fresh frozen plasma.
- Hypotension: dose-related, more common with streptokinase and anistreplase.
- Allergic reactions: rare and usually only with streptokinase and anistreplase due to their bacterial origin.

CLINICAL USES OF THROMBOLYTIC AGENTS

- Treatment of acute myocardial infarction (Chapter 6).
- Treatment of pulmonary embolism or venous thrombosis. Anticoagulant drugs are the treatment of choice in most situations, but thrombolytic treatment can be used for severe venous thromboembolic disease.
- Treatment of peripheral arterial thrombo-embolic disease either in native vessels or in arterial grafts.
- Restoration of patency of intravenous catheters after clot-related occlusion.

ANTIFIBRINOLYTIC AGENTS

Examples: tranexamic acid, aprotinin.

Mechanisms of action

Aprotinin and tranexamic acid produce competitive inhibition of the activation of plasminogen to plasmin, binding to the active site on plasmin that interacts with fibrin. Aprotinin is a polypeptide and tranexamic acid is a synthetic amino acid.

An additional action of aprotinin is inhibition of plasma kallikrein. This is involved in the coagulation cascade, at the stage of activation of factor XII (Fig. 10.1).

Pharmacokinetics

Tranexamic acid is incompletely absorbed from the gut. It has a short half-life and is excreted unchanged by the kidney. Aprotinin is not absorbed orally and is given intravenously. It has an intermediate half-life and is metabolized in the kidney.

Unwanted effects

The theoretical risk of a thrombotic tendency does not appear to be a clinical problem. Unwanted effects are rarely seen.

CLINICAL USES OF ANTIFIBRINOLYTIC AGENTS

- Prevention of bleeding after surgery, especially of the prostate.
- Treatment of menorrhagia (tranexamic acid).

- Reduction of bleeding during cardiovascular surgery with extracorporeal circulation (aprotinin).

PLATELETS

PLATELET FUNCTION

When vascular endothelium is damaged, platelets adhere to the subendothelial surface. Aggregation of platelets at the site of the breached endothelium then initiates or enhances the coagulation cascade leading to the deposition of fibrin. Platelets also inhibit fibrinolysis. Aggregates of platelets and fibrin thrombi can embolize and occlude more distal parts of the circulation.

Platelet adhesion occurs when glycoprotein ligands such as collagen and fibronectin in the subendothelium are exposed to platelet adhesion receptors. Platelet aggregation then occurs via activated surface receptors (known as the glycoprotein 11b/111a complex) binding to fibrinogen which cross-links between platelets. Expression of these surface receptors is triggered by several physiological agonists such as ADP, adrenaline, thrombi and collagen. These work partially by direct receptor activation and partially via release of arachidonic acid in the platelet leading to the production of thromboxane A_2 (Chapter 30) which enhances expression of the surface receptors. Both the direct and thromboxane-mediated activation of cell surface receptors can be inhibited by increasing the concentration of cyclic AMP in the platelet; this is the mechanism by which prostacyclin (Chapter 30) released from vascular endothelium inhibits platelet aggregation. The platelet thromboxane produced from the polyunsaturated fatty acids in fish oils causes less platelet aggregation than thromboxane A_2 from arachidonic acid: the corresponding endothelial-derived prostacyclins are equally inhibitory so that a high intake of fish oils shifts the balance to become less pro-aggregatory (see also Chapter 51).

Thromboxane A_2, in addition to promoting platelet aggregation, mobilizes intracellular calcium which leads to the secretion of platelet granules. These contain several active substances such as platelet factor 4, β-thromboglobulin, ADP and 5HT which impede prostacyclin production by vascular endothelium, neutralize heparin produced by the same cells and induce further platelet aggregation.

ANTIPLATELET AGENTS

ASPIRIN

Mechanism of action on platelets

Inhibition of thromboxane A_2 synthesis by aspirin reduces platelet aggregation but does not eliminate it. The direct pathway for surface receptor activation and expression still functions. The antiplatelet action occurs at very low doses that have no analgesic or anti-inflammatory action. Full details of the pharmacology of aspirin are found in Chapter 31.

DIPYRIDAMOLE

Mechanism of action

Dipyridamole inhibits the enzyme phosphodiesterase and this increases intracellular cyclic AMP concentrations. In the platelet, this inhibits activation and expression of cell surface receptors for adhesion and aggregation.

Dipyridamole also blocks the cellular uptake of adenosine which is released by hypoxic tissue, especially the heart. The excess adenosine acts on specific receptors in the coronary circulation to produce vasodilation. However, since the vascular action occurs in small resistance vessels which are maximally dilated in ischaemic tissue, the drug has no useful antianginal action, and may even divert blood away from ischaemic tissue by dilating vascular beds in non-ischaemic myocardium.

Pharmacokinetics

Dipyridamole is absorbed variably from the gut and is metabolized in the liver. It has an intermediate half-life.

Unwanted effects

- Headache.

EPOPROSTENOL (PROSTACYCLIN)

Mechanism of action

Epoprostenol increases platelet cyclic AMP which at low concentrations inhibits platelet aggregation and at higher concentrations reduces adhesion. It also has vasodilator properties in peripheral arterial beds.

Pharmacokinetics

Epoprostenol is given by intravenous infusion. Unlike most prostaglandins it is not inactivated in the lung but is rapidly metabolized by hydrolysis in peripheral tissues. The half-life is less than 3 min.

Unwanted effects

- Facial flushing.
- Headache.
- Hypotension.

CLINICAL USES OF ANTIPLATELET AGENTS

- Prevention of embolic stroke and transient ischaemic attacks (especially aspirin).
- Secondary prevention of myocardial infarction (aspirin) (Chapter 6).
- Prevention of myocardial infarction in patients with stable angina (aspirin). The evidence for a role in primary prevention in healthy individuals who do not have evidence of established coronary artery disease is inconclusive.
- Treatment of unstable angina to reduce the risk of myocardial infarction (Chapter 6) (aspirin, alone or with the anticoagulant heparin).
- Slowing of the progression of peripheral vascular disease (aspirin alone or with dipyridamole).
- As an anticoagulant in extracorporeal circulations, for example cardiopulmonary by-pass, and renal haemodialysis (epoprostenol).
- Peripheral vasodilation in Raynaud's phenomenon or peripheral vascular disease (epoprostenol).
- Dipyridamole is sometimes used as a pharmacological stress of the coronary circulation to detect myocardial ischaemia in patients who are unable to exercise.

Respiratory System

11

Asthma

Reversible airways obstruction is the characteristic feature of asthma (which can co-exist with underlying irreversible chronic airways obstruction). The pathogenesis of asthma involves several processes. Chronic inflammation of the bronchial mucosa is prominent with infiltration of activated T-lymphocytes and eosinophils. This leads to subepithelial fibrosis and the release of several powerful chemical mediators which can damage the epithelial lining of the airway. Many of these mediators are released following activation and degranulation of mast cells in the bronchial tree. This occurs in response to a variety of immunological or irritant insults to the airway. The mediators act as chemotactic agents for other inflammatory cells, produce mucosal oedema and stimulate smooth muscle contraction which leads to bronchoconstriction. Prostaglandins, platelet activating factors and particularly leukotrienes appear to be prominent amongst the mediators. Excessive production of mucus can cause further airway obstruction by plugging the bronchiolar lumen.

Viral upper respiratory tract infections exacerbate the mucosal inflammatory process while exposure to a variety of allergens (such as pollen or house-dust mite faeces), irritants (such as dust or gases), or exercise can cause bronchoconstriction in sensitive airways. Attacks of asthma rapidly follow exposure to a provoking agent. However, initial recovery may be followed some 4–6 hours later by a late phase bronchoconstrictor response, which can leave the bronchi hyper-reactive to various irritants for several weeks.

The most common symptoms of asthma are wheeze and breathlessness. In younger patients cough, especially at night, may be the only symptom. Treatment has two aims:

- Relief of symptoms.
- Reduction of airway inflammation.

SYMPTOM-RELIEVING DRUGS

β_2-ADRENOCEPTOR AGONISTS

Examples: salbutamol, salmeterol.

Mechanism of action and effects

The airways are rich in β_2-adrenoceptors, and stimulation produces bronchodilation (Chapter 4) via generation of intracellular cyclic AMP. In addition, β_2-adrenoceptor agonists prevent activation of mast cells, thus reducing mediator release, and may stimulate release of relaxant factors from bronchial epithelial cells. Selectivity of an agonist for the β_2-adrenoceptor is desirable to minimize systemic unwanted effects from stimulation of β_1-adrenoceptors.

Pharmacokinetics

The selectivity of β_2-adrenoceptor agonists is dose-dependent. Inhalation of drug delivers small but effective doses to the airways and minimizes systemic exposure. A metered-dose aerosol inhaler is prescribed most frequently but good co-ordination of inhalation and activation of the device is essential. Even if co-ordination is optimal, about 80% of the aerosol is deposited in the oropharynx and then swallowed. If co-ordination is poor there are several alternative strategies which will aid drug delivery. Attaching a large plastic reservoir (a "spacer" device) to the inhaler permits inhalation of drug after delivering the aerosol dose into the chamber. Alternatively, breath-activated devices are available which deliver the agonist in powder or aerosol form. To deliver larger doses, a solution of drug can be nebulized by bubbling air or oxygen through it, and then inhaled via a face mask.

After inhalation, the onset of drug action is rapid, often within 5 min. Agents such as salbutamol are short-acting (producing an effect for up to about 6 h), but have a far longer duration than the natural agonists adrenaline and noradrenaline. Their chemical structure prevents neuronal uptake and reduces their affinity for COMT (Chapter 4). The long-acting agent salmeterol produces prolonged bronchodilation by virtue of a long lipophilic side-chain on the molecule which binds to a site adjacent to the receptor active site. It is no more effective than salbutamol.

β_2-Adrenoceptor agonists can also be given orally (as conventional or modified-release formulations), subcutaneously or by intravenous infusion. However, larger doses are required to deliver an adequate amount to the lungs by any of these routes and consequently the selectivity for β_2-adrenoceptors is reduced and systemic effects can be troublesome.

Unwanted effects

- Skeletal muscle tremor from β_2-adrenoceptor stimulation.
- Tachycardia and arrhythmias from both β_1- and β_2-adrenoceptor stimulation with high doses of inhaled drug or after oral or parenteral administration.

- Concern has been expressed that regular use of inhaled β_2-adrenoceptor agonists, especially at high dosages may be linked with asthma deaths. One proposed mechanism is precipitation of serious arrhythmias. Alternatively, use of these drugs might allow patients to tolerate initial exposure to higher doses of allergens or irritants which then produce an enhanced late asthmatic response. The link remains controversial and should not detract from their use, although if large doses of β_2-adrenoceptor agonists are needed, then use of an anti-inflammatory agent is recommended (see below).
- Salmeterol produces headache in about 10% of patients.

METHYLXANTHINES

Examples: theophylline, aminophylline.

Mechanism of action and effects

Methylxanthines are a group of naturally occurring substances found in coffee, tea, chocolate and related foodstuffs (Table 11.1). Theophylline and its ester derivative aminophylline are the only compounds in clinical use. The precise mechanisms of action of methylxanthines remain obscure. Known actions include:

- Inhibition of the enzyme phosphodiesterase (PDE) which degrades intracellular cyclic AMP, producing bronchodilation. Until recently it was believed that this did not occur at therapeutic concentrations of theophylline, but tissue cyclic AMP concentrations do rise to a potentially useful degree. Theophylline appears to preferentially inhibit the PDE type IV isoenzyme which is found in bronchial smooth muscle and several inflammatory cells, including mast cells.

  Intracellular cyclic AMP is also increased in cardiac muscle which stimulates both the force

Table 11.1 A comparison of the relative potency of methylxanthines at effector sites

Methylxanthine	Common sources	Bronchi	Heart	CNS
Caffeine	Coffee, tea, cola, cocoa	+	+	+++
Theophylline	Tea	+++	++	++
Theobromine	Cocoa	Of little clinical relevance		

and rate of contraction (Chapter 8). This increases the cardiac output which produces a rise in glomerular filtration rate (GFR) and consequent diuresis. Additional effects of methylxanthines on the renal tubule reduce tubular sodium reabsorption. These actions can be useful for enhancing diuresis in heart failure.

- Release of calcium from intracellular stores and enhanced extrusion from the cell. Influx of calcium into the cell may also be reduced. Both effects will aid smooth muscle relaxation.
- Adenosine receptor antagonism. This enhances smooth muscle relaxation and reduces neurotransmitter release. Interference with the effects of adenosine is believed to be responsible for CNS stimulation and gastrointestinal irritation. Initial CNS effects include improved mental performance and alertness, particularly if these are impaired by tiredness or boredom.

A comparison of the pharmacological effects of dietary methylxanthines is shown in Table 11.1.

Pharmacokinetics

Theophylline is absorbed erratically from the gut and has an irritant action on the stomach. It can be given as a more soluble inactive ester aminophylline which is hydrolysed rapidly to theophylline and ethylenediamine after absorption. Aminophylline can also be given by intravenous infusion. The short plasma half-life after oral administration has resulted in the widespread use of modified-release formulations. Theophylline has a narrow therapeutic index and since different formulations have widely varying release characteristics, they are not readily interchangeable. Measurement of blood theophylline concentrations is valuable as a guide to effective dosing.

Unwanted effects

Most are dose-related and can occur within the accepted therapeutic plasma concentration range:

- Gastrointestinal upset: nausea, vomiting, diarrhoea.
- CNS stimulation: insomnia, irritability, headache. Fits can occur at very high concentrations.

- Cardiovascular effects: these occur at high blood concentrations and include hypotension from peripheral vasodilation. Unlike other peripheral vessels, cerebral arteries are constricted by methylxanthines. Cardiac stimulation produces various arrhythmias.
- Tolerance to the beneficial effects of methylxanthines can occur.

ANTICHOLINERGIC DRUGS

Example: ipratropium.

Mechanism of action and effects

Muscarinic receptors for acetylcholine in bronchial smooth muscle are linked to cyclic-GMP-mediated contractile events. Inhibition produces bronchodilation. Ipratropium may have some selectivity for the M_3 subtype of muscarinic receptors but local delivery to the lung is mainly responsible for the lack of many of the unwanted effects characteristically associated with atropine (Chapter 4).

Pharmacokinetics

Ipratropium is a quaternary amine which is poorly absorbed from the gut and is given exclusively by inhalation from a metered-dose aerosol or a nebulizer. It has a slower onset and a longer duration of action than salbutamol, probably due to its slow absorption from the airway.

Unwanted effects

- Dry mouth.
- Exacerbation of glaucoma if delivered to the eye.

ANTI-INFLAMMATORY DRUGS

"MAST CELL STABILIZERS"

Examples: sodium cromoglycate, nedocromil sodium.

Mechanisms of action and effects

- Sodium cromoglycate was originally introduced as a "mast cell stabilizer". This may be achieved by the drug enhancing phosphorylation of a protein which acts as a substrate for the intracellular enzyme protein kinase C. The end result of this interference with the normal signal transduction process is reduced release of histamine, PGD_2 and LTC_4 from mast cells (Chapter 40) which probably explains the protective action of these drugs on immediate bronchoconstriction induced by allergen, exercise or cold air.

- Inhibition of sensory C-fibre neurones is probably responsible for protection against bronchoconstriction produced by irritants such as sulphur dioxide.
- Inhibition of accumulation of eosinophils in the lungs and reduced activation of eosinophils, neutrophils and macrophages in inflamed lung tissue. This may be important in preventing the "late phase" response to allergen and the development of bronchial hyperreactivity.

A single dose of either nedocromil sodium or sodium cromoglycate will prevent the early phase bronchoconstrictor response to allergen, but treatment for 1–2 months may be necessary to block the late-phase reaction. Only about one-third of patients benefit from treatment with these agents, which are generally less effective than inhaled corticosteroids, but are associated with few side-effects.

Pharmacokinetics

Both compounds are highly ionized and poorly absorbed across biological membranes. They are therefore retained at the site of action on bronchial mucosa after inhalation as a powder or from a metered-dose aerosol inhaler. Swallowed drug is voided in the faeces.

Unwanted effects

- Cough and wheeze may be provoked transiently following inhalation.

CORTICOSTEROIDS

Examples: beclomethasone dipropionate, budesonide, hydrocortisone, fluticasone, prednisolone.

Mechanism of action and effects

Intracellular events involved in the action of corticosteroids are detailed in Chapter 47. Powerful glucocorticoids, devoid of significant mineralocorticoid activity are usually used. They are the most effective class of drug in the treatment of chronic asthma.

Following a delay of 6–12 h several anti-inflammatory actions are produced which may be important in asthma. These include immediate anti-inflammatory effects of:

- Reduced mucosal oedema and decreased local generation of prostaglandins and leukotrienes (see Chapter 30).
- Reduced inflammatory cell activation.
- Adrenoceptor upregulation which restores responsiveness to β_2-adrenoceptor agonists.

Long-term anti-inflammatory effects include:

- Reduced T-cell lymphokine production (Chapter 40).
- Reduced eosinophil and mast cell deposition in bronchial mucosa.

Pharmacokinetics

Corticosteroids can be used intravenously or orally in severe asthma. However, whenever possible they are given by inhalation of an aerosol or dry powder to minimize systemic unwanted effects, although about 80% of drug delivered from a metered-dose inhaler is swallowed. Desirable properties of an inhaled corticosteroid include low absorption from mucosal surfaces and rapid inactivation once absorbed. Beclomethasone dipropionate fulfils the former condition, but is hydrolysed after absorption to active beclomethasone. This has ready access (albeit in small quantities) to the systemic circulation where it is only slowly inactivated. Budesonide and to a greater extent fluticasone fulfil both properties and may be preferred if high doses of inhaled drug are needed, or for the treatment of children.

Unwanted effects

The unwanted effects of oral or parenteral corticosteroids are described in Chapter 47. Inhaled steroids only have systemic actions when given in high doses. This is partly due to swallowed drug, the amount of which can be minimized by using a plastic spacer between the aerosol and the mouth; large aerosol particles which would otherwise be deposited on the oropharyngeal mucosa are trapped in the spacer, and only the smaller particles are inhaled. Specific problems with inhaled steroids include:

- Dysphonia due to deposition on vocal cords. This may be less troublesome with breath-activated delivery since the method of inspiration leads to protection of the vocal cords by the false cords.
- Oral candidiasis. This can be reduced by using a spacer device or by gargling after use of the inhaler.

MANAGEMENT OF ASTHMA

THE ACUTE ATTACK

Mild infrequent attacks can often be controlled by occasional use of an inhaled β_2-adrenoceptor agonist. Anticholinergic agents are most effective when asthma co-exists with chronic obstructive airways disease. Inhaled drugs are usually preferred to oral administration. A comparison of oral and inhaled therapy is shown in Table 11.2.

More severe attacks, including status asthmaticus which is a medical emergency, require intensive treatment with bronchodilators and systemic corticosteroids. A β_2-adrenoceptor agonist such as salbutamol, perhaps supplemented by an anticholinergic agent, should be given via a nebulizer. Salbutamol can also be given intravenously by slow injection, followed by a constant infusion. Intravenous aminophylline is sometimes used, but its narrow therapeutic index makes it a less satisfactory choice. Corticosteroids are almost always required. Intravenous hydrocortisone is often given initially, followed by oral prednisolone, although there is a delay in the onset of action by both routes. Additional measures such as humidified oxygen and antibiotics for bacterial infections should supplement this treatment. In the most severely ill, assisted ventilation is required to give time for resolution of the acute inflammatory changes.

PROPHYLAXIS OF RECURRENT ATTACKS

An initial attempt should be made to identify and exclude precipitating factors, for example allergens and β-adrenoceptor antagonists (including eye drops). Anti-inflammatory drugs should be used if inhaled β_2-adrenoceptor agonists are used more than once each day, if sleep is disturbed or if there is regular exercise-induced asthma. Inhaled corticosteroid is the treatment of first choice, initially using a low dose but if necessary high doses can produce additional benefit. Sodium cromoglycate or nedocromil sodium can be

Table 11.2 Comparison of aerosol and oral therapy for asthma

	Aerosol	Oral
Ideal pharmacokinetics	Slow absorption from the lung surface	Good oral absorption
	Rapid systemic clearance	Long systemic action
Dose	Low dose delivered direct to target	High systemic dose necessary to achieve an appropriate concentration in the lung
Systemic drug concentration.	Low	High
Incidence of unwanted effects	Low	High
Distribution in the lung	Reduced in severe disease	Unaffected by disease
Compliance	Good with bronchodilators Poor with anti-inflammatories	Good
Ease of administration	Difficult for small children and infirm patients	Good
Effectiveness	Good in mild to moderate disease	Good even in severe disease

used as a substitute or additional treatment if control is inadequate or unwanted effects of corticosteroids are a problem. Nocturnal symptoms or early morning bronchospasm (morning "dipping" of peak expiratory flow rate) are often helped by a sustained-release oral or a long-acting inhaled β_2-adrenoceptor agonist or by a modified-release theophylline derivative given before retiring. These can also be added in cases of poor control during the day. If all alternative approaches to treatment still leave the patient with inadequately controlled symptoms, then long-term oral corticosteroids should be used.

12

Respiratory Stimulants

These have a limited place in chronic respiratory failure. By producing an increase in respiratory drive they may enable a patient to cough and clear excessive mucus, thus improving ventilation:

- Nikethamide and doxapram stimulate the medullary respiratory centre by a direct action and through the carotid body. Given by intravenous injection, their action is very brief.

Doxapram can be given by a maintenance infusion since its therapeutic index is greater than nikethamide. Both rate and depth of ventilation are improved, but restlessness, twitching and vomiting are common, while fits occur with overdose.

- Acetazolamide (Chapter 15) stimulates respiration by creating a mild metabolic acidosis.

13

Cough

The cough reflex is initiated by sensory receptors located at the epithelial surface of airway mucosa. Receptors are found at and below the oropharynx and in the external auditory meatus and tympanic membrane in the ear. Afferent fibres travel in the vagus nerve to the medullary cough centre. Efferent fibres pass in somatic nerves to respiratory muscles. The cortex can also directly initiate cough, by-passing the medullary centre.

A cough is initiated by a rapid inspiration followed by closure of the glottis. Forced expiration against the closed glottis raises intrathoracic pressure, and sudden opening of the glottis expels air with secretions and debris. Flow rates can approach the speed of sound, producing vibration of upper respiratory structures and the typical sound of cough.

Cough can be a symptom of various respiratory disorders. In some situations it can be considered useful, and clears excess secretions and inhaled foreign matter. In others it is unproductive and has no useful function. It is important to remember that asthma can present with nocturnal cough as the only symptom.

ANTITUSSIVES

Cough suppressants fall into three classes.

Centrally acting

These increase the threshold for stimulation of neurones in the medullary cough centre. Weak opiate analgesics (Chapter 20) are most commonly used, especially codeine and pholcodeine. They are less addictive than more powerful opiates which are reserved for terminal conditions.

Peripherally acting

Local anaesthetics such as lignocaine are used to reduce cough during bronchoscopy. Sprays or lozenges are also given to reduce oropharyngeal stimulation of the cough reflex, but inhaled local anaesthetics produce too many unwanted effects for routine use. Bronchodilators (see above) are the treatment of choice for cough associated with asthma. Antihistamines reduce postnasal drip from allergic rhinitis which can stimulate cough, but probably have little direct antitussive activity.

Locally acting

Demulcents line the surface of the airway above the larynx, reducing local irritation. The syrup in simple linctus acts by this mechanism. Inhalation of a water aerosol may be useful if the cough arises below the larynx.

EXPECTORANTS AND MUCOLYTICS

Expectorants

Expectorants such as iodide, guaiacols, squill and creosotes are given to improve clearance of mucus from the airways. They are claimed to act by irritating the gastric mucosa; a reflex response via the vagus then stimulates bronchial secretions from goblet cells and submucous glands. There is no evidence of their clinical value.

Mucolytics

Mucolytics such as acetylcysteine and bromhexine act to reduce the viscosity of bronchial secretions by breaking disulphide cross-linking between molecules. Acetylcysteine may also bind irritant chemicals from cigarette smoke. Bromhexine is given orally, acetylcysteine by mouth or by inhalation. The value of mucolytics is uncertain and they do not always improve lung function. They may make clearance of mucus easier, but they may be no more effective than hydration from inhaling water vapour.

MANAGEMENT OF COUGH

Cough should be treated only if it is unproductive or excessive. The most common cause of cough is a self-limiting viral illness for which simple linctus or a weak opiate should be used. Any cough still present after 14 days should be investigated further to identify an underlying cause. Specific treatment for left ventricular failure or asthma will eliminate the cough associated with those conditions. Mucolytics are occasionally useful in chronic bronchitis or bronchiectasis. It should be remembered that cough is a side-effect of ACE inhibitors (Chapter 7) which is found in up to 10% of patients.

Kidney and Urinary Tract

Functions of the Kidney

The kidney has several important functions. These include:

- Regulation of plasma electrolyte concentrations.
- Regulation of acid–base balance.
- Elimination of waste products.
- Conservation of essential nutrients.

MAINTENANCE OF SALT AND WATER BALANCE

A healthy adult will filter some 200 l of fluid at the glomerulus each day. Since urine output is only 1–2 l in 24 h, most of the filtrate undergoes reabsorption along the nephron. The processes of salt and water handling differ in the various segments of the nephron (Fig. 14.1).

- In the proximal tubule (site I) sodium reabsorption is driven by active sodium transport across the basolateral membrane into the pericapillary space. The transfer of three sodium ions occurs in exchange for only two potassium ions. This ATP-dependent process creates an electrochemical gradient across the tubular membrane which favours reabsorption of sodium from the tubular filtrate. Sodium passage across the tubular membrane is mainly passive diffusion accompanied by chloride ions but may also involve facilitated diffusion by a co-transport system using glucose. Some active reabsorption is associated with the action of carbonic anhydrase involving a sodium–hydrogen counter-transport. This enzyme has a major role in conservation of filtered bicarbonate and excretion of hydrogen ions in addition to its effect on sodium. Between 60 and 80% of filtered sodium is reabsorbed in the proximal tube.

- The descending limb of the loop of Henle is permeable to water (which leaves the tubule in response to the osmotic gradient between the tubule and the interstitium) but not to sodium. By contrast, the ascending limb of the loop (site II) is impermeable to water. Reabsorption of chloride occurs here accompanied by sodium, driven by the basolateral membrane sodium–potassium exchange pump. This produces a hypotonic filtrate and increases the tonicity of the interstitial environment. Up to 30% of filtered sodium can be reabsorbed at this site. Sodium and chloride transfer from the long loops of Henle associated with juxtamedullary nephrons creates a medullary tonicity gradient. Along with the associated blood vessels, the vasa recta, this forms a countercurrent multiplier and exchanger system that generates the conditions for producing hypertonic urine in the collecting ducts.

- In the cortical diluting segment of the early distal tubule (site III) again sodium, but not water, is reabsorbed. Sodium and chloride are absorbed here against an electrochemical gradient for both ions by using a co-transporter. The active sodium–potassium

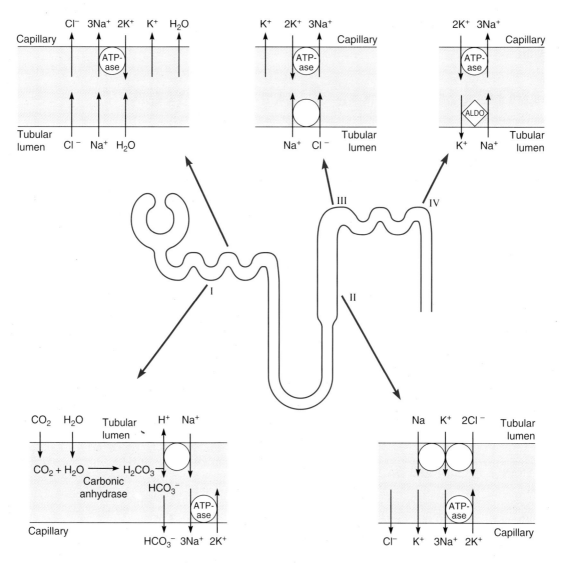

Figure 14.1 Sodium reabsorption from the nephron. ATP-ase, sodium pump; ALDO, protein induced by the action of aldosterone; ◯, co-transporter/counter-transporter; I, proximal convoluted tubule; II, ascending limb of the loop of Henle; III, proximal part of the distal convoluted tubule; IV, distal part of the distal convoluted tubule.

exchange pump on the basolateral membrane is also the driving force for this transfer. The mechanism is inefficient since the transport creates an unfavourable concentration gradient for sodium between the tubular lumen and the cell; only about 5% of the filtered sodium load can be reabsorbed at this site. However, the rich blood supply prevents the interstitium from becoming hypertonic.

- In the late distal convoluted tubule (site IV) further sodium reabsorption occurs with chloride and in exchange for potassium and hydrogen ion loss. This exchange is dependent on the presence of the mineralocorticoid aldosterone. A protein produced by the action of aldosterone increases the permeability of the luminal membrane of the tubule to sodium, which is then actively pumped across the basolateral membrane. The potassium that accumulates in the cell as a consequence of this active counter-transport is extruded into the tubular urine. Overall excretion of potassium is regulated by two further factors. A separate potassium–

chloride co-transport system reabsorbs potassium from the tubule and tends to counteract the loss into urine. The mechanism that predominates will depend on the plasma potassium concentration. If this is low, it will inhibit the basolateral sodium pump and potassium will be conserved. Only about 3% of the filtered sodium can be reabsorbed at this site.

- In the collecting ducts water continues to be absorbed if antidiuretic hormone (ADH) is present. ADH increases tubular permeability and the hypertonic interstitium favours transfer of water out of the tubule.

Diuretics

Any compound that increases urinary excretion of water is a diuretic. Most useful diuretics primarily enhance sodium excretion with the excess tubular solute producing diuresis by osmotic action, that is, they are also natriuretic agents. The effectiveness of a diuretic is determined partly by its effect on the kidney but also by compensatory homeostatic mechanisms in the body. Protective responses to excess salt and water excretion include activation of the renin–angiotensin–aldosterone system, release of antidiuretic hormone and inhibition of atrial natriuretic peptide which will limit the depletion of intravascular volume. Diuretics are conveniently classified by their site of action in the kidney (Fig. 15.1). Since progressively less salt is reabsorbed in the more distal parts of the nephron, drugs have a less powerful natriuretic potential if they act on the distal tubule than those acting on the loop of Henle.

OSMOTIC DIURETICS

Example: mannitol.

Mechanism of action

Osmotic diuretics are filtered at the glomerulus and exert osmotic activity within the renal tubule. This limits passive tubular water reabsorption that is normally driven by the osmotic gradient created by active transport of sodium throughout the nephron. Water loss is accompanied by a variable natriuresis, a consequence of the gradient between diluted sodium in tubular fluid and that in the tubular cells. Expansion of plasma and extracellular fluid volume limits the clinical uses of osmotic diuretics.

Pharmacokinetics

Mannitol is given by intravenous infusion, and has a fairly short duration of action. It is excreted unchanged at the glomerulus.

Unwanted effects

- Expansion of plasma volume can precipitate heart failure.

PROXIMAL TUBULAR DIURETICS (CARBONIC ANHYDRASE INHIBITORS)

Example: acetazolamide.

Mechanism of action

Acetazolamide interferes with the small proportion of sodium reabsorbed in the proximal tubule by exchange with H^+ ions (Fig. 14.1). The ensuing mild metabolic acidosis produced by carbonic anhydrase inhibition soon leads to tolerance to the diuretic action.

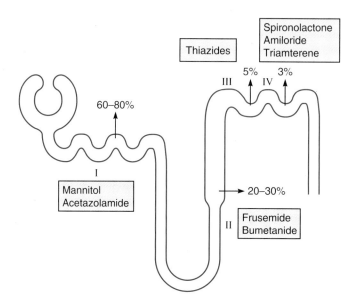

Figure 15.1 The site of action of diuretics showing maximum percentage of filtered sodium reabsorbed at each site. % = %Na$^+$ reabsorbed.

Pharmacokinetics

Acetazolamide is well absorbed from the gut and is eliminated unchanged by the kidney. Its duration of action is short.

Unwanted effects

- Parasthesiae.
- Hypokalaemia (see loop diuretics).
- Drowsiness.

LOOP DIURETICS

Examples: frusemide, bumetanide.

Mechanism of action and effects

Loop diuretics act from inside the kidney tubule. They compete with chloride ions for binding to the sodium–potassium:2 chloride co-transporter complex at the luminal border of the thick ascending limb of the loop of Henle. The drugs compete with chloride for binding to the transporter; inhibition of chloride transport reduces sodium reabsorption by diminishing the electrochemical gradient across the cell. They do not affect the basolateral active transport of sodium. Loop diuretics are powerful, "high ceiling", diuretics which can inhibit reabsorp-tion of up to 30% of sodium that appears in the glomerular filtrate. The dose–response curve is steep, and they are effective even in advanced renal failure.

Intravenous injection of a loop diuretic releases prostaglandins in peripheral veins producing dilation. Pooling of blood in the capacitance vessels reduces central blood volume, which can be useful in acute left ventricular failure. Arterial vasodilation also occurs (see thiazide diuretics) but because of the short duration of action of these drugs, they are not widely used to treat hypertension.

Pharmacokinetics

Frusemide is moderately well absorbed orally and partially metabolized by glucuronide conjugation, principally in the kidney. Bumetanide is more completely absorbed and partially metabolized in the liver. In plasma, these drugs are highly protein bound, and little is filtered at the glomerulus. Unmetabolized drug is secreted into the proximal tubular lumen via the anion transport mechanism (Chapter 2). The rate of sodium excretion is directly related to the urinary excretion of the diuretic. Diuresis begins about 30 min after an oral dose and lasts 4–6 h. A more rapid effect can be achieved by intravenous injection, with an onset of diuresis within minutes, lasting about 2–3 h.

Unwanted effects

- Hypokalaemia. Urinary potassium loss is increased due to the higher urine flow rate. In addition, delivery of excess sodium to the lumen of the distal tubule stimulates renin release, producing hyperaldosteronism. Aldosterone enhances sodium reabsorption in the distal tubule at the expense of increased potassium excretion. Urinary chloride loss creates a mild metabolic alkalosis favouring intracellular accumulation of potassium in exchange for hydrogen ions, which exacerbates the hypokalaemia. Magnesium depletion may accompany the hypokalaemia and make its correction more difficult. Treatment of hypokalaemia is discussed below.

- Salt and water depletion can produce hypotension and hyponatraemia.

- Incontinence due to rapid increase in urine volume. In older males with prostatic hypertrophy, retention of urine can occur.

- Hyperuricaemia. This is due to competition between uric acid and the diuretic for tubular secretion and to reduced filtration of uric acid following contraction of plasma volume. Gout can occur, but is less common than with thiazide diuretics.

- Increased urinary calcium excretion by inhibition of tubular reabsorption.

- Ototoxicity: cochlear damage can produce deafness, especially in the presence of renal failure or when very large doses are used. Vertigo may result from vestibular damage. Both are more common with frusemide, and usually reversible.

THIAZIDE DIURETICS AND THIAZIDE-LIKE DIURETICS

Examples: hydrochlorothiazide, bendrofluazide, chlorthalidone, metolazone.

Mechanisms of action and effects

The thiazides (or more correctly benzothiadiazines) are related to sulphonamides. They act at the cortical diluting segment of the distal convoluted tubule to inhibit sodium and chloride cotransport. Although structurally different, the thiazide-like drugs chlorthalidone and metolazone share this site of action. Thiazides have a lower "ceiling" effect than loop diuretics, achieving a maximum natriuresis of about 5% of the filtered sodium load; the dose–response curve is flat. The onset of diuresis is slow, and they also have a longer duration of action than loop diuretics which varies among the drugs; bendrofluazide produces a natriuresis over 6–12 h, chlorthalidone over 48–72 h. Most thiazide diuretics are ineffective in renal failure (that is creatinine clearance below $20\,ml\,min^{-1}$). Metolazone has a higher ceiling effect than other thiazide diuretics, probably due to an additional effect on the proximal tubule; it also works in advanced renal failure.

Arterial vasodilation occurs during long-term use of thiazides which produces a useful hypotensive effect (Chapter 7). The vascular action appears at lower dosages than are required for diuresis. The mechanism is obscure but may involve synthesis of local vasodilators or increased responsiveness of vascular smooth muscle to these agents.

Pharmacokinetics

The thiazides and related drugs are fairly well absorbed from the gut and extensively metabolized in the liver. They are highly protein-bound and little is filtered at the glomerulus. Thiazides act from the renal tubular lumen after secretion of the parent drug via the proximal tubule anion transport mechanism (Chapter 2).

Unwanted effects

- Hypokalaemia (see loop diuretics). The greatest reduction occurs within 2 weeks of starting treatment.

- Salt and water depletion. The combination of a thiazide with amiloride is particularly associated with hyponatraemia. This is usually a dilutional phenomenon due to sodium loss in excess of water loss but without true sodium depletion.

- Nocturia and urinary frequency due to prolonged diuresis.

- Hyperuricaemia: (see loop diuretics). Gout occurs infrequently and is less common in women.

- Decreased urinary calcium excretion (in contrast to loop diuretics). The mechanism is not well understood.

- Glucose intolerance: a dose-related, progressive increase in plasma glucose can occur during treatment with thiazides. The mechanism is in part due to prolonged hypokalaemia, with the consequent low intracellular potassium inhibiting insulin synthesis. The glucose intolerance usually reverses over several months if treatment is stopped.

- Hyperlipidaemia: thiazide diuretics produce a dose-related increase in low density lipoprotein cholesterol and triglycerides. The long-term effects are small but may increase atherogenic risk (Chapter 51).

- Impotence is reported in up to 10% of middle-aged hypertensive males treated with high dose thiazides.

POTASSIUM-SPARING DIURETICS

Examples: spironolactone, amiloride, triamterene.

Mechanism of action and effects

These drugs act at the aldosterone-sensitive site in the late distal convoluted tubule and cortical collecting duct. The maximum natriuresis will be small (less than 5% of filtered sodium). Spironolactone and its active metabolite, canrenone, have a steroid structure and are specific competitive aldosterone receptor antagonists. Thus they enter the tubular cell and bind to the cytosolic steroid receptor (see Chapter 47). Sodium and water loss is accompanied by preservation of plasma potassium. Amiloride and triamterene act at the same site but do not competitively antagonize aldosterone; they may interfere with luminal sodium channels in the tubule.

When used with thiazide or loop diuretics, potassium-sparing diuretics reduce or eliminate urinary potassium loss, and produce a small additional natriuresis.

Pharmacokinetics

Spironolactone is metabolized in the wall of the gut and the liver to canrenone, which is probably responsible for most of the diuretic effect. Triamterene is also extensively metabolized but tubular secretion of the parent compound is responsible for the diuretic action. Amiloride is excreted unchanged. All three drugs are given orally, but potassium canrenoate (the salt of canrenone) is available for intravenous use.

The onset of action of amiloride and triam-terine is rapid but that of spironolactone is slow, over several days.

Unwanted effects

- Hyperkalaemia: more common in the presence of pre-existing renal disease, in the elderly and during combination treatment with ACE inhibitors (Chapter 7). Magnesium retention also occurs, in contrast to the thiazides and loop diuretics.

- Spironolactone has oestrogenic effects producing gynaecomastia and impotence in males. Menstrual irregularities can occur in women.

- Hyponatraemia: more common with thiazide-amiloride combinations.

- Spironolactone is carcinogenic in rats. It is, therefore, no longer licenced for use in hypertension, when treatment may be required for long periods.

MANAGEMENT OF DIURETIC-INDUCED HYPOKALAEMIA

A modest reduction in plasma potassium is common during treatment with loop or thiazide diuretics. Marked hypokalaemia (below $3.0\,mmol\,l^{-1}$) predisposes to cardiac rhythm disturbances, particularly in the presence of acute myocardial ischaemia, during treatment with digitalis glycosides (Chapter 8) or with anti-arrhythmic agents that prolong the Q–T interval on the ECG (Chapter 9). It may also precipitate encephalopathy in patients with liver failure. The risk of hypokalaemia is greatest with:

- Thiazide rather than loop diuretics due to their longer duration of action.
- Low oral intake of potassium.
- High doses of diuretic.
- High aldosterone production, for example hepatic cirrhosis and nephrotic syndrome.

Both the treatment and prevention of diuretic-induced hypokalaemia can be achieved by using either potassium chloride supplements or a potassium-sparing diuretic.

- Potassium supplements are less effective unless used in large quantities, when they often produce gastric irritation. Modified-release tablets, effervescent formulations and intravenous solutions are available.

Supplements of greater than 30 mmol potassium daily are usually needed. Most oral formulations of potassium contain no more than 8 mmol in each tablet or sachet.

- Intravenous supplements are rarely needed unless there is severe potassium depletion. Rapid injection can produce potentially lethal hyperkalaemia (provoking serious cardiac arrhythmias). A maximum infusion rate of $10–20$ mmol h^{-1} is recommended, with hourly monitoring of plasma potassium.

Potassium-sparing diuretics are widely used in combination with thiazide or loop diuretics, often as fixed-dose combinations. While these combinations are convenient, they lack the facility for flexible dose adjustments. Routine prescribing of a potassium-sparing diuretic should not be necessary in most patients. A pragmatic approach would be to reserve them for patients in high-risk categories or those who develop significant hypokalaemia during regular diuretic treatment.

MAJOR USES OF DIURETICS

(1) Control of oedema in heart failure (Chapter 8), nephrotic syndrome and hepatic disease.

In renal failure large doses of loop diuretic may be required. For ascites associated with hepatic disease, spironolactone is often used alone or in combination with a loop diuretic to counteract the secondary hyperaldosteronism.

(2) Hypertension (Chapter 7). Thiazide diuretics are usually used.

(3) Hypercalcaemia (Chapter 45) can be treated with a loop diuretic.

(4) Hypercalciuria with renal stone formation. Thiazides can be used to reduce urinary calcium excretion.

(5) Glaucoma: acetazolamide can be used to reduce intraocular pressure by reducing formation of HCO_3^- and secretion of aqueous humour in the anterior chamber of the eye. Tolerance does not occur.

(6) Raised intracranial pressure: an osmotic diuretic is occasionally useful, for example postneurosurgery.

(7) Acute renal failure: a loop or an osmotic diuretic may prevent incipient acute renal failure from becoming established. The mechanism of action in this situation is unknown.

(8) Stimulation of respiration by acetazolamide (Chapter 12).

16

Bladder Dysfunction

CHAPTER SUMMARY

The urinary bladder is a smooth muscle organ composed chiefly of the detrusor muscle, which relaxes to allow bladder filling. A smaller muscle, the trigone, is found between the ureteric orifices and bladder neck. The external urethral sphincter is formed from striated muscle which in the male sits below the prostate; constriction prevents bladder emptying. The bladder relaxes to accommodate urine by stimulation of β_2-adrenoceptors via the sympathetic nervous system, which also inhibits parasympathetic ganglia innervating the detrusor.

The detrusor contracts in response to parasympathetic (muscarinic) stimulation. This is co-ordinated with inhibition of α_1-adrenoceptor activity in the external sphincter and bladder neck and with contraction of the diaphragm and abdominal muscles, which combine to promote micturition. Co-ordination of these activities is a function of the hind-brain.

Several abnormalities of bladder function are recognized. These usually require sophisticated studies of bladder function for accurate classification.

DETRUSOR INSTABILITY

Abnormalities of bladder function include detrusor instability producing uncontrolled contractions and urge incontinence. Most cases are idiopathic, but upper motor neurone lesions, for example stroke or multiple sclerosis, or, in the male, prostatic hypertrophy can be the cause.

Treatments which decrease bladder activity include:

- Anticholinergic drugs (Chapter 4), for example propantheline. Anticholinergic unwanted effects may limit tolerability, and the clinical response is unpredictable.

- Tricyclic antidepressants, for example imipramine (Chapter 23). Although anticholinergic effects contribute to the action of these drugs, an additional local anaesthetic or membrane stabilizing action on bladder smooth muscle may be important.

- α-Adrenoceptor antagonists (Chapter 7), for example prazosin. These produce relaxation of urethral muscles which is of greatest benefit if there is underlying prostatic hypertrophy.

- Antispasmodic muscle relaxants, for example oxybutinin. Drugs in this group act directly on the detrusor muscle, but anticholinergic and local anaesthetic actions also contribute to their effectiveness. The anticholinergic unwanted effects can be troublesome.

- Calcium antagonists, for example nifedipine (Chapter 6). These agents produce muscle relaxation *in vitro* in mammalian bladder, but studies demonstrating clinical efficacy in man are lacking.

HYPOTONIC BLADDER

Hypotonic bladder is due to lower motor neurone lesions or bladder distension from chronic urinary retention. This leads to incomplete bladder emptying. Treatment is usually only successful for limited periods using:

- Cholinergic agonists (Chapter 4), which can be either an anticholinesterase, for example distigmine, or a direct-acting agonist, for example bethanechol. These drugs increase the force of detrusor contraction and should not be used in the presence of urinary outflow obstruction.

URETHRAL SPHINCTER INCOMPETENCE

Urethral sphincter incompetence produces stress incontinence in women or sphincter weakness incontinence in men. The most common cause in women is loss of collagenous support in the pelvic floor or perineum; other causes are pelvic trauma or in males prostatectomy. Drug treatment is not appropriate, except for oestrogen replacement in postmenopausal women, topically or as HRT (Chapter 48), to restore urethral secretions and possibly alter mucosal receptor responsiveness.

The Nervous System

17

Introduction to the Nervous System

The concept of synaptic transmission has been introduced for noradrenaline and acetylcholine in relation to the autonomic nervous system (Chapter 4). However, the central nervous system (CNS) is of far greater complexity than the autonomic nervous system with respect to anatomical structure, inter-neuronal connections, feedback mechanisms and the range of compounds utilized as neurotransmitters.

The human brain contains approximately 10^{12} neurones, each of which may have hundreds or even thousands of interconnections. The neurones and interconnections may occur in well-defined areas or tracts and control specific functions or activities, but some areas of the brain represent a diffuse network, for example the cerebral cortex.

The greatest opportunity for selective therapeutic intervention occurs when specific activities are linked to the use of a particular neurotransmitter. However, modification of the activity of a neurotransmitter within the CNS will usually affect all areas or aspects controlled by that neurotransmitter. In many cases the side-effects of a drug can be anticipated from the roles of the neurotransmitter affected. Selectivity of therapeutic effect, within the spectrum of possible actions mediated by the "target" neurotransmitter, may be possible if the dose is adjusted carefully to correct an underlying pathophysiological imbalance while at the same time not creating an imbalance within normally func-

tioning tracts. However, in many cases the dose–response relationships for therapeutic and unwanted effects are very close and toxicity is inevitable to some degree in a proportion of patients (see Chapter 56). This is illustrated well in the case of dopamine since psychotic changes and nausea may accompany attempts to increase dopaminergic activity to treat Parkinson's disease (Chapter 25) while Parkinsonian-like side-effects are frequently encountered when dopamine antagonists are used in the treatment of psychotic disorders (Chapter 22) or given as antiemetics (Chapter 34).

The composition of the "internal environment" of the brain is controlled by the blood–brain barrier (Chapter 2) which limits the entry of potentially neuroactive compounds such as catecholamines, amino acids and peptides (see below), as well as polar therapeutic drugs.

The CNS shows a far greater range of types of inter-neuronal junctions compared with the simplified schemes for noradrenaline and acetylcholine given in Chapter 4. These may be subdivided based on the site of the synapse on the neurone, the electrophysiological effect and the neurotransmitter involved.

TYPES OF INTER-NEURONAL JUNCTION

These may be subdivided into three main types (see Fig. 17.1).

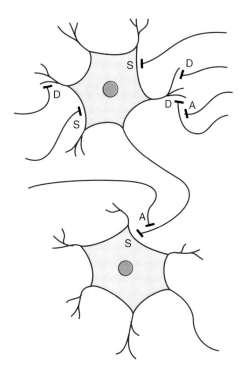

Figure 17.1 Types of inter-neuronal synapses present in the central nervous system. D, axo-dendritic; S, axo-somatic; A, axo-axonal.

- *Axo-dendritic* — the axon of the transmitting (innervating) cell forms a synaptic knob with the dendrite of the receiving (innervated) cell; account for 98% of synapses in the cortex.
- *Axo-somatic* — the synapse is on the cell body.
- *Axo-axonal* — the synapse is on the axon and usually serves to alter the local release of neurotransmitter from the receiving cell (see opiate analgesics, Chapter 20).

Synapses and interconnections are so numerous that about 50% of the total surface area of neuronal cells, and their processes, is covered by synapses.

ELECTROPHYSIOLOGICAL EFFECTS

These may be subdivided into 2 main types:

- *Excitatory* — binding of the neurotransmitter to the postsynaptic membrane receptors causes depolarization of the membrane. The current inflow from a single synaptic knob is insufficient to cause generalized depolarization but serves to increase the excitability of the inner-

vated neurone, that is, it is an *excitatory post-synaptic potential* (EPSP). EPSPs decay rapidly and therefore summation of the effects of a number of synaptic knobs within a certain time is necessary for the action potential to be transmitted to the innervated or receiving neurone. The main ionic mechanism for an EPSP is the opening of a Na^+ channel (Chapter 1); the closing of a K^+ channel will also cause an EPSP (see Fig. 17.2).

- *Inhibitory* — binding of the neurotransmitter to the postsynaptic receptor hyperpolarizes

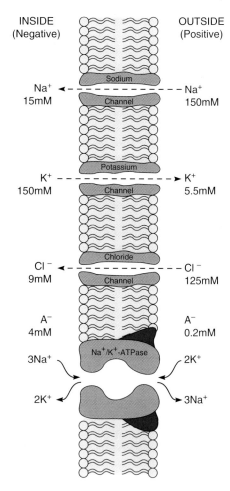

Figure 17.2 Factors influencing the resting potential. A^- is protein anion. The inside of the cell membrane is negative with respect to the outside because the diffusion of potassium down its concentration gradient (out of the cell) exceeds that of sodium (into the cell). The concentration gradients are maintained by the Na^+/K^+-ATPase. Hyperpolarization of the cell may arise from the opening of potassium or chloride channels or from the activation of the Na^+/K^+-ATPase.

the innervated neurone and thereby reduces its excitability, that is it causes an *inhibitory postsynpatic potential* (IPSP). The main ionic mechanism is the opening of chloride (Cl^-) channels so that Cl^- ions diffuse down their concentration gradient into the cell; the opening of a K^+ channel will also cause an IPSP. Enhancing the opening of Cl^- channels is an important mechanism of action of a number of anti-epilepsy drugs (Chapter 24). Axo-axonal synapses frequently inhibit neurotransmitter release from the receiving cell by the generation of an IPSP (see opiate analgesics, Chapter 20).

NEUROTRANSMITTERS

There are four major classes of transmitters based on their chemical structure:

ESTERS

- *Acetylcholine*, the only physiological example, has been discussed in Chapters 1 and 4. Both muscarinic and nicotinic (N_1) receptors are present in many parts of the brain. Muscarinic and nicotinic agonists cause tremor. Muscarinic antagonists, which are able to cross the blood–brain barrier, are used as antiemetics (Chapter 34) and in movement disorders (Chapter 25).

AMINES

- *Noradrenaline* has been discussed in Chapter 4. Neither noradrenaline nor its precursor, dopamine, crosses the blood–brain barrier (Chapter 2) and they are synthesized within the neurone from tyrosine (Chapter 4). Noradrenaline is found in high concentrations in many parts of the brain and is involved in the central control of sympathetic tone (and hence vasoconstriction and blood pressure, Chapters 4 and 7), behavioural aspects (such as mood, emotion and vigilance) and thermoregulation in the hypothalamus. Both pre- and postsynaptic α- and β- adrenoceptors are present within the brain.
- *Dopamine* is synthesized from levodopa and stored by neurones lacking dopamine β-

hydroxylase (Chapter 4). There are two major types of central dopamine receptors (D_1 and D_2): D_1 receptors occur in the nigrostriatal and mesolimbic pathways and act by stimulating adenylate cyclase; D_2 are found both presynaptically (on dopaminergic neurones where they modulate transmitter release) and postsynaptically (in striatal pathways where they produce an IPSP by opening K^+ channels); D_2 receptors are also present in the anterior lobe of the pituitary gland. Dopamine agonists are used in the treatment of Parkinson's disease (Chapter 25) and antagonists are useful antipsychotic drugs (Chapter 22) and antiemetics (Chapter 34). D_3 receptors have been described recently but their physiological role remains uncertain.

- *5-Hydroxytryptamine (5HT)* — (see Chapter 1 for structure) — is synthesized from tryptophan by decarboxylation and aromatic hydroxylation. It shares a number of characteristics with the other amine neurotransmitters: it does not readily cross the blood–brain barrier, it is removed from the synapse by a specific reuptake mechanism and loss of the amino group (by MAO; Chapter 4) produces an inactive metabolite (5-hydroxyindoleacetic acid, 5HIAA). 5HT is present in numerous pathways and is important in sleep/wakefulness, mood, feeding and thermoregulation. There are a number of receptor subtypes (five identified in man at present) of which $5HT_{1A}$, $5HT_{1B}$ and $5HT_{1D}$ are largely presynaptic, $5HT_2$ are the principal postsynaptic receptors acting via Cl^- channels, and $5HT_3$ are important in emesis (Table 17.1). 5HT receptor antagonism and reuptake inhibition are important in the central actions of some antidepressants (Chapter 23), antiemetics (Chapter 34) and drugs of abuse (e.g. LSD; Chapter 58); 5HT receptor agonists are used in the treatment of migraine (Chapter 26).

- *Histamine* — (see Chapter 1 for structure) — histamine-containing neurones are found in the brain, particularly in the brain stem with pathways projecting into the cerebral cortex. H_1 receptors are probably important in these pathways since sedation is a serious problem with H_1 receptor antagonists (Chapter 41) which are able to cross the blood–brain barrier (Chapter 2). H_1 receptors are also involved in emesis (Chapter 34). H_2 receptors are present in the brain and are probably

Table 17.1 Location, function and drug effects at 5HT receptors

Receptor	Response	Agonist	Antagonist	Chapter
$5HT_{1A}$	Presynaptic autoreceptors which inhibit neurotransmitter release in dorsal raphe, hippocampus and cerebral cortex. Postsynaptic receptors at several sites including hippocampus	Ergotamine Buspirone	—	26 21
$5HT_{1C}$	Central neuronal depolarization	—	Mianserin	23
$5HT_{1D}$	Vasoconstriction in some cranial vascular beds, e.g. carotid artery, pial and dural vessels. Also found as inhibitory presynaptic autoreceptors which reduce 5HT release	Sumatriptan		26
$5HT_2$	Platelet aggregation. Vasoconstriction, bronchoconstriction. Postsynaptic receptors mediate central and peripheral neuronal depolarization	—	Methysergide, pizotifen, mianserin	26 26 23
$5HT_3$	Central and peripheral neuronal depolarization. Vomiting via sensory nerve terminals of the vagus	—	Ondansetron	34

responsible for the confusional state associated with the use of the H_2-receptor antagonist cimetidine (Chapter 35).

AMINO ACIDS

(See Chapter 1 for structures).

- *Glutamate* and *aspartate* are normal dietary and plasma constituents which enter the brain by a controlling transport process. They are widely distributed within the CNS and have a generalized excitatory effect rather than being linked with synaptic vesicles or with specific neurones or neuronal tracts. There are three major receptor subtypes based on their ligand binding characteristics: (i) NMDA (*N*-methyl-D-aspartate) receptors which are primarily for aspartate; (ii) quisqualate receptors which are primarily for glutamate; and (iii) kainate receptors for which the primary endogenous ligand is not known. Administration of glutamate or aspartate causes CNS excitation, tachycardia, nausea and headache (Chinese Restaurant Syndrome) and convulsions at very high doses. Hyperactivity at glutamate receptors has been proposed as a factor in the generation of epilepsy (Chapter 24).

- *γ-Aminobutyrate (GABA)* is synthesized from glutamate by glutamic acid decarboxylase within neurones in the CNS. Although it is not stored in vesicles it is released by a Ca^{2+}-dependent process. It is inactivated by both reuptake and metabolism via a transaminase enzyme (GABA-T). GABA receptors are closely linked with and activate Cl^- channels thereby producing hyperpolarization (IPSP). The receptor may be either postsynaptic ($GABA_A$) possibly axo-dendritic and axo-somatic or act presynaptically (mainly $GABA_B$) to inhibit transmitter release locally, that is axo-axonal. The actions of GABA via its receptor may be enhanced by benzodiazepines and barbiturates and GABA is critical in the mechanisms of action of these drugs (Chapters 21 and 24).

- *Glycine* is released in response to nerve stimulation and acts as an inhibitory transmitter in the spine, lower brain stem and retina. It is inactivated by a high affinity uptake process. It is the inhibitory neurotransmitter acting on motor neurones. Therapeutic agonists or antagonists are not known; strychnine is a glycine antagonist.

PEPTIDES

The importance of peptides has been appreciated in recent years with the development of histochemical techniques allowing their detection and measurement. Unlike other classes of neurotransmitter, peptides are synthesized in the cell body as a precursor which is transported down the axon to its site of storage. An action potential causes the release of the peptide from its precursor; inactivation is probably via hydrolysis by a local peptidase (cf. ACh and AChE; see Chapter 4).

Peptide neurotransmitters are often found stored in the same nerve endings as other transmitters and undergo simultaneous release.

Peptides do not cross the blood–brain barrier readily and a major problem for exploiting our increasing knowledge in this field is delivering the products of molecular biology to the sites within the brain where they can have an effect.

- *Substance P* is released from C-fibres (Chapter 19) by a Ca^{2+}-linked mechanism and is the principal neurotransmitter for sensory afferents in the dorsal horn. It is present in the substantia nigra associated with dopaminergic neurones and may be involved in the control of movement.

- *Opioids* are a range of peptides which are the natural ligands for the "morphine receptor" which has been recognized for many years in brain and gastrointestinal tract. These are discussed in Chapter 20.

- *Other peptides*. A number of other peptides are detectable in the CNS which can produce physiological effects if given by intrathecal injection. A number of these peptides detected in the brain are also present in high concentrations in the hypothalamus and/or pituitary (e.g. neurotensin, oxytocin, somatostatin, TRH, vasopressin; see Chapter 46) or in the gastrointestinal tract (e.g. cholecystokinin (CCK), vasoactive intestinal peptide (VIP)).

General Anaesthetics

General anaesthesia is the loss of awareness of general sensory inputs and includes analgesia, amnesia and loss of consciousness. It may also be associated with muscle relaxation and loss of homeostatic control of respiration and cardiovascular function. An adequate level of general anaesthesia is essential for major surgical procedures. General anaesthesia was introduced into clinical practice last century with the use of volatile liquids such as diethyl ether and chloroform. Major drawbacks with such compounds include the time taken to cause loss of consciousness and unpleasant taste and irritant properties. Cardiac and hepatic toxicity also limited the usefulness of chloroform. Modern general anaesthetic agents allow the rapid and smooth induction of surgical anaesthesia with a rapid recovery phase.

Anaesthesia was originally induced and maintained by inhalation of a volatile agent. If this method is used, several phases of general anaesthesia are passed through during induction and recovery. These are shown in Table 18.1. An ideal agent would give rapid induction of surgical anaesthesia with a minimal excitation stage, a rapid recovery with minimal hangover and have a wide safety margin (large therapeutic index). No single anaesthetic possesses all of these properties and it is now usual practice to use a combination of agents. To avoid the initial phases, anaesthesia is induced with a non-volatile agent given as an intravenous bolus

Table 18.1 The stages of anaesthesia

Stage	Description	Effects produced
I	Analgesia	Analgesia without amnesia or loss of touch sensation; consciousness retained
II	Excitation	Excitation and delirium with struggling; respiration rapid and irregular; frequent eye movements with increased pupil diameter; amnesia
III	Surgical anaesthesia	Loss of consciousness; subdivided into four levels or planes of increasing depth; *plane I* shows a decrease in eye movements and some pupillary constriction; *plane II* shows loss of corneal reflex; *planes III and IV* show increasing loss of pharyngeal reflex, and a progressive decrease in thoracic breathing and general muscle tone
IV	Medullary depression	Loss of spontaneous respiration and progressive depression of cardiovascular reflexes; should be considered as an overdose requiring respiratory and circulatory support

dose and anaesthesia is subsequently maintained by a gaseous anaesthetic.

Surgical procedures are usually associated with multiple drug therapy since in addition to the anaesthetic agent(s) the patient will normally be given a premedication which may include an opiate analgesic (Chapter 20), anti-muscarinic (Chapter 4) and a benzodiazepine (Chapter 21) or neuroleptic (Chapter 22) to provide post-operative pain relief, dry secretions and to reduce anxiety and produce amnesia. In addition, an antiemetic such as metoclopramide (Chapter 36) may be given. A neuromuscular blocking drug (Chapter 28) is given after tracheal intubation for some procedures.

MECHANISM OF ACTION

General anaesthesia can be produced by compounds of widely differing chemical structure:

Simple gases   — e.g. nitrous oxide N_2O

Organic liquids — e.g. isoflurane

$$F-\underset{\underset{F}{|}}{\overset{\overset{F}{|}}{C}}-\underset{\underset{Cl}{|}}{\overset{\overset{H}{|}}{C}}-O-\underset{\underset{F}{|}}{\overset{\overset{F}{|}}{C}}-H$$

Complex drugs — propofol

$$(CH_3)_2HC \overset{OH}{\diagup\diagdown} CH(CH_3)_2$$

Despite this diversity of chemical structure, all general anaesthetics interfere with the propagation of nerve impulses by a non-specific mechanism involving the cell membrane. General anaesthesia is characterized by a number of properties:

(1) Anaesthetic potency of different agents is proportional to their lipid solubility.
(2) Anaesthesia is produced when the concentration of the compound in the cell membrane is about 0.05 M irrespective of the agent.
(3) Anaesthesia is reversed if the body is subjected to a high atmospheric pressure (50 atmospheres).
(4) The potency ranking of different agents is consistent across organisms of widely different phylogenetic origins (e.g. protozoa to humans).
(5) Different stereoisomers (where these occur) show the same potency.

Anaesthetic potency is measured as the MAC, which is the minimum alveolar concentration of an agent necessary to immobilize 50% of subjects exposed to a noxious stimulus (which in man is a surgical skin incision). Thus, MAC is the equivalent of the ED_{50} (the 50% effective dose) for other drugs (Chapter 1). The MAC for inhaled anaesthetics correlates closely with their lipid solubility or oil:gas partition coefficient (see Table 18.2).

Properties (1), (2) and (3) above led Meyer and Overton at the turn of century to propose that general anaesthetics were simply incorporated into the lipid membrane and at a critical

Table 18.2 Inhalation anaesthetics

Compound	Blood:gas partition coefficient	Oil:gas partition coefficient	Induction time (min)	MAC (%)	Metabolism (%)
Nitrous oxide	0.5	1.4	2–3	>100	0
Isoflurane	1.4	91	—	1.2	0.2
Enflurane	1.9	96	—	1.7	2–10
Halothane	2.3	224	4–5	0.8	15
Diethyl ether*	12.1	65	10–20	2	5–10

Induction time: inhalation time necessary if used as the sole anaesthetic; correlates with blood:gas coefficient.
MAC: minimum alveolar concentration necessary for surgical anaesthesia (equivalent to potency); correlates inversely with oil:gas coefficient.
Metabolism: percentage eliminated as urinary metabolites; most of the remainder is eliminated in the expired air; influenced by volatility and blood:gas coefficient.
*No longer available for clinical use.

concentration caused sufficient disruption to interfere with impulse conduction. Hyperbaric conditions reverse the increased membrane fluidity. Properties (4) and (5) are consistent with this proposal since they indicate that a specific site of action such as a protein receptor or enzyme is not involved. The original hypothesis was subsequently refined to take into account the molecular volume of the anaesthetic since property (2) was far more consistent if molar volume rather than molar concentration was considered. This hypothesis, based on *membrane expansion*, is consistent with the electrophysiological changes produced, that is an increase in the threshold for firing and a reduction in the slope of the action potential. This indicates interference with the opening of sodium channels (perhaps due to distortion).

Such an action would be generalized and would be expected to affect to all excitable membranes. The different stages of anaesthesia (Table 18.1) probably arise from the accessibility and size of different neurones. A rapid action on small neurones in the dorsal horn (nociceptive impulses, Chapter 19) and inhibitory cells in the brain (cf. effects of alcohol, Chapter 58) would give the early analgesia and excitation phases. In contrast, neurones of the medullary centres are relatively insensitive and are affected last.

The non-specific membrane expansion mechanism described above is possibly involved in the anaesthesia produced at the site of administration by some local anaesthetics (Chapter 19). General anaesthetics can be grouped according to their route of administration:

- Intravenous anaesthetics.
- Inhalation anaesthetics.

INTRAVENOUS ANAESTHETICS

Examples: propofol, thiopentone.

Pharmacokinetics

Thiobarbiturates, such as thiopentone, have a very rapid onset of action (about 10 s) due to their high lipid solubility and ease of passage across the blood–brain barrier. The delay in onset is largely due to the circulation time between the site of injection in the arm and the brain. The duration of action is very short

(about 2–5 min) due to redistribution from rapidly equilibrating tissues (including the brain) into more slowly equilibrating tissues such as muscle (Fig. 18.1; see pharmacokinetics, Chapter 2). Anaesthesia could be maintained by continuous infusion but for thiopentone this would allow the blood and slowly equilibrating tissues to reach equilibrium during anaesthesia; the cessation of anaesthetic action would then depend on the elimination half-life (12 h for thiopentone) not the distribution half-life (about 3 min). Therefore after induction of anaesthesia with thiopentone, an inhaled agent is used for maintenance of anaesthesia.

Propofol has a slightly slower onset of action (about 30 s) compared with thiopentone; its duration of action is limited either by redistribution if given as a bolus dose or by rapid hepatic clearance (half-life 1–2 h) if given as an infusion for total intravenous anaesthesia. Propofol is useful for day-surgery due to its rapid elimination and

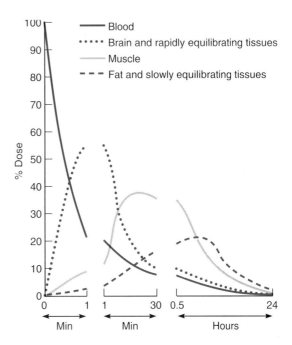

Figure 18.1 The amounts of thiopentone in blood, brain (and other rapidly equilibrating tissues), muscle and adipose tissue (and other slowly equilibrating tissues). NB: the time axis is not linear; the continued uptake into muscle between 1 and 30 min lowers the concentration in the blood and in all rapidly equilibrating tissues (including the brain); the terminal elimination slopes are parallel for all tissues; metabolism removes about 15% of the body load per hour.

absence of hangover effects and it has tended to replace the thiobarbiturates in recent years.

Unwanted effects

- Some are related to the mechanism of action, such as respiratory and cardiovascular depression. All intravenous anaesthetics (except ketamine — see below) also have a negative inotropic effect on the heart. Such effects are particularly likely if there is pre-existing circulatory failure in which case the distribution rate is reduced and may lead to prolonged high concentrations of the drug.

- Some intravenous anaesthetics such as propofol are lipid soluble and therefore are given in a complex vehicle, the intravenous injection of which may be associated with pain and possibly thrombophlebitis. Thiobarbiturates and ketamine are produced in aqueous solution.

ALTERNATIVE INTRAVENOUS AGENTS

- Ketamine is an anaesthetic drug which has some advantages over thiopentone for minor procedures. It produces analgesia unlike all other available intravenous anaesthetics. The duration of action is about 15 minutes, and it allows the maintenance of pharyngeal tone. However there are some disadvantages, for example hallucinations during recovery, and a slow recovery time after repeated administration. Cardiac stimulation with tachycardia and increased blood pressure may also occur.

- Opiate analgesics (Chapter 20): in recent years there has been increased use of intravenous doses of potent opiate analgesics, such as fentanyl, to produce anaesthesia. Respiratory depression and postoperative recall can occur although these can be minimized if modest doses of fentanyl are given in combination with benzodiazepines (Chapter 21) or other anaesthetics such as nitrous oxide or thiopentone.

INHALATION ANAESTHETICS

Examples: isoflurane, enflurane, halothane, nitrous oxide.

The concentration of anaesthetic used (potency) and the duration of inhalation necessary to give the concentration within the membranes of the CNS causing general anaesthesia depend on the relationships shown in Fig. 18.2. There are four factors which are important:

(1) The rate of absorption across the alveolar membranes. This depends on both the concentration in the inspired air and the rate of delivery, that is, the rate and depth of inspiration. Conditions such as pulmonary emphysema which give poor alveolar ventilation will slow the induction of anaesthesia; premedication with drugs which depress respiration rate (e.g. opiate analgesics; Chapter 20) may increase the duration of induction.

(2) The rate at which the concentration in blood reaches equilibrium with that in the inspired air. An important variable in this context is the solubility of the anaesthetic in blood and rapidly equilibrating tissues which include the brain. A high solubility in blood will be associated with a slow attainment of equilibrium. Anaesthesia could be attained more rapidly if the concentration inhaled during induction was higher than the maintenance concentration, since this would be equivalent to a "loading dose" (see Chapter 2).

(3) The cardiac output, which will determine circulation time and drug delivery to the brain.

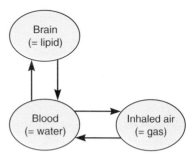

Figure 18.2 Equilibration of inhaled general anaesthetics between air, blood and brain. The concentration ratio in blood and air at equilibrium is indicated by the blood:gas partition coefficient. The concentrations in brain and blood at equilibrium reflect the different affinities of the two media for general anaesthetics. The brain:blood ratio is 1–3:1 for all commonly used anaesthetics. The concentration in the inspired air to give the necessary concentration in brain membranes is an indication of the potency of the compound.

(4) The relative concentrations in the brain and blood at equilibrium, that is, the partition coefficient. The rate of entry into the brain is not limiting because for lipid-soluble drugs which are relatively insoluble in blood, the brain is part of the rapidly equilibrating central compartment. The rate-limiting step is the rate of delivery via the inhaled gas compared with the total amount in the body at equilibrium.

The time to onset of anaesthesia and maintenance concentrations for a range of anaesthetic compounds are given in Table 18.2. This table also contains data on:

The blood:gas partition coefficient which indicates the relative solubility in blood (or water) and gas. A high solubility in water, and therefore all rapidly equilibrating body tissues, means that a greater amount of the agent will need to be administered before the partial pressure of the agent in the blood equilibrates with that in the inspired air. Diethyl ether, although no longer available, has been included in Table 18.2 since this illustrates well the relationship between a high blood:air partition coefficient and a long induction period. (Note: the data in Table 18.2 conform to the basic pharmacokinetic principle that compounds with a large apparent volume of distribution take longer to reach steady state during a constant rate of drug input.)

The oil:gas partition coefficient which reflects the ratio between the concentration in the brain lipid membranes and the inhaled concentration. Since all agents require approximately the same concentration in the brain membrane lipids (see above) the higher the partition coefficient the lower will be the concentration of gas required to maintain anaesthesia. This is illustrated by the data in Table 18.2. Nitrous oxide is of such low potency that surgical anaesthesia requires its use in combination with another agent. It has the advantage in this situation of providing analgesia (which is not produced by the other inhalational anaesthetics) and reducing the required dose of the other agent.

Pharmacokinetics

The major route of elimination of inhaled anaesthetics is via the airways. Factors that influence the duration of induction, such as ventilation rate and the blood:gas partition coefficient, will also affect the time taken to eliminate the anaesthetic, and thus the recovery. The recovery time may also depend on the duration of inhalation since this may affect the extent of entry into slowly equilibrating tissues, elimination from which may delay recovery. During recovery the depth of anaesthesia changes from III to I to consciousness and a rapid recovery which minimizes stage II is beneficial. Comparing the data in Table 18.2, it is hardly surprising that diethyl ether is no longer used.

General anaesthetics are also partly eliminated by metabolism — the extent of which depends on the time that the agent is retained in the body and available to the metabolizing enzymes. Thus exhalation and metabolism can be regarded as alternative pathways, the extents of which are determined largely by the volatility of the agent and its blood:gas partition coefficient (see Table 18.2). The formation of reactive metabolites of halothane has been linked to hepatotoxicity (see below).

Inhaled anaesthetics are given with oxygen to avoid the risk of hypoxia during anaesthesia. Halothane, isoflurane and enflurane are usually given in combination with nitrous oxide.

Unwanted effects

A number of effects are common to most clinically useful inhaled anaesthetics; however each agent also shows a unique profile of unwanted effects. These are summarized below in relation to the major organ systems and effects which may be seen following the normal production of stage III anaesthesia. General comments apply particularly to halothane, isoflurane and enflurane.

Cardiovascular system — most agents are negatively inotropic and depress myocardial function; this produces a decrease in mean arterial pressure especially when the compound also produces a decrease in systemic vascular resistance (e.g. isoflurane). Nitrous oxide is less depressant and its use in combination with other agents may reduce their dosage and therefore their depressant effect on the heart. There is often an increase in cerebral blood flow which may exacerbate an elevated intracranial pressure.

Respiratory system — most agents depress the response of the respiratory centre in the medulla to CO_2 and cause a decrease in tidal volume and an increase in respiratory rate.

Depression of mucociliary function may lead to increased risk of mucous pooling in the lung.

- CNS — mild seizure-like activity on the electroencephalogram may occur with high doses. This is seen at clinically used doses of enflurane, which should be avoided in epileptic patients.

- Liver — there is a decrease in liver blood flow. About 1 in 10 000 patients treated with halothane develop hepatitis especially after repeat exposure. Obese patients, and those who become hypoxic during anaesthesia appear to be at greatest risk. This toxic effect has resulted in the decreased use of halothane.

- Kidney — both renal blood flow and renal vascular resistance decrease resulting in a decrease in glomerular filtration rate and an increase in filtration fraction.

- Uterus — there is relaxation of the uterus which may increase risk of haemorrhage if used in labour. Nitrous oxide has little activity on uterine muscle compared with the other agents.

- Skeletal muscle — unlike diethyl ether, modern agents do not produce clinically useful muscle relaxation although there may be a weak effect which enhances the activity of neuromuscular blocking drugs (Chapter 28).

19

Local Anaesthetics

LOCAL ANAESTHETICS

Local anaesthetics are drugs which reversibly prevent the transmission of pain stimuli locally at their site of administration. The clinical uses and responses depend both on the drug selected and the site of administration.

Examples: lignocaine, cocaine, bupivacaine.

Mechanism of action

The main effect of local anaesthetics is to block the ion fluxes which accompany an action potential; particularly the very rapid influx of sodium ions via the opening of sodium channels as well as the slower efflux of potassium ions. Because local anaesthetics act on such a generalized mechanism they inhibit both afferent and efferent pathways as well as neuroeffector systems such as the neuromuscular junction. The effect is most rapid and intense on small diameter and/or myelinated fibres such as pain afferents and such fibres also show the greatest duration of effect. This apparent selectivity is probably related to the ease of entry of the compound into the neurone based on its surface area/volume relationship. Thus, pain pathways are considerably more sensitive to blockade by local anaesthetics than the larger fibres involved in touch or pressure (Table 19.1).

It is probable that local anaesthesia may be produced by a variety of different mechanisms acting on nerve transmission:

- Non-specific membrane effects — local anaesthesia can be produced by a wide range of compounds including acidic, basic and neutral molecules. Many drugs which act at specific receptors, for example atropine and propranolol, are also potent local anaesthetics. The structural requirements for local anaesthetic activity appear to involve:

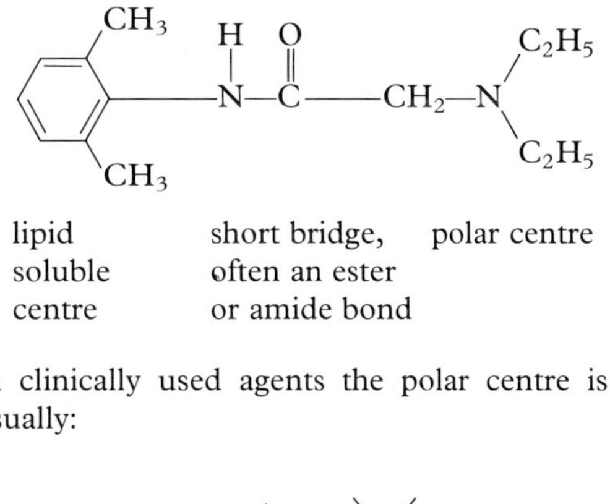

lipid	short bridge,	polar centre
soluble	often an ester	
centre	or amide bond	

In clinically used agents the polar centre is usually:

a secondary amino

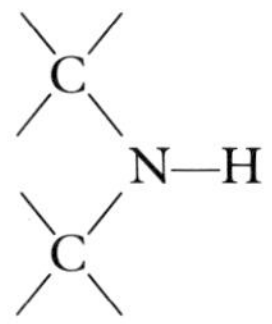

or a tertiary amino

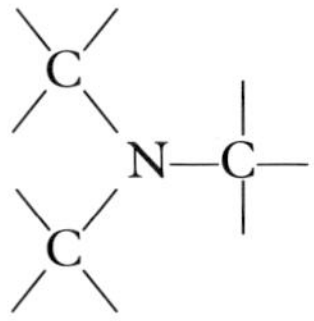

group but it may also be a weakly acidic function. Given this low substrate specificity it is probable that local anaesthesia may be produced by a non-specific mechanism such as changes in the fluidity of the ring of lipid immediately surrounding ion channels.

Table 19.1 Nerve fibres and their responsiveness to local anaesthetics

Type	Site	Myelination	Diameter (μm)	Sensitivity to anaesthesia
A - α	Motor	+	12–20	+
- β	Touch/pressure	+	5–12	+
- γ	Muscle spindle	+	3–6	++
- δ	Pain pathways	+	2–5	+++
B	Preganglionic autonomic	(+)	1–3	+++
C	Dorsal horn	−	0.4–1.2	+++
	Postganglionic	−	0.3–1.3	+++

- Specific intraneuronal receptor activity — most local anaesthetics are weak bases and there is evidence that different stereoisomers of some therapeutic compounds show different potencies.

The principal site of action of local anaesthetics is the sodium channel and their effectiveness is dependent on the frequency of firing of the neurone. The open sodium channel has a much higher affinity for local anaesthetics than the resting channel. These facts, combined with the observation that quaternary analogues of local anaesthetics are active within the cytoplasm of the neurone but not if placed externally, has given rise to the concept of binding of the ionized (protonated) form of the local anaesthetic to an intraneuronal "receptor" which is accessible when the channel is open (Fig. 19.1). Once the local anaesthetic has bound to the channel, the influx of sodium is blocked but the channel remains inactivated and only slowly reverts to the resting state with its loss of local anaesthetic binding. In view of this proposed mechanism of action it is not surprising that there is a faster onset of local anaesthesia in rapidly firing neurones.

Pharmacokinetics

The duration of action of local anaesthetics is dependent on their rate of removal from the site of administration rather than their systemic elimination by metabolism. Therefore, the duration of action as well as potency of local anaesthetics are proportional to their lipid solubility with the larger, lipid soluble drugs such as bupivacaine having a longer duration of action than simpler drugs such as lignocaine.

The duration of action is also affected by the extent of vasodilation locally at the site of administration. Thus procaine (no longer used clinically), which produces local irritation and vasodilation, increases its own removal from the site of action, thereby reducing its duration of action. In contrast cocaine (restricted use), which blocks noradrenaline reuptake (uptake 1, Chapter 4) by noradrenergic neurones, produces vasoconstriction and has a longer duration of action than would be expected given its polarity.

The duration of action of any local anaesthetic can be extended considerably by co-administration of a vasoconstrictor such as an α_1-adrenoceptor agonist, for example noradrenaline or methoxamine. There are numerous local anaesthetic preparations available as combinations of a local anaesthetic and a vasoconstrictor.

Once the local anaesthetic has diffused away from the site of administration it enters the general circulation and undergoes elimination from the body. Because local anaesthetics are lipid-soluble molecules they are eliminated by metabolism, mainly in the liver, which frequently involves the hydrolysis of the central ester or amide bond. The half-life within the circulation varies from short (lignocaine) to intermediate (bupivacaine).

Unwanted effects

- *Local effects* at the site of administration such as irritation and inflammation; local hypoxia if co-administered with a vasoconstrictor; tissue damage/necrosis following inappropriate administration (e.g. accidental intra-arterial administration or spinal administration of an epidural dose).

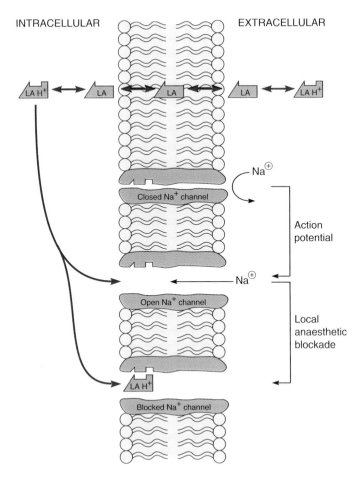

Figure 19.1 Site and mechanism of action of local anaesthetics. Weakly basic local anaesthetics exist as an equilibrium between ionized (LAH$^+$) and unionized (LA) forms. The ionized form binds to the intracellular receptor and the unionized form is lipid soluble and crosses the axonal membrane. Local anaesthesia may also result from incorporation of the compound into a ring of lipid around the sodium channel which becomes rigid and prevents channel opening.

- *Systemic effects — related to the local anaesthetic action.* High systemic doses may affect other excitable membranes such as the heart (see antiarrhythmic action of lignocaine, Chapter 9; excessive amounts may cause cardiovascular collapse; cardiotoxicity with serious arrhythmias is a particular problem with bupivicaine) and the CNS (giving rise to either sedation and loss of consciousness or generalized excitation and convulsions). Because of its pronounced CNS effects cocaine has restricted use as a local anaesthetic.

- *Systemic effects — unrelated to the primary action —* such as methaemoglobinaemia with prilocaine and possible interference with sulphonamide therapy by benzocaine

due to hydrolysis to *p*-aminobenzoic acid (Chapter 54).

CLINICAL USES

The extent of local anaesthesia depends largely on the technique of administration:

- *Surface administration —* high concentrations (up to 10%) of the free base in an oily vehicle can slowly penetrate the skin to give a small localized area of anaesthesia; but the same effect can be produced more efficiently by infiltration anaesthesia. Benzocaine is a relatively non-polar local anaesthetic which produces useful anaesthesia of mucous membranes such as the throat and is included in some throat pastilles. Cocaine is restricted to ophthalmological procedures (where it combines anaesthesia with mydriasis due to the inhibition of reuptake of noradrenaline by sympathetic nerve terminals) and for nasal surgery (to produce vasoconstriction and reduce mucosal bleeding).

- *Infiltration anaesthesia* — a local injection of an aqueous solution of a water soluble salt of the base (such as the hydrochloride); sometimes used with a vasoconstrictor; produces a local field of anaesthesia.

- *Nerve trunk block anaesthesia* — injection of an aqueous solution similar to that described above around a nerve trunk to produce a field of anaesthesia distal to the site of injection.

- *Epidural anaesthesia* — injection or slow infusion of an aqueous solution adjacent to the spinal column but outside the dura mater. This produces anaesthesia both above and below the site of injection, the extent of which depends on the volume of anaesthetic administered. This technique is used extensively in obstetrics. The concentration used is the same as that for spinal anaesthesia, but the volume and therefore the dose is greater.

- *Spinal anaesthesia* — injection of an aqueous solution into the lumbar subarachnoid space, usually between the third and fourth lumbar vertebrae. The spread of anaesthetic within the subarachnoid space can be altered depending on the density of the solution (a solution in 10% glucose is more dense than CSF) and the posture of the patient during the first 10–15 min while the solution flows up or down the subarachnoid space. Sympathetic fibres are particularly sensitive to local anaesthetics which may result in cardiovascular complications, particularly hypotension.

20

Narcotic or Opiate Analgesics

PAIN AND PAIN PERCEPTION

Pain is a complex phenomenon which involves both the generation of pain stimuli and the response of the patient to that pain. Non-steroidal anti-inflammatory drugs (NSAIDs) (Chapter 31) and opiates act at different levels in the production and recognition of pain as indicated in Fig. 20.1. Sharp pain stimuli are transmitted to the CNS by the neospinothalamic pathway, while chronic visceral pain is transmitted by the paleospinothalamic pathway.

- NSAIDs: act mainly in the periphery to block the generation of the original nociceptive impulses. These drugs are most effective against peripheral pain of musculo-skeletal origins, and act by reducing both inflammation and the production of prostaglandins which increase the sensitivity of nerve endings to agents such as bradykinin.

- Opiates: act at the level of the spinal cord especially in the dorsal horn pathways associated with the paleospinothalamic pathway. They also have important supra-spinal actions and the thalamus is a major site of action. The perception of pain is affected, thereby altering the effective response to the stimulus. Opiates act on specific receptors affecting the neuronal pathway from periphery to CNS.

Pain spontaneously generated from within damaged neurones (neuralgia) responds poorly to both classes of pain killers.

A narcotic analgesic is literally a "stupor-inducing pain killer". Morphine, the archetypal drug in this class is an active ingredient in the exudate of the seed head of the poppy *Papaver somniferum* which has been used for centuries in crude preparations, such as the alcoholic extract laudanum. Morphine was isolated as a pure compound by Serturner in 1803 who described its pharmacological actions; it has a complex structure which exists as stereoisomers of which the L-form is pharmacologically active.

OPIATE ANALGESICS

Examples: morphine, diamorphine (heroin), buprenorphine, pethidine, codeine, pentazocine.

Mechanism of action

Opiate analgesics are sometimes referred to as opioid analgesics because they act at opioid receptors. In this chapter "opioid" is used for the receptors and their natural ligands and "opiates" for drugs such as morphine and its synthetic analogues. Opiates show a range of specific effects both in the CNS and periphery (see below). These drugs are extremely potent and show stereospecific, high-affinity reversible binding to brain membranes; this suggests a mechanism of action involving a specific membrane-bound receptor. Minor modifications

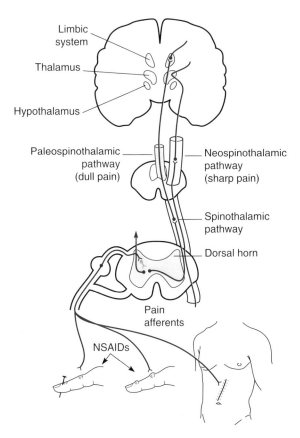

Figure 20.1 Pathways of pain perception. Shaded areas are rich in opioid receptors. In addition to the ascending afferent pathways shown in the diagram there are descending tracts which modulate the nociceptive inputs at the level of the dorsal horn. Neurones of the periaqueductal grey matter, which receive inputs from the thalamus and spinomesencephalic pathway, act on the raphe magnus nucleus via the release of enkephalins. This activates the descending raphe-spinal pathway which stimulates interneurones in the substantia gelatinosa of the dorsal horn to release enkephalins which then inhibit the pain afferent pathways (see Figure 20.2).

to the structure of morphine changes the compound from an agonist into an antagonist. Antagonists, such as naloxone (Fig. 20.2), do not produce analgesia but can block the actions of morphine or precipitate withdrawal in an opiate dependent subject.

The mystery of why the brain should contain receptors for the exudate of a poppy plant was resolved in 1975 when researchers in Aberdeen identified two pentapeptides present in normal brain tissue which showed morphine-like effects that could be blocked by drugs such as naloxone. These peptides contain *tyr-gly-gly-phe*

linked to either *leucine* or *methionine* and were called leu- and met-enkephalin. The brain shows a regional distribution of these enkephalins with high concentrations in the limbic system and spinal cord; this distribution is similar to that previously described for "morphine receptors". These regions also contain high concentrations of a neutral endopeptidase (enkephalinase) which rapidly hydrolyses the pentapeptides into inactive fragments (i.e. analogous to ACh and AChE; see Chapter 4). The enkephalins are thought to act as neurotransmitters at the "enkephalin receptors" on the presynaptic membrane of the main pain pathways; the presence of an agonist (morphine or enkephalin) inhibits the release of the neurotransmitter for the main pain pathway (Fig. 20.2).

The enkephalin pentapeptides are members of a group of neuropeptides, the endorphins, which are formed from larger precursor peptides. The biochemistry of the endorphins is complex and members of the group are found in both brain and pituitary tissue. It is unclear at present which is the most important peptide in the group for morphine-like effects; a prime candidate is β-endorphin, an extremely potent 31-amino acid peptide with met-enkephalin at its carboxyl end. It is possible that met-enkephalin is a breakdown product of β-endorphin which retains partial activity. Alternatively met-enkephalin may be a separate active metabolite of an active precursor (cf. dopamine and noradrenaline). Recent studies on receptor subtypes support the latter possibility.

Three major subclasses of opioid receptors have been identified which produce distinct effects:

- μ (mu) — analgesia at a supraspinal level, euphoria, respiratory depression, dependence.
- κ (kappa) — analgesia at a spinal level, miosis, sedation.
- δ (delta) — analgesia, euphoria, respiratory depression and constipation.

In addition, distinct σ (sigma) binding sites mediate effects of opiate analgesics such as dysphoria and hallucinations, but are not true opioid receptors.

The different endogenous peptides show different binding affinities, for example β-endorphin, mainly μ and δ; dynorphin, κ; and the enkephalins, δ. Therapeutic agents also show receptor selectivity:

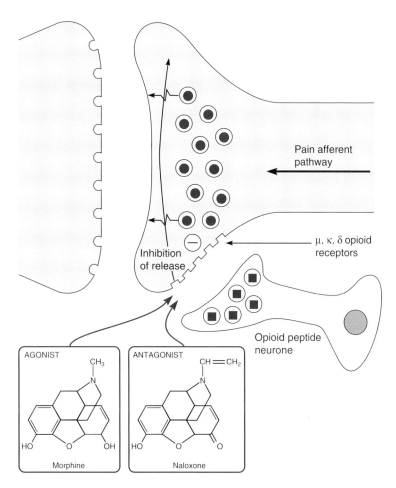

Figure 20.2 Action of opiates via opioid peptide receptors. Opiates (☐) act as agonists on the opioid peptide receptor (↴↲) of which there are three main types. Activation of the receptor inhibits the release of the neurotransmitter (●; substance P) in the main pain afferent pathway. Different opioid receptor subtypes may act via different mechanisms; μ receptors increase resting K^+ efflux thereby reducing Ca^{2+} influx; κ receptors directly inhibit voltage dependent Ca^{2+} influx. Release of enkephalins in the dorsal horn is stimulated by descending pathways which activate the opioid peptide neurone by the release of 5HT.

- μ *agonists* — morphine, heroin, pethidine, codeine, dextropropoxyphene.
- μ *partial agonist* — buprenorphine.
- κ-*agonist* — nalbuphine (which is also a μ-receptor antagonist and σ binding site agonist).
- κ *partial agonist* — pentazocine (which is also a μ-receptor antagonist and σ binding site agonist).

Morphine, the original opiate, has effects on both the CNS and peripheral tissues. They are used to illustrate the actions of this group of drugs. Details of other opiates are given in Table 20.1.

EFFECTS AND CLINICAL USES

CNS depression

- *Analgesia* — the paleospinothalamic pathway and limbic system are rich in opioid receptors; thus the analgesia produced by morphine is most effective for chronic visceral pain and alters the patient's perception of the pain rather than removing the pain signals. Opiates have no anti-inflammatory effect and may even release the inflammatory mediator histamine locally at the site of an injection. The analgesia is often associated with an elevated sense of well being (euphoria) whereas opiate administration to a pain-free

Table 20.1 Opiate analgesics

Compound	Pharmacokinetics	Analgesic potency	Tolerance and dependence	Clinical uses
Morphine	Short half-life; poor oral bioavailability; metabolized by glucuronidation (morphine-6-glucuronide retains analgesic action)	+++	+++	See text
Diamorphine (heroin)	Diacetylmorphine readily crosses blood–brain barrier where it is converted to morphine; very short half-life; very poor oral absorption intact but is effective orally	++++	++++	Clinical uses restricted due to high abuse potential; given orally or by infusion for the pain of terminal cancer; given for acute severe pain, e.g. myocardial infarction
Buprenorphine	Short half-life that does not reflect duration of therapeutic response which is 6–8 h; well absorbed orally or sublingually	++++	++	Used as an alternative to morphine for analgesia, but nausea may limit its tolerability
Codeine	Short half-life; undergoes O-demethylation to morphine which is responsible for the analgesia; good oral bioavailability	+	+	See text; also used when the non-analgesic effects such as antitussive or anti-diarrhoeal actions are needed. Produces little respiratory depression
Pethidine	Short half-life; incomplete (50%) oral absorption; eliminated by hydrolysis and oxidation	++	+	Main opiate used for obstetrics; not useful for antitussive or antidiarrhoeal effects
Pentazocine	Short half-life; rapid absorption but low bioavailability from the gut; eliminated by oxidation and conjugation	+++	++ (but not cross-tolerance to morphine)	See text; will provoke a withdrawal syndrome in a morphine-dependent subject, due to a weak antagonist or partial agonist action on μ receptors
Methadone	Very long half-life; high oral efficacy	+++	++	Major use is for withdrawal from morphine/heroin dependence
Dextro-propoxyphene	Intermediate half-life; good oral absorption	(+)	+	Widely used for mild analgesia (usually in combination with paracetamol as co-proxamol despite its low therapeutic index; reports of fatalities with overdose, especially when taken with alcohol)

subject can produce the opposite effect (dysphoria).

μ-Receptor full agonists are the most powerful analgesics; the ceiling effect of partial agonists is lower. However, some μ-receptor full agonists are less effective analgesics either because unwanted effects prevent the use of high enough doses (e.g. codeine) or the affinity of the drug for the receptor is low (e.g. dextropropoxyphene).

If a person receiving high doses of a potent μ-receptor full agonist is given a μ-receptor partial agonist (e.g. buprenorphine) or an antagonist (e.g. pentazocine), then the latter will displace some of the full agonist molecules from receptor sites, and the level of analgesia may be reduced. In dependent patients, withdrawal symptoms can also be produced (see below).

- *Respiratory depression* — the sensitivity of the respiratory centre to CO_2 is reduced, which decreases the respiratory rate. Respiratory paralysis is a common cause of death in opiate overdose. The effect on respiratory rate may be of clinical benefit when intravenous morphine relieves the dyspnoea associated with acute pulmonary oedema; the mechanism for this effect may involve a lowering of the respiratory drive thereby reducing the stress and anxiety associated with the feeling of breathlessness.

- *Suppression of the cough centre* — opiates possess a useful antitussive action. Compounds such as codeine and dextromethorphan are useful for cough suppression despite having relatively weak analgesic effects (Chapter 13).

- *Sleep* — opiates are not hypnotics, but often the relief of pain is associated with relaxation so that sleep is an indirect consequence of opiate administration.

CNS excitation

- *Vomiting* — opiates stimulate the chemoreceptor trigger zone (Chapter 34); emesis is more common in ambulatory patients.

- *Miosis* — stimulation of the third nerve nucleus results in pupillary constriction. A pin-point pupil, together with coma and slow respiration, are signs of opiate overdose (Chapter 57).

- *Convulsion* — is a very rare effect.

Peripheral effects

- *Gastrointestinal tract* — there is a general increase in resting tone of the gut wall and sphincters, but a decrease in propulsive activity. Thus opiate administration is associated with constipation and an increase in biliary pressure. Because opiates slow gastrointestinal transit they are useful in the treatment of diarrhoea (Chapter 37); opiates may exacerbate biliary colic (especially at low doses); pethidine shows less activity in the gastrointestinal tract than equi-analgesic doses of morphine.

- *Cardiovascular system* — opiates have limited effects on the heart or blood vessels; hypotension may occur, possibly due to histamine release or an action on the baroreceptor reflex.

- *Other systems* — opiates have minor effects on other systems, for example there is an increase in tone of the bladder wall and sphincter with possible urinary retention. Changes in the release of some pituitary hormones may be mediated via interference with the actions of opioid peptide hormones.

Tolerance and dependence

Tolerance and dependence are inter-related phenomena probably resulting from changes in the functioning of opioid receptors during continuous opiate administration. The exact mechanism is not known but may involve decreases in the numbers of receptors and/or their affinity for agonists ("down-regulation" Chapter 1). Consequences of these adaptive changes are that more drug is necessary to produce the same effect (tolerance) and withdrawal of the drug produces adverse physiological effects (dependence).

Tolerance occurs rapidly on initiation of chronic opiate administration and is not associated with changes in pharmacokinetics (e.g. induction of microsomal metabolism). Tolerance develops to analgesia, euphoria, respiratory depression and emesis but not to the gastrointestinal effects or miosis. A high degree of cross-tolerance is shown by many opiates, that is a patient who develops tolerance to one opiate will be tolerant to another opiate; however, not all opiates show cross-tolerance.

The non-uniform nature of tolerance and cross-tolerance may be due to the multiplicity of opioid receptors.

Dependence manifests itself as a withdrawal syndrome if patients who are receiving chronic opiate therapy (or are abusing the drug) have their intake stopped or are given an opiate antagonist or partial agonist. The effects during the first 12 h after drug withdrawal — such as nervousness, sweating and craving — are largely psychological since they may be alleviated by the administration of a placebo. Following this period the effects of physiological dependence manifest themselves, for example dilated pupils, anorexia, weakness, depression, cramps in the intestinal tract and skeletal musculature, increased respiratory rate, elevated temperature and diarrhoea. The time course for the development and loss of these symptoms varies among the opiates. In the case of morphine the maximum withdrawal effects occur quickly (about 1–2 days) and subside rapidly (about 5 days) but the intensity of the symptoms may be intolerable. In contrast, withdrawal from methadone is a slow process due to its very long half-life but the effects are far less intense (peak effect at almost 1 week and symptoms persist for about 3 weeks). Therefore, morphine- or heroin-dependent subjects are often transferred from their drug of abuse to methadone, which does not initiate withdrawal but does not produce the euphoria of drugs with a high abuse potential. After a period of chronic methadone treatment to allow the methadone to replace the morphine, the methadone dosage is gradually reduced and the patient undergoes a more tolerable withdrawal.

Pharmacokinetics of individual agents

The properties of individual opiate analgesics in addition to those general effects given above are summarized in Table 20.1. Opiates may be given either parenterally by intramuscular or subcutaneous injection, or orally. Some opiates, for example morphine, show a low and variable oral bioavailability so that they are usually given by injection for treatment of acute pain, for example postoperative pain. Oral treatment with larger doses of opiates such as morphine and heroin is mainly to establish adequate control of severe chronic pain. Due to the short half-life of morphine, a modified-release formulation is often used when it is given for long-term pain control.

Unwanted effects

The unwanted effects of opiates are due to their actions on opioid receptors which are not the primary site for therapeutic benefit. For example, respiratory depression and constipation are unwanted effects when an opiate is used as an analgesic. Tolerance and dependence can also be regarded as unwanted problems associated with chronic administration. However, concerns about tolerance and dependence should not inhibit the administration of adequate analgesia for patients with severe chronic pain, for example the pain of terminally ill cancer patients.

DRUG THERAPY IN PAIN MANAGEMENT

Appropriate treatment for pain depends on its origin and severity. Minor pain can be effectively treated with a peripherally acting analgesic such as paracetamol or aspirin (Chapter 31). If there is an inflammatory component, for example soft tissue injuries, then a drug with combined anti-inflammatory and analgesic properties from the non-steroidal anti-inflammatory (NSAID) class (Chapter 31) will be particularly useful. More severe pain may require centrally acting drugs, for example opiates either alone or in combination with peripherally acting compounds.

ACUTE PAIN

For rapid pain relief in a self-limiting condition, for example migraine, a readily absorbed, short-acting drug will be appropriate. For more protracted conditions, for example sprains, a long-acting drug may be helpful to improve compliance by reducing the frequency of administration. More severe acute pain can be treated with a combination of an NSAID and a weak opiate, such as codeine. Very severe pain, for example myocardial infarction, will require a strong opiate such as morphine. This should be given parenterally for rapid effect.

Intramuscular injection should be avoided since the peripheral vasoconstriction that is often produced by sympathetic nervous system stimulation in severe pain can delay absorption.

CHRONIC PAIN

Non-pharmacological or local treatments are often appropriate for disorders associated with chronic pain. Examples include:

- Surgery for neoplastic, structural or ischaemic disorders.
- Physical methods such as acupuncture, transcutaneous electrical nerve stimulation (TENS), local anaesthetic nerve block.
- Behavioural modification, for example biofeedback, relaxation techniques, hypnosis.

If a drug is needed, peripherally acting analgesics, for example paracetamol or NSAIDs, will often be adequate. NSAIDs are preferred when there is an inflammatory component. Opiates are used for many severe chronic conditions, not just for the pain of terminal illness. Dependence is unusual when they are given for pain relief. The dose should be rapidly increased to control symptoms and to allay the anxiety that often exacerbates pain. Once control is achieved and the drug concentration is at "steady state", then gradual dose reduction can be considered. Oral administration should be used whenever possible. If parenteral treatment is needed, then portable infusion pumps can be used to deliver subcutaneous opiates or segmental analgesia achieved via an epidural catheter. In some situations combination treatment with an opiate and an NSAID can be beneficial, for example pain from bony metastases when the NSAID may reduce osteolysis. Combinations of different opiates are usually not advisable since the weaker of the two drugs will reduce the receptor occupancy of the stronger agent, especially if high doses of the latter have been used.

Pharmacological adjunctive treatments for chronic pain include:

- Tricyclic antidepressants (Chapter 23), which are particularly useful for "burning" neurological pain produced by deafferentation, for example diabetic neuropathy, post-herpetic neuralgia and trauma.
- Anticonvulsants, for example sodium valproate, carbamazepine (Chapter 24) which are useful for "stabbing" neurological pain.
- Corticosteroids which have a co-analgesic action in advanced cancer. Dexamethasone (Chapter 47) is often advocated.

21

Anxiolytics, Sedatives and Hypnotics

There is considerable overlap in the pharmacology of drugs which comprise these categories. Compounds with sedative properties at low dosages often have hypnotic (sleep-inducing) effects at high doses. In addition, sedative drugs may have anxiolytic properties at doses that are too small to produce sedation. However, compounds such as buspirone have been developed which have anxiolytic properties but do not sedate.

BENZODIAZEPINES

Examples: diazepam, temazepam.

Mechanism of action and effects

Benzodiazepines act at specific binding sites which are closely linked to both the presynaptic and postsynaptic gamma-aminobutyric acid (GABA)-receptor subtype (Chapter 17). GABA is a CNS inhibitory neurotransmitter which acts at a specific protein complex in the cell membrane. Postsynaptic $GABA_A$ receptors control the influx of chloride into the cell; stimulation opens the ion channel leading to membrane hyperpolarization and decreased cell excitability. Presynaptic GABA autoreceptors open potassium channels in the nerve terminal, leading to a loss of intracellular potassium. This hyperpolarizes the nerve terminal and inhibits neurotransmitter release. Benzodiazepines act only in the presence of GABA to enhance GABA-mediated opening of the channels; they have no direct action (Fig. 21.1). The increased inhibitory neurotransmission produces several potentially useful effects:

- Sedation due to reduced sensory input to the reticular activating system. At higher concentrations, sleep is induced.
- Anxiolysis as a consequence of actions on the limbic system and hypothalamus.
- Anticonvulsant activity (Chapter 24).

Pharmacokinetics

Most benzodiazepines are well absorbed from the gut. Many, including diazepam, are subsequently metabolized to active compounds which contribute to a prolonged duration of action through relatively slow elimination from the body. For a few drugs, for example temazepam, metabolism produces inactive derivatives. The pharmacokinetics of individual benzodiazepines determine their major clinical uses.

Hypnotic benzodiazepines are rapidly absorbed and their lipid solubility ensures good entry into the brain. This produces a fast onset of sedation, then sleep. A brief duration of action is desirable to avoid hangover sedation in the morning; this can be achieved by inactivation in the liver (e.g. temazepam) or by rapid redistribution to peripheral tissues (e.g. diazepam). Repeated dosing, particularly with

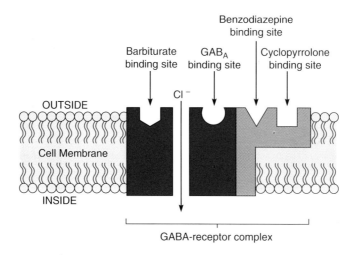

Figure 21.1 The relationship between the GABA binding site on the postsynaptic neuronal membrane and those for benzo-diazepines and cylopyrrolones (e.g. zopiclone). Occupation of the drug binding sites potentiates the action of GABA which increases the frequency of chloride channel opening and leads to hyperpolarization of the neuronal membrane. Barbiturates activate the chloride channel even in the absence of GABA.

diazepam, increases the risk of accumulation with a prolonged sedative effect.

The anxiolytic properties of benzodiazepines are best exploited by using a compound with a long duration of action. Smaller doses can then be used to minimize sedation, and the rebound in anxiety symptoms that can occur between doses of a short-acting drug is avoided.

Diazepam and some other benzodiazepines can also be given by intravenous injection for rapid onset of effect. Diazepam is available in solution for rectal administration.

Unwanted effects

- Drowsiness, which may cause problems with driving or operating machinery.
- Confusional states especially in the elderly.
- Impaired memory.
- Incoordination or ataxia.
- Dependence with physical and psychological withdrawal symptoms during long-term treatment. The risk is highest in patients with personality disorders, a previous history of dependence on alcohol or drugs and if high doses of benzodiazepine are used. Restricting their use to 6 weeks maximum duration of treatment will minimize the risk. With long-acting drugs symptoms may be delayed by several days after withdrawing treatment. Anxiety is the most frequent symptom and

may take up to a month to resolve. Insomnia, depression or abnormalities of perception such as altered sensitivity to noise, light or touch can all occur. Gradual withdrawal of the drug over 6–8 weeks is desirable after long-term use. Lorazepam is a potent benzodiazepine with a relatively short action that proves particularly difficult to stop. Substitution by the longer-acting drug diazepam may be helpful before withdrawal is attempted. There are no proven treatments for reducing symptoms of withdrawal, but β-adrenoceptor antagonists (Chapter 6) and sedative antidepressants (Chapter 23) have been used.

- Tolerance to the therapeutic effects of benzo-diazepines is common. Hypnotic effects are lost quite early but rebound insomnia on withdrawal can perpetuate benzodiazepine use.
- Potentiation by other CNS depressant drugs, for example alcohol, can be troublesome.

CYCLOPYRROLONES

Example: zopiclone.

Mechanism of action and effects

Zopiclone interacts with the $GABA_A$ receptor on postsynaptic neuronal membranes but at a binding site distinct from that for benzodiaze-pines. Like the benzodiazepines, zopiclone increases chloride influx into the cell which inhibits neurotransmission, and produces a marked hypnotic effect. Although it possesses anxiolytic and anticonvulsant activity, its short duration of action makes it unsuitable for these indications.

Pharmacokinetics

The rapid absorption and short half-life of zopiclone make it ideally suited to its role as a hypnotic. Metabolism in the liver is responsible for elimination.

Unwanted effects

- Bitter metallic taste.
- Drowsiness, headache and fatigue.

There is only anecdotal evidence for tolerance, dependence or withdrawal symptoms but experience with zopiclone is limited compared to benzodiazepines.

CHLORMETHIAZOLE

Mechanism of action, effects and clinical uses

Chlormethiazole is structurally similar to thiamine (vitamin B_1). It probably enhances GABA receptor activity by interaction with the barbiturate binding site (Fig. 21.1 and Chapter 24). Chlormethiazole has sedative, hypnotic and anticonvulsant properties. Clinical uses include the management of alcohol withdrawal (Chapter 58), status epilepticus (Chapter 24) and control of confusion in the elderly.

Pharmacokinetics

Chlormethiazole is readily absorbed from the gut, but undergoes extensive first-pass metabolism in the liver. The half-life is short. It can also be given in smaller doses by continuous intravenous infusion which avoids first-pass metabolism.

Unwanted effects

- Nasal and conjunctival irritation early in use.
- Dependence is common.
- Hangover effects occur.
- Respiratory depression in overdose, especially if taken with alcohol.

CHLORAL DERIVATIVES

Examples: chloral betaine, chloral hydrate.

Mechanism of action and effects

The metabolite, trichloroethanol, is mainly responsible for the hypnotic effects of chloral derivatives. The mechanism of action is obscure. The narrow therapeutic index means that chloral derivatives are not ideal hypnotic drugs.

Pharmacokinetics

Chloral is a prodrug which is well absorbed from the gut, then rapidly metabolized to trichloroethanol by alcohol dehydrogenase. The drug competes with ethanol for metabolism.

Unwanted effects

- Gastric irritation (less with chloral betaine).
- Rashes.
- Hangover effects, tolerance and dependence are frequent, as with benzodiazepines.
- Respiratory and myocardial depression can occur in overdose.

AZAPIRONES

Example: buspirone.

Mechanism of action and effects

Unlike many anxiolytics, buspirone has no effect on GABA receptors. It is a partial agonist (Chapter 1) mainly at the $5HT_{1A}$ receptor which is found on presynaptic neurones (see Table 17.1). These receptors act by negative feedback to inhibit neurotransmitter release. Initial exacerbation of anxiety may be due to postsynaptic 5HT receptor stimulation. The onset of action of buspirone is slow over several days and it is relatively ineffective in patients who have previously been treated with benzodiazepines. It has no sedative action.

Pharmacokinetics

Buspirone is well absorbed from the gut and undergoes extensive first-pass metabolism in the liver. The half-life is short.

Unwanted effects

- Gastrointestinal upset.
- Dizziness and headache.

Neither tolerance nor dependence have been reported.

MANAGEMENT OF ANXIETY

Symptoms of anxiety, if mild, may respond to counselling and relaxation training. If they are more severe or persistent, benzodiazepines are the most effective drugs, with a rapid onset of action over a few minutes. Problems with dependence should limit their use to a maximum of 6 weeks, and the dose should be gradually reduced after the first 2 weeks. Buspirone is equally effective but the slow onset of action over 3 weeks makes it less versatile for managing anxiety. It is of no use in patients who have previously been ·treated with benzodiazepines. Somatic symptoms of anxiety (e.g. tremor, palpitations) are often helped by β-adrenoceptor antagonists (Chapter 6). Anxiety frequently co-exists with depression and antidepressants (Chapter 23) provide a useful alternative in this situation. In particular, the selective 5HT re-uptake inhibitor antidepressants (SSRIs)may be more effective than benzodiazepines, although their onset of action is delayed by up to 2 weeks.

HYPNOTICS AND SLEEP PATTERN

The ideal hypnotic will induce good quality prolonged sleep without disturbance of the normal sleep pattern. It should have a rapid onset of action, with no "hangover" sedation in the morning and not produce tolerance or dependence. Few drugs have this ideal profile. Benzodiazepines reduce sleep latency (the time between settling down and falling asleep) and prolong sleep duration. However, the structure of sleep is disturbed, with loss of rapid eye movement (REM) sleep, which normally occurs every 1.5 h and lasts for some 20 min. Progressive shortening of the deeper stages of sleep (associated with "slow waves" on the electroencephalogram) is also seen.

Of the other hypnotic drugs, zopiclone may produce less disturbance of sleep "architecture", having little effect on REM sleep and increasing the duration of slow-wave sleep.

MANAGEMENT OF INSOMNIA

Drugs play only a small part in the treatment of insomnia. Explanation of the normal variations in sleep patterns and avoidance of diuretics or of drinks containing caffeine or alcohol in the hours before retiring can help. Avoiding excessive noise or heat in the bedroom and encouraging regular exercise in the day may also be useful. Hypnotic drugs are reserved for when abnormal sleep markedly disrupts the patient's life. They should usually be used for short periods and intermittently if possible. Tolerance frequently occurs after 2 weeks but if used continuously for 4–6 weeks rebound insomnia is common when the drug is stopped, due to mild dependence. Benzodiazepines are widely used since they are safe in overdose. Short-acting benzodiazepines may produce wakefulness early in the morning, but longer-acting drugs carry the risk of hangover effects the following day. There is little experience with zopiclone. Of the other hypnotics, chloral derivatives can be useful in the elderly while sedative antihistamines (Chapter 41) are useful in children. Sedative tricyclic antidepressants (Chapter 23) should be considered if there is an underlying depressive illness. Compounds such as barbiturates (Chapter 24) and chlormethiazole are best avoided because of dependence.

22

Psychotic Disorders

CHAPTER SUMMARY

PSYCHOTIC DISORDERS AND CNS DOPAMINE RECEPTORS

Psychoses are characterized by delusions, hallucinations, grossly disordered thought or marked cognitive impairment such as disorientation and profound memory loss. They can be classified as organic (e.g. acute delerium and chronic dementia) or functional. Functional psychoses include depressive psychosis, mania, schizophrenia and paranoia.

Psychotic disorders are believed to result from dopaminergic over-activity in the mesolimbic system of the dominant hemisphere. This includes the amygdala, nucleus accumbens and frontal cortex, which receive innervation from the ventral tegmental area (Fig. 22.1). The mesolimbic system is believed to be involved in the control of behaviour, emotion and mood. Several receptors for the neurotransmitter, dopamine are found in the brain (Chapter 17), which are structurally distinct from peripheral dopamine receptors (Chapter 8). The main subtypes are known as D_1, D_2 and D_3 with the former two having further variants; additional subtypes may also exist. D_2 and D_3 receptors appear to be particularly involved in mesolimbic function.

Recent evidence also implicates abnormalities of 5HT neurotransmission in the production of

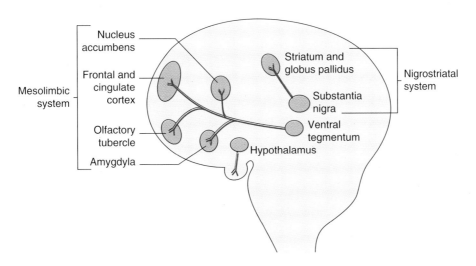

Figure 22.1 Major dopaminergic pathways in the central nervous system.

some features of psychotic illness, particularly the "negative" symptoms of blunted affect, poverty of thought and speech and loss of volition.

ANTIPSYCHOTIC DRUGS

CLASSIFICATION

Antipsychotic drugs (also known as neuroleptics or major tranquillizers) belong to various chemical classes.

- *Phenothiazines* which have a tricyclic structure and a side-chain. According to the nature of the side-chain they are subdivided into:
    aliphatic, e.g. chlorpromazine;
    piperidine, e.g. thioridazine;
    piperazine, e.g. fluphenazine.
- *Thioxanthenes* which also have a tricyclic structure but a different side-chain, e.g. flupenthixol.
- *Butylpiperidines* which have a different core structure:
    butyrophenones, e.g. haloperidol;
    diphenylbutylpiperidines, e.g. pimozide.
- *Other unrelated compounds:*
    substituted benzamides, e.g. sulpiride;
    dibenzodiazepines, e.g. clozapine;
    benzisoxazoles, e.g. risperidone.

The first three groups are most widely used. They differ mainly in the degree of associated or unwanted effects.

Mechanism of action and effects

This appears to involve blockade of CNS dopamine receptors in mesolimbic and mesocortical pathways. Blockade of D_2 receptors and possibly the recently discovered D_3 receptor may be particularly important. Most antipsychotic drugs are not site-selective and also block dopamine receptors elsewhere in the brain, including the hypothalamus, basal ganglia (Chapter 25) and the chemoreceptor trigger zone (CTZ) in the brain stem (Chapter 34). These actions are responsible for many of the unwanted effects of the drugs, or in the case of the CTZ, for anti-emetic activity. Various antipsychotic drugs show different affinity for CNS dopamine receptor subtypes. Chlorpromazine binds equally to D_1 and D_2 receptors; clozapine binds more tightly to D_1 receptors, but also shows preferential binding at mesolimbic dopamine receptors. Risperidone is relatively selective for D_2 receptors.

Some newer antipsychotics, for example risperidone, also bind to $5HT_2$ receptors (see Table 17.1) which makes them more effective in controlling the "negative" symptoms of schizophrenia.

Many antipsychotic drugs also act as antagonists at several other receptors including muscarinic, α_1-adrenergic and histamine H_1 receptors. In this respect they resemble tricyclic antidepressants. These actions do not influence their efficacy in psychotic illness but can produce unwanted effects, the severity of which varies considerably among the different individual drugs.

The clinically useful effects produced by antipsychotic drugs include:

- A depressant action on conditioned responses and emotional responsiveness. In psychoses this is particularly helpful for management of thought disorder, abnormalities of perception and delusional beliefs.

- A sedative action which is used for treatment of restlessness and confusion. Sensory input into the reticular activating system is reduced by blockade of collateral fibres from the lemniscal pathways but spontaneous activity is preserved. Arousal stimuli, therefore, produce less response.

- An anti-emetic effect through dopamine blockade at the CTZ which is useful to treat vomiting associated with drugs (e.g. cytotoxics, opiate analgesics), uraemia and several other disorders. They are also effective in motion sickness through muscarinic receptor blockade (Chapter 34).

- Antihistaminic activity produced by H_1 receptor blockade is useful in allergic reactions (Chapter 41).

Pharmacokinetics

Antipsychotics are rapidly absorbed from the gut, but undergo extensive first-pass metabolism, involving up to 90% of the parent drug. The circulating concentrations of active drug (including metabolites) can vary some 10-fold among individuals. However, the relationship between plasma drug concentration and clinical response is not close. The half-lives vary widely, for example, that of chlorpromazine is short while that of risperidone is long.

Since compliance with treatment is often poor in psychotic disorders, depot formulations of many antipsychotics have been developed. They are given by intramuscular injection in an oily base which slowly releases the drug over several days. Depot preparations are given in smaller doses than oral treatment due to lack of first-pass metabolism.

Unwanted effects

The profile of unwanted effects varies widely among the different groups of drug (see Table 22.1).

- Extrapyramidal effects such as akathisia (motor restlessness), dystonia (tongue protrusion, torticollis, oculogyric crisis) or Parkinsonism arise from dopaminergic blockade in the nigrostriatal pathways. They are usually reversible if the drug is stopped. If treatment is continued, Parkinsonism is best treated with anticholinergic drugs (Chapter 25) rather than dopamine agonists. With prolonged use tardive dyskinesias can develop due to dopamine receptor up-regulation. These consist of choreo-athetoid and repetitive orofacial movements which may only occur after months or years of continued treatment and often do not resolve when the drug is withdrawn. Clozapine appears to have limited potential to cause extrapyramidal effects, and is often termed an "atypical" antipsychotic agent.
- Apathy and lassitude can occur as a result of dopamine receptor blockade.
- Galactorrhoea, amenorrhoea and infertility

result from dopamine receptor blockade in hypothalamic pathways, leading to hyperprolactinaemia and reduced gonadotrophin secretion.
- Anticholinergic effects (Chapter 4). In addition to the peripheral anticholinergic actions, CNS muscarinic receptor blockade predisposes to acute confusional states.
- α_1-Adrenoceptor blockade produces postural hypotension, nasal stuffiness and impaired ejaculation.
- Hypersensitivity reactions include cholestatic jaundice (chlorpromazine), skin reactions and agranulocytosis. The last is a particular problem with clozapine and regular blood tests are mandatory during treatment.
- Hypothermia as a consequence of depressed hypothalamic function. Altered 5HT activity may be responsible.
- Increased risk of seizures.
- Sudden withdrawal after long-term use can produce a prolonged syndrome of insomnia, sweating and dyskinesias.

MANAGEMENT OF PSYCHOTIC DISORDERS

In acute organic psychosis with decreased short-term memory, visual hallucinations and focal neurological deficits it is important to make a thorough search for a remediable underlying cause. Sedative drugs, for example benzodiazepines (Chapter 21), chlormethiazole (Chapter 21) or phenothiazines may be helpful.

Table 22.1 Consequences of receptor antagonist activity among antipsychotic drugs

	Sedative	Anticholinergic	Extrapyramidal	Hypotension
Phenothiazines				
Aliphatic	+++	++	++	+++
Piperidine	++	+++	+	++
Piperazine	++	+	+++	+
Thioxanthenes	+	+	+++	+
Butylpiperidines	+	+	+++	+
Other agents				
Substituted benzamides	+	+	○	○
Dibenzodiazepines	++	+	○	+
Benzisoxazoles	+	+	+	+

+++, high risk; ++, moderate risk; +, low risk; ○, minimal risk.

For chronic organic psychosis (dementia) sedative compounds should usually be avoided since they can worsen the mental state.

The management of depressive psychosis is similar to that of severe depression (Chapter 23) although the addition of a specific antipsychotic drug such as thioridazine to a tricyclic antidepressant has been advocated.

Mania can be controlled by a sedative antipsychotic, often in large doses. Carbamazepine (Chapter 24) can also be used to abort the manic episode or to reduce the risk of recurrence. Lithium (Chapter 23) is also very effective for reducing relapse, but is usually too slow acting to be useful for treatment of acute symptoms.

Schizophrenia and persecutory delusions (paranoia) are treated acutely with oral antipsychotic drugs. The choice for most patients is dictated by unwanted effects rather than differences in efficacy. However, risperidone may be useful if "negative" symptoms predominate. Long-acting depot preparations are almost always used for prophylaxis to improve compliance and to maintain prolonged remission. Clozapine has a particular role for treatment-resistant schizophrenia, but its use requires close hospital supervision and regular blood tests.

Treatment can be gradually withdrawn after several months of remission especially following the first psychotic episode, although relapse is very common.

23

Depression

Clinical depression is characterized by diverse psychological symptoms such as sadness, and a sense of guilt and worthlessness. These are frequently accompanied by physical symptoms including sleep disturbance, weight loss and loss of libido. If severe, there may be marked suicidal tendencies. The cause of depression is unknown but current views centre around the "monoamine hypothesis". Depletion of CNS monoamines such as noradrenaline and 5-hydroxytryptamine (5HT) with reduced central monoaminergic tone is believed to underlie depressive disorders. There is particularly strong evidence that 5HT deficiency is involved in depression.

Evidence in support of this includes:

- The ability of drugs that deplete CNS mono-amines (e.g. reserpine) to cause depression.
- Suicide victims have low CNS levels of 5HT.
- Depressed patients have low cerebrospinal fluid concentrations of the 5HT metabolite 5-hydroxyindole acetic acid (5HIAA), and sometimes of noradrenaline metabolites as well.

However, amine concentrations are only part of the story; adaptive changes occur in response to amine depletion. Inactivation of reuptake sites may be one attempt to compensate for reduced release of neurotransmitter. Compensatory changes in the entry of monoamine precursors into the neurone and adaptive changes in biosynthetic enzymes will also influence the amount of stored neurotransmitter. Postsynaptically, monoamine receptors appear to up-regulate (Chapter 1) in response to neuro-transmitter deficiency. At present it is unclear how these various homeostatic mechanisms interact.

TRICYCLIC ANTIDEPRESSANT DRUGS AND RELATED COMPOUNDS

Examples—tricyclic compounds: amitriptyline, imipramine, nortriptyline, lofepramine
—non-tricyclic compounds: mianserin.

Mechanism of action

The detailed mechanisms by which this class of drugs produce symptomatic improvement in depression is not well understood. All act rapidly to increase the synaptic concentrations of monoamine neurotransmitters in the CNS. However, the delay of 2–3 weeks after starting treatment before symptoms improve indicates that the response is more complex.

Older compounds have a triple carbon ring structure (tricyclic antidepressants). Many newer drugs are structurally unrelated to tricyclic compounds despite having the same mechanism of action. These include bicyclic, tetracyclic and non-cyclic structures.

Most tricyclic antidepressants and related drugs inhibit the reuptake of neurotransmitter by the presynaptic neurone, by competitive inhibition of the ATPase in the membrane pump (Fig. 23.1). Some show little monoamine selectivity while newer compounds are highly selective for noradrenaline (Table 23.1). However the specificity has not been shown to influence the efficacy of the drug.

Several postsynaptic receptors are also blocked to varying degrees by these drugs, for example muscarinic, histamine H_1 or α_1-adrenergic receptors. This does not influence their anti-

depressant action but contributes to their unwanted effects.

One compound, the tetracyclic drug mianserin, is believed to have a distinct mechanism of action. It appears to increase monoamine release from the neurone by blocking presynaptic α_2-adrenoceptors and $5HT_{1c}$ receptors, thus reducing negative feedback control (Chapter 4).

Pharmacokinetics

All are well absorbed from the gut, and are highly protein bound in plasma. Tertiary amines, for example imipramine and amitripty-

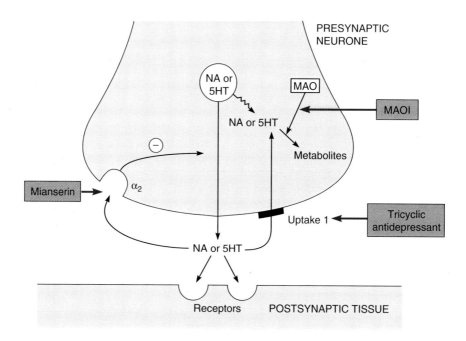

Figure 23.1 Site of action of antidepressants on CNS neurotransmitter regulation.

Table 23.1 Comparative properties of some commonly used antidepressants

	Active metabolites	Activity	Anticholinergic	Sedative	Stimulant	Epileptogenic	Toxicity in overdose
Amitriptyline	Yes	5HT > NA	+++	+++	○	++	+++
Imipramine	Yes	5HT > NA	+++	++	○	++	+++
Nortriptyline	No	NA > 5HT	++	○	+	+	++
Mianserin	Yes	NA > 5HT	++	+	○	+	++
Lofepramine	Yes	NA	+	+	○	○	○
Fluoxetine	No	5HT	○	○	○	○	○

+++, high risk; ++, moderate risk; +, low risk; ○, minimal risk.

line, undergo extensive first-pass metabolism by demethylation in the liver. Active secondary amines such as desipramine and nortriptyline are formed and contribute to a long duration of action. Half-lives vary from long, for example the active metabolite of imipramine, to up to 4 days, for example nortriptyline.

Unwanted effects are dose-related but there is no clear relationship for therapeutic effects. This may reflect the considerable interindividual variability in first-pass metabolism of most tricyclic antidepressants, and the difficulty in quantifying the contribution of both parent drug and active metabolites to the clinical response. Plasma concentrations of the parent drug show up to a 40-fold variation among individuals. Because of these differences, dose titration is usual to optimize the therapeutic response; this should be gradual to minimize unwanted effects. However, the need for routine use of maximally tolerated doses is not universally accepted.

Unwanted effects

The incidence and nature of unwanted effects vary widely among the different drugs. In general, tertiary amine tricyclic drugs have greater α_1-adrenoceptor, histamine and cholinergic-receptor blocking activity. Tricyclic compounds tend to be cardiotoxic. These differences are outlined in Table 23.1 which compares the profile for selected compounds.

- Sedation. Some compounds are highly sedative, for example amitriptyline, and others neutral, for example imipramine. Sedation is due to histamine H_1 receptor blockade (Chapter 17). It can be useful to help restore sleep patterns in depressed patients by using a larger dose at night, but can be troublesome or dangerous in the day. Protriptyline probably has mild stimulant effects which could be useful in retarded patients. Doses should be given early in the day to avoid sleep disturbance.

- Anticholinergic effects (see Chapter 4). These are common with older drugs, especially dry mouth. Tolerance can occur and gradual increases in dose may reduce these problems.

- Postural hypotension produced by peripheral α_1-adrenoceptor blockade (Chapter 7).

- Epileptogenic effects. Fits can be provoked even when there is no previous clinical history.

- Cardiotoxicity in overdosage. Several tricyclic drugs depress myocardial contractility or produce tachycardia and severe arrhythmias when taken in overdosage. Anticholinergic effects and excessive noradrenergic stimulation both contribute to the genesis of arrhythmias. Lofepramine appears to be the safest drug after overdosage.

- "Sudden withdrawal syndrome". During long-term treatment, doses should be progressively reduced to avoid headache, malaise and gastrointestinal upset which accompany sudden withdrawal of treatment in some patients.

- Weight gain. Appetite stimulation is common with tricyclic drugs.

- Drug interactions. Several important drug interactions are recognized. The antihypertensive action of adrenergic neurone blockers (Chapter 7) is prevented since tricyclic antidepressants block their uptake into the neurone. Direct-acting sympathomimetics are potentiated and indirect-acting sympathomimetics (Chapter 4) attenuated by the same mechanisms. Dangerous interactions can result from giving a monoamine oxidase (MAO) inhibitor (see below) and a tricyclic antidepressant together. Potentiation arises from the prolonged action of excess noradrenaline released from the neurone. The long duration of MAO inhibition means that the interaction can occur up to 2 weeks after stopping an MAO inhibitor.

SELECTIVE SEROTONIN (5HT) REUPTAKE INHIBITORS (SSRIs)

Examples: fluoxetine, paroxetine.

Mechanism of action

Unlike the tricyclic antidepressants, the SSRIs reduce the neuronal reuptake of 5HT but have no effect on noradrenaline reuptake. Their efficacy is similar to that of tricyclic antidepressants but they have a more favourable profile of unwanted effects.

Pharmacokinetics

They are well absorbed from the gut and metabolized in the liver. Fluoxetine has a very long half-life of 2 days while that of its active metabolite norfluoxetine is 7 days. Paroxetine has a long half-life. The half-life of fluoxetine can be a disadvantage if a monoamine oxidase inhibitor is subsequently used (see below).

Unwanted effects

In contrast to the tricyclic antidepressants, SSRIs have few anticholinergic effects, cause little sedation or weight gain and are not cardiotoxic in overdose.

- Nausea can be frequent, diarrhoea less so.
- Sedation with paroxetine, insomnia with fluoxetine.
- Anxiety and agitation, especially with fluoxetine.
- Drug interactions: the most potentially serious is with monoamine oxidase inhibitors (see tricyclic antidepressants above).

CLASSICAL (NON-SELECTIVE) MONOAMINE OXIDASE INHIBITORS (MAOIs)

Examples: phenelzine, tranylcypramine.

Mechanism of action

The way these drugs act is probably complex. However, their "primary" action is to inhibit intracellular MAO which is responsible for degrading free dopamine, noradrenaline and 5HT. The accumulation of monoamine neurotransmitters in the presynaptic neurone leads to increased release when the nerve is stimulated (Fig. 23.1). Two forms of MAO isoenzymes have been identified. MAO-A preferentially deaminates noradrenaline, and to a lesser extent 5HT. MAO-B is mainly responsible for deamination of phenylethylamine. Both enzymes deaminate dopamine and tyramine. MAO-B is the predominant enzyme in many parts of the brain, but MAO-A is present in noradrenergic and serotoninergic neurones, especially in the locus coeruleus and other cells of the brain stem, as well as being the main enzyme in peripheral tissues. Most MAO inhibitors (MAOIs) are not selective, although MAO-A inhibition in the brain produces the therapeutic effects. MAO-A inhibition in the gut wall and liver also has important consequences (see below). MAOIs also inhibit drug-metabolizing enzymes in the liver, which predisposes to drug interactions while not contributing to clinical efficacy.

Pharmacokinetics

All drugs in this group are well absorbed from the gut. Structurally, they are either derivatives of hydrazine (e.g. phenelzine) or similar to amphetamine (e.g. tranylcypramine). They are irreversible enzyme inhibitors so that the short half-life of the drugs, due to extensive liver metabolism, has no influence on their duration of action. Withdrawal is followed only gradually by restoration of normal MAO activity as new enzyme is synthesized.

Unwanted effects

Compared to tricyclic drugs, anticholinergic effects are unusual and there is no predisposition to fits.

- Postural hypotension. This is dose-related and, unlike the tricylic compounds, tolerance does not occur. The mechanism may involve conversion of tyramine (normally degraded by MAO) to octopamine, a false neurotransmitter which competes with noradrenaline at sympathetic nerve terminals.
- CNS stimulation with tranylcypramine leading to irritability and insomnia. These are amphetamine-like actions (Chapter 58) and doses should be given early in the day to avoid disturbing sleep.
- Hepatitis. This is a rare idiosyncratic reaction to hydrazine derivatives.
- Acute overdose produces delayed toxic effects after some 12 h. Excessive adrenergic stimulation leads to chest pain, headache and hyperactivity, progressing to confusion and severe hypertension with eventually profound hypotension and fits.
- Food interactions. MAO in the gut wall and liver usually prevents the absorption of natural amines, particularly tyramine which is an indirect-acting sympathomimetic (Chapter 4). If food containing tyramine, for example cheese, yeast extracts, pickled herrings, chianti and caviare, or broad bean pods (which contain L-dopa), is eaten the increased release of noradrenaline produces vasoconstriction and hypertension which can

lead to subarachnoid or intracerebral haemorrhage. A warning card should be supplied to patients.

- Drug interactions. Indirect-acting sympathomimetics (Chapter 4) in cold remedies (e.g. ephedrine, phenylpropanolamine) and amphetamine (Chapter 58) will be potentiated. Levodopa given for Parkinson's disease (Chapter 25) will also be more active.

The combination of MAOIs with tricyclic antidepressants (see above) can be dangerous. Other important interactions are due to impaired hepatic metabolism of drugs, especially opiate analgesics.

REVERSIBLE INHIBITORS OF MONOAMINE OXIDASE-A (RIMAs)

Example: moclobemide.

Mechanism of action and effects

Moclobemide is a selective inhibitor of the MAO-A isoenzyme which is responsible for the antidepressant action of classical MAOIs. If tyramine is absorbed from the gut, MAO-B is able to degrade it and the "cheese reaction" seen with classical MAOIs is very unlikely to occur. The action of moclobemide on the enzyme is reversible and high concentrations of tyramine will displace the drug from MAO-A, further facilitating tyramine degradation. Enzyme inhibition by moclobemide lasts less than 24 h after a single dose.

Unlike classical MAOIs, moclobemide has a broad spectrum of antidepressant activity, with efficacy similar to that of tricyclic antidepressants.

Pharmacokinetics

Oral absorption is good but there is substantial first-pass metabolism, partially to an active metabolite. Extensive hepatic metabolism means that the half-life is short.

Unwanted effects

- CNS stimulation can produce sleep disturbance.
- Nausea.
- Dizziness.

- Drug interactions: inhibition of cytochrome P450 activity with cimetidine (Chapter 2) substantially reduces the metabolism of moclobemide and smaller starting doses are recommended in this situation.

LITHIUM

Mechanism of action

This is not well understood. Lithium enhances neurotransmitter reuptake in the CNS, and produces changes in electrolyte fluxes across cell membranes which reduce intracellular sodium accumulation. The synthesis of intracellular second messengers such as phosphatidylinositides (Chapter 1) is reduced which may decrease the sensitivity of neurones to neurotransmitters.

Pharmacokinetics

Lithium is given as a salt which is rapidly absorbed from the gut. To avoid high peak plasma concentrations (which are associated with unwanted effects), modified-release formulations are normally used. Lithium is widely distributed but enters the brain slowly. It is selectively concentrated in bone and the thyroid gland. Excretion is by glomerular filtration with 80% reabsorbed in the proximal tubule by the same mechanism as sodium. There is no reabsorption from more distal parts of the kidney. When the body is depleted of salt and water, for example by vomiting, or hypovolaemia following the use of a potent diuretic, enhanced reabsorption of sodium in the proximal tubule is accompanied by lithium reabsorption which can produce acute toxicity. Lithium has a long half-life of about 1 day and has a narrow therapeutic index. Regular monitoring of plasma concentrations (which should be measured 12 h after dosing to avoid the absorption and distribution phases) is mandatory at least every 3 months during long-term treatment.

Unwanted effects

- Nausea and diarrhoea can occur at low plasma concentrations.
- CNS effects, including tremor, giddiness, ataxia and dysarthria, occur commonly with moderate intoxication.

- Severe intoxication produces coma, convulsions, and profound hypotension with oliguria.
- Hypothyroidism due to interference with thyroxine synthesis during long-term treatment.
- The distal renal tubule becomes less responsive to antidiuretic hormone. This occasionally produces reversible nephrogenic diabetes insipidus with polyuria.
- Drug interactions: diuretics (especially loop diuretics) can reduce lithium excretion by producing dehydration (see above).

TREATMENT OF DEPRESSION

Drugs form only part of the management of the depressed patient but are usually necessary for moderate, severe or protracted symptoms lasting 2 weeks or more. All antidepressant drugs have a delayed onset of action and severely ill patients should be considered for electroconvulsive therapy. Tricyclic antidepressants or related compounds are still considered by many psychiatrists to be the drugs of choice for initial management. About 70% of patients can be expected to respond, compared to about half that number taking placebo. Responders show an initial improvement in sleep pattern within a few days. Psychomotor retardation responds more gradually over several days and the patient becomes more involved with everyday activities and begins to enjoy life. Improvement in the depressed mood is delayed, beginning up to 2 or more weeks after treatment with adequate doses. The response of most symptoms tends to be erratic with "good and bad" days.

Persuading patients to comply with treatment may initially be difficult since unwanted effects can be troublesome before any benefit is perceived. Introducing a small dose with gradual titration is desirable. Older tricyclic antidepressants with cardiotoxic effects when taken in overdose should usually be avoided when treating patients with a high risk of suicide. The newer drugs, for example specific 5HT reuptake inhibitors, are no more effective and do not work any faster, but are better tolerated and safer when treating patients with a high risk of suicide.

Treatment with adequate doses of an antidepressant should be given for 6 weeks before the patient is considered to be a non-responder. If a good response is seen the dose can usually be reduced but maintenance treatment should be continued for at least 4 months to minimize the risk of relapse.

Classical MAOIs are usually reserved for "atypical" depression with hypochondriacal and phobic symptoms, or when tricyclic-type antidepressants have failed. The place of the RIMA moclobemide in therapy is yet to be fully established. Small doses of a phenothiazine such as flupenthixol (Chapter 22) are often recommended for elderly depressed patients. Evidence for a true antidepressant effect is slight but some symptoms undoubtedly do improve.

Lithium is reserved for patients with severe recurrent depressive episodes and for those with "bipolar" mood swings between depression and mania (Chapter 22). The effect of lithium can take several months to become fully established.

24

Epilepsy

NEUROTRANSMITTERS AND EPILEPSY

Co-ordinated activity among neurones depends on a controlled balance between excitatory and inhibitory influences on the cell membrane. Amino acids are involved in both forms of neurotransmission. Excitatory amino acids, aspartate and glutamate are found only in the CNS. An important inhibitory transmitter is gamma aminobutyric acid (GABA), which acts both inside and outside the CNS.

The pathophysiology of epilepsy probably involves a local imbalance among neurotransmitters which leads to an unstable neuronal membrane. Spontaneous repetitive firing of this focus is maintained by a feedback mechanism known as post-tetanic potentiation (see Chapter 28). Most evidence suggests that there is abnormal activity at a specific receptor for glutamate on the postsynaptic neuronal membrane. Activation of the receptor opens a transmembrane ion channel through which sodium and calcium pass inwards and potassium out. This depolarizes the cell membrane and will produce an action potential if the threshold potential in the cell is reached. The ion channel is blocked in the resting state by magnesium ions, which inhibit the response to glutamate. If another stimulus depolarizes the cell, there is less negative charge inside the channel to attract magnesium and the response

to glutamate is restored. This process is believed to be involved in the burst of firing that produces epileptiform activity, and which most antiepileptic drugs are believed to suppress.

Seizures may be focal or generalized, depending on the spread of the abnormal discharge. Further subdivision is broadly based on the clinical manifestations of the seizure.

ANTIEPILEPTIC DRUGS

SODIUM VALPROATE

Mechanism of action

This is poorly understood but is probably related to increasing the concentration of the inhibitory amino acid, GABA, or perhaps to decreasing the amount of the excitatory aspartate.

Pharmacokinetics

Sodium valproate is well absorbed from the gut. To reduce the risks of gastric upset, conventional tablets should be taken with food or enteric coated tablets can be given. Protein binding is high, but the proportion of free (and therefore active) drug rises with increasing blood concentration. Drug concentration in plasma does not correlate well with therapeutic effect and routine monitoring is only useful to assess compliance or to avoid toxic concentrations. Sodium valproate is extensively metabolized in the liver. The dose should be increased slowly to minimize unwanted effects. The half-life is long.

Unwanted effects

- Gastrointestinal upset. These include nausea, vomiting, anorexia, abdominal pain, bowel disturbance.
- Weight gain.
- Transient hair loss.
- Thrombocytopenia.
- Tremor and ataxia.
- Rarely, severe hepatotoxicity especially in children under age 2 years receiving multiple drug therapy for seizures.
- Inhibition of hepatic drug-metabolizing enzymes (Chapter 2).

CARBAMAZEPINE

Mechanism of action

Inhibition of repetitive neuronal firing is produced by reduction of transmembrane sodium influx, but the mechanism is unknown. Reduced calcium influx produced by interaction with benzodiazepine binding sites or adenosine receptor antagonism may contribute.

Pharmacokinetics

Absorption is slow and incomplete after oral administration. The major epoxide metabolite, produced in the liver, is also active but present in lower concentrations than the parent drug. The half-life of carbamazepine is initially very long at about 1.5 days but decreases by two-thirds over the first 2–3 weeks of treatment due to "autoinduction" of its own metabolizing enzymes in the liver. Seizure control may then require an increase in dose. During chronic therapy the half-life is extremely variable among individuals. The plasma concentration of carbamazepine correlates well with its clinical efficacy and measurement can be useful in monitoring treatment. Salivary concentrations are an alternative guide.

Unwanted effects

- Nausea and vomiting, especially early in treatment.
- CNS toxicity: double vision, dizziness, drowsiness. Ataxia occurs at high doses.
- Transient leucopenia is common, especially early in treatment, but severe bone marrow depression is rare.
- Hyponatraemia, due to potentiation of the action of antidiuretic hormone which can lead to water intoxication.
- Induction of hepatic drug-metabolizing enzymes (Chapter 2).

PHENYTOIN

Mechanism of action

Phenytoin has "membrane stabilizing" activity which is due to inhibition of sodium influx across the cell membrane (Chapter 9). This probably explains its antiepileptic activity by reducing the spread of seizure discharges, rather than preventing their initiation.

Pharmacokinetics

Phenytoin is absorbed slowly from the gut. Slow intravenous injection can be used if a rapid onset of action is needed. Intramuscular injection should be avoided since absorption is erratic and unpredictable and muscle damage can occur. Extensive metabolism by liver microsomal enzymes is responsible for the elimination of almost all phenytoin at lower doses. However, the enzyme is saturable at plasma drug concentrations near the lower end of the therapeutic range. The pharmacokinetics then change from first order (linear) kinetics to zero order (Chapter 2) (Fig. 24.1) when the enzyme is saturated. When the plasma concentration is close to or within the therapeutic range, a small change in dose produces a large change in plasma concentration. The half-life is similarly lengthened four-fold to almost 2 days. Plasma concentrations are closely related to effect and their measurement is useful as a guide to dosing. Salivary concentrations measure free drug concentration and are useful if protein binding is altered (e.g. pregnancy, renal failure; Chapter 2) or in children.

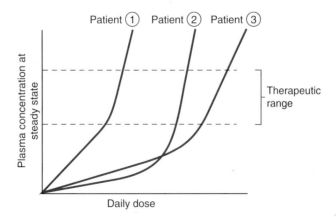

Figure 24.1 Phenytoin pharmacokinetics showing typical interindividual variation. Linear (first-order) kinetics would give a linear increase in plasma concentration with increase in daily dose.

Unwanted effects

- Impaired brain stem and cerebellar function producing nystagmus, double vision, vertigo, ataxia and dysarthria.
- Chronic connective tissue effects: gum hyperplasia, coarsening of facial features and hirsutism. For this reason it is usual to avoid phenytoin in young women.
- Skin rashes including acne.
- Induction of hepatic drug-metabolizing enzymes (Chapter 2).
- Teratogenic effects including facial and digital malformations and which occur in up to 10% of pregnancies.
- Folate deficiency producing macrocytic anaemia.
- Vitamin D deficiency producing osteomalacia.

ETHOSUXIMIDE

Mechanism of action

This may be due to antagonist activity in cell membrane T-type calcium channels (distinct from the L-type channel blocked by cardiovascular-active calcium antagonists: Chapter 6) found in high density in thalamic neurones. These channels may contribute to the generation of thalamocortical activity in absence seizures.

Pharmacokinetics

Absorption from the gut is almost complete. Metabolism in the liver is extensive and the half-life is very long at 2–3 days. Plasma concentrations correlate well with control of seizures, as do salivary concentrations; either can be used to monitor treatment.

Unwanted effects

- Nausea, vomiting, anorexia. These are less frequent if the drug is taken with food and if the dose is gradually increased.
- Drowsiness and headaches.

PHENOBARBITONE AND PRIMIDONE

Mechanism of action

Three separate actions have been proposed to contribute to the effectiveness of phenobarbitone in epilepsy. A presynaptic effect which reduces calcium influx into the neurone may reduce neurotransmitter release. There is also a postsynaptic action, leading to opening of the transmembrane chloride channel. This effect is partly a direct one and partly via potentiation of the inhibitory amino acid GABA on the chloride channel (Fig. 23.1). The direct action of barbiturates produces more widespread effects in tissues with chloride channels than benzodiazepines (see also Chapter 21). There may also be a third separate action on transfer of sodium and potassium across cell membranes.

The action of primidone may be due in part to its conversion to phenobarbitone.

Pharmacokinetics

Oral absorption of phenobarbitone is almost complete. Elimination is mainly by hepatic metabolism but up to 40% is excreted unchanged by the kidney. The half-life is very long, ranging between 2 and 6 days.

Primidone is well absorbed orally and converted in the liver to two active metabolites, phenobarbitone and phenylethylmalonamide, producing rather more of the former. Enzyme induction increases the conversion to phenobarbitone.

The plasma concentrations of phenobarbitone and primidone are not closely related to control of seizures. They are only useful as a guide to compliance with treatment; control of seizures or unwanted effects should determine doses.

Unwanted effects

- CNS effects: sedation, unsteadiness, giddiness. Hyperactivity and other behavioural disturbances can occur in children. Poor memory and depression are also seen.
- Nausea and vomiting (especially after the first dose of primidone).
- Induction of hepatic drug-metabolizing enzymes (Chapter 2).
- Tolerance to both toxic and therapeutic effects tends to occur during long-term administration.
- Dependence with a physical withdrawal reaction is seen after long-term treatment.

VIGABATRIN

Mechanism of action

Vigabatrin is a structural analogue of GABA and produces irreversible inhibition of the enzyme which inactivates GABA (GABA-T, gamma-aminobutyric acid transaminase). The increase in CNS concentrations of GABA inhibits the spread of epileptic discharges.

Pharmacokinetics

Vigabatrin is rapidly absorbed from the gut and excreted unchanged by the kidney. The half-life is short but irreversible binding to the enzyme results in a long duration of action which is unrelated to the plasma drug concentration. Blood concentration monitoring is therefore of no value.

Unwanted effects

- Sedation and fatigue.
- Psychotic reactions, especially in patients with a history of psychiatric disorder.
- Weight gain.

LAMOTRIGINE

Mechanism of action

Lamotrigine is believed to inhibit release of the excitatory neurotransmitter glutamate.

Pharmacokinetics

Lamotrigine is well absorbed orally and extensively metabolized in the liver. The half-life is long.

Unwanted effects

- Skin rashes.
- CNS reactions, similar to phenytoin.

GABAPENTIN

Mechanism of action and effects

Although designed as a structural analogue of GABA, gabapentin does not mimic GABA in the brain. Specific binding sites are present in the superficial neocortex and hippocampus but how these produce an anticonvulsant effect is unclear. Its major efficacy is in partial seizures.

Pharmacokinetics

Gabapentin is incompletely absorbed from the gut and excreted unchanged by the kidney. It has a short half-life.

Unwanted effects

- CNS effects including drowsiness, dizziness, ataxia, fatigue and diplopia.

BENZODIAZEPINES

Examples: clonazepam, diazepam.

Mechanism of action

These drugs enhance the action of GABA (Chapter 21).

Pharmacokinetics

These are considered fully in Chapter 21. Clonazepam is used orally for prophylaxis while diazepam is usually used intravenously or rectally to control individual fits.

Unwanted effects

These are discussed in Chapter 21. Partial or complete tolerance to the anticonvulsant action often occurs after about 4–6 months of continuous treatment.

DRUG INTERACTIONS AMONG ANTICONVULSANTS

Since many anticonvulsants affect drug metabolizing enzymes in the liver, interactions are frequent. They have major clinical implications when more than one anticonvulsant is used concurrently.

- Sodium valproate inhibits hepatic drug metabolism and may increase phenobarbitone concentrations. It can displace phenytoin from plasma protein binding sites, but also inhibits phenytoin metabolism. The net result is a reduction in total phenytoin plasma concentration but an increase in the active free component.
- Carbamazepine, phenytoin and phenobarbitone all enhance hepatic drug metabolism and decrease plasma concentrations of each other when given together. Other clinically important interactions produced by this effect on liver enzymes are reduction in the efficacy of warfarin (Chapter 10) and oestrogen-containing contraceptive pills (Chapter 48).

- Vigabatrin reduces plasma phenytoin concentrations by an unknown mechanism.

MANAGEMENT OF EPILEPSY

TREATMENT OF INDIVIDUAL SEIZURES

Prolonged or repetitive seizures (status epilepticus) usually require parenteral treatment. Diazepam is the drug of choice given either intravenously or as a rectal solution. Intravenous phenytoin or chlormethiazole (Chapter 21) are alternative choices.

PROPHYLAXIS FOR SEIZURES

A diagnosis of epilepsy requires two or more spontaneous seizures. After a single event, less than one-third of patients will have a second fit within 2 years. If a predisposing cause cannot be avoided (e.g. alcohol withdrawal, photosensitive epilepsy precipitated by viewing a television from too close a distance) drug treatment will usually be started after the second fit. Treatment should begin with a single drug, the choice depending on the type of epilepsy and relative toxicity of the drugs. The usual first-line drugs are carbamazepine or sodium valproate which will give long-term control in up to 80% of patients. If fits are not controlled with the first choice drug, a second single drug should be tried while the first is gradually withdrawn (Table 24.1). Multiple drug treatment should be reserved for patients resistant to two or three single agents. Drugs like vigabatrin, lamotrigine or gabapentin are only used in this situation.

It is not usually necessary to monitor plasma drug concentrations to determine whether the drug concentration is within the "therapeutic range" unless seizure control is poor or if poor

Table 24.1 Choice of drug for different forms of epilepsy

	First choice	Second choice
Partial seizures	Carbamazepine	Valproate/phenytoin
Generalized seizures		
Absence (petit mal)	Vaproate/ethosuximide	Clonazepam
Benign myoclonic	Valproate	Clonazepam
Tonic and/or clonic	Valproate	Carbamazepine/phenytoin

compliance or toxicity are suspected. Many patients will achieve good control at plasma drug concentrations which are below conventional "therapeutic" levels, and an increase in dose will not be necessary unless there are recurrent fits. Conversely, other patients may need concentrations above the "therapeutic range" if there is no evidence of toxic effects. Once started, treatment should usually be continued for at least 2–3 years after the last fit. If there is a continuing predisposing condition or the patient wishes to drive, treatment should probably be life-long.

ANTICONVULSANTS IN PREGNANCY

No anticonvulsant has a proven safety record in pregnancy. Fetal abnormalities are most common with phenytoin or if combinations of drugs are used. Either carbamazepine, valproate or ethosuximide, used as single drug therapy, are believed to be the least likely to produce teratogenic effects in the fetus. These are the anticonvulsants of choice if the patient is attempting to become pregnant. If a patient becomes pregnant while taking an alternative treatment, then the drug therapy should probably not be changed.

25

Extrapyramidal Movement Disorders and Spasticity

The neuronal connections of the area of the brain known as the basal ganglia are intimately involved in the co-ordination of motor function in conjunction with the motor cortex, cerebellum and spinal cord. Several major neurotransmitters are involved in regulating the function of the basal ganglia (Fig. 25.1) and altered concentrations of these neurotransmitters are responsible for the extrapyramidal movement disorders. Treatment for these disorders is directed at restoring the balance among the neurotransmitters.

PARKINSON'S DISEASE

Parkinson's disease is a disorder characterized by a triad of resting tremor, skeletal muscle rigidity and bradykinesia (poverty of movement). The underlying pathology involves degeneration of the cells in the substantia nigra which use dopamine as a neurotransmitter. The cause for the progressive degeneration of the neurones is not known; it may be related to the production of free radicals during dopamine biosynthesis and metabolism, or to the presence of environmental toxins. The cells in the striatum which receive impulses from the substantia nigra remain intact, as do their dopamine receptors. Most of these cells use GABA as a neurotransmitter. The result of the relative dopamine deficiency in the substantia nigra is that there is an impaired inhibition of the cholinergic input to the striatum which then

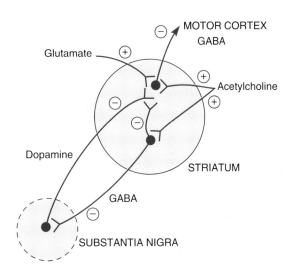

Figure 25.1 Outline of the major neurotransmitter pathways controlling the function of the basal ganglia. ⊕, Excitatory; ⊖, inhibitory.

produces the typical symptoms. In some conditions which have similarities to Parkinson's disease, for example the Steele–Richardson and Shy–Drager syndromes, the GABA neurones also degenerate which explains the poor response of these conditions to treatment with dopamine replacement.

Drugs can also produce a Parkinsonian-type syndrome by blockade of striatal dopamine receptors. Antipsychotic drugs (Chapter 22) most commonly produce this syndrome, which also responds poorly to dopamine replacement therapy.

Treatment of Parkinson's disease involves either enhancing dopaminergic activity (Fig. 25.2) or inhibiting cholinergic activity.

DOPAMINERGIC DRUGS

LEVODOPA

Mechanism of action

Dopamine cannot be given to replace the deficiency in the basal ganglia since it does not cross the blood–brain barrier. However, the large neutral amino acid, levodopa, can enter the brain, after which it is taken up into dopaminergic neurones, and converted

to dopamine by L-aromatic amino acid decarboxylase (Chapter 4).

Pharmacokinetics

Levodopa is absorbed from the small intestine by an active transport mechanism for large neutral amino acids. A similar transport system is used to cross the blood–brain barrier. However, decarboxylation of levodopa occurs extensively in peripheral tissues such as the gut wall and liver. This reduces the amount of levodopa that reaches the brain and generates substantial amounts of extracerebral dopamine which produces unwanted effects. Therefore levodopa is usually given in combination with a peripheral decarboxylase inhibitor (carbidopa or benserazide) that does not cross the blood–brain barrier. About 80% of the peripheral metabolism of levodopa can be inhibited, reducing dosage requirements by about the same amount.

The half-life of levodopa is short. In the early stages of the disease, storage of dopamine in striatal neurones can ensure a stable response despite infrequent doses. Modified-release formulations are also available, and are more useful later in the disease to provide a continuous supply of drug to the neurones. Transition from conventional to a modified-release formulation may be difficult since the latter has a

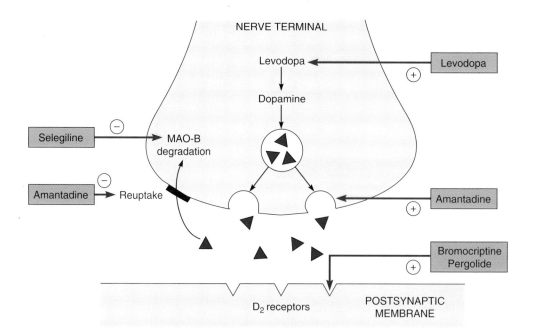

Figure 25.2 Major effects of drugs on the dopaminergic nerve terminal in the basal ganglia. ⊕, Stimulation; ⊖, inhibition.

lower bioavailability which makes dosage estimations difficult.

Unwanted effects

Unwanted effects fall broadly into two categories:

- Those arising mainly from peripheral dopamine generation (which will be reduced by a peripheral decarboxylase inhibitor). Nausea and vomiting are due to stimulation of the chemoreceptor trigger zone (CTZ) of the medullary vomiting centre which lies outside the blood–brain barrier (Chapter 34). Postural hypotension is produced by vasodilation.
- Those arising from excessive central dopamine generation: dyskinetic involuntary movements, especially of the face and neck, or akathisia (restlessness): psychological disturbance including hallucinations, confusion.

DOPAMINE RECEPTOR AGONISTS

Examples: bromocriptine, pergolide.

Mechanism of action

In contrast to levodopa, these drugs act as direct agonists of central dopaminergic receptors. They have a longer duration of action than levodopa, and are selective for the inhibitory dopamine D_2 receptor subtype, showing little activity at excitatory D_1 receptors (see Chapter 17).

Pharmacokinetics

Bromocriptine is incompletely absorbed from the gut and undergoes extensive presystemic metabolism in the liver. It has a long half-life.

Unwanted effects

- Constipation, at low doses.
- Peripheral vasospasm. These drugs are structurally related to ergot alkaloids (Chapter 26).
- Other unwanted effects are similar to those of levodopa. Pergolide produces less nausea and postural hypotension than bromocriptine.

AMANTADINE

Mechanism of action

Amantadine was introduced originally as an antiviral drug. It is believed to act in Parkinson's disease by stimulating release of dopamine stored in nerve terminals and by reducing reuptake of released dopamine into the presynaptic neurone. Its usefulness tends to be short-lived, due to the development of tolerance.

Pharmacokinetics

Amantadine is well absorbed from the gut and has a variable but long half-life. It is excreted unchanged by the kidney.

Unwanted effects

- Ankle swelling.
- Confusion with high doses.
- Livedo reticularis: skin vasoconstriction due to local catecholamine release.

SELECTIVE MONOAMINE OXIDASE-B INHIBITORS

Example: selegiline.

Mechanism of action

Selegiline inhibits the enzyme monoamine oxidase (MAO) which is responsible for the intraneuronal degradation of monoamine neurotransmitters (Chapter 4). It is selective at low doses for the enzyme subtype found in the striatum, called MAO-B. This enzyme is distinct from MAO-A found in the gut wall and other peripheral tissues, so interactions with drugs and foods that are found with conventional non-selective monoamine oxidase inhibitor antidepressants do not occur (Chapter 23). Selegiline prolongs the duration of action of levodopa and reduces the levodopa dosage requirement by about one-third. It produces a small degree of clinical benefit when used alone. It may reduce the production of toxic free radicals in the striatum but it remains unproven whether this will alter progression of the disease.

Pharmacokinetics

Selegiline is completely absorbed from the gut and has a variable but long half-life. It is extensively metabolized in the liver, in part to amphetamine metabolites.

Unwanted effects

- Transient nausea, dizziness or lightheadedness are common.
- Abdominal pain or dry mouth.
- Insomnia, confusion, hallucinations are due to production of active amphetamine metabolites.

ANTICHOLINERGIC DRUGS

Examples: benzhexol, procyclidine.

Mechanism of action

These drugs block central muscarinic receptors (Chapter 4) and restore the balance between cholinergic and dopaminergic activity by reducing the former.

Pharmacokinetics

Oral absorption is almost complete, and most of these drugs undergo extensive hepatic metabolism. High lipid solubility ensures ready transfer across the blood–brain barrier.

Unwanted effects

- These are predictable and due to blockade of peripheral muscarinic receptors (Chapter 4). Reduced saliva production can be helpful in some Parkinsonian patients, in whom sialorrhoea is a problem.
- Blockade of CNS muscarinic receptors can produce confusion in the elderly.

MANAGEMENT OF PARKINSON'S DISEASE

Levodopa (with a peripheral decarboxylase inhibitor) is the mainstay of treatment and is particularly useful for reducing bradykinesia. Clinical response is achieved in about 70% of patients with idiopathic Parkinson's disease; those with drug-induced Parkinsonism respond poorly. Frequent doses may be needed especially in advanced disease to prevent the response "wearing off". A further problem late in the disease is the "on–off" phenomenon with rapid swings between severe bradykinesia and toxic dyskinesias. Fluctuating delivery of levodopa to the striatum is believed to be responsible; there are too few surviving neurones to store dopamine and smooth out the response when delivery of levodopa is not constant. Modified-release formulations of levodopa, combining levodopa with selegiline or the addition of a dopamine receptor agonist may be helpful in some patients.

Anticholinergic agents are less widely used. They are most effective against tremor and rigidity, but have little effect on bradykinesia. They can be helpful in reducing excessive salivation. Amantadine is well tolerated but effective only in mild Parkinsonism, with rapid loss of clinical benefit after a few weeks.

Combinations of drugs are sometimes used but unwanted effects can be troublesome: confusion is a particular problem, especially in the elderly.

Drugs improve symptoms and quality of life but they do not appear to alter the underlying rate of neuronal degeneration. However, early treatment with levodopa may delay the onset of motor disability. Initial encouraging evidence that selegiline might delay the neuronal degeneration of Parkinson's disease has not been confirmed by a more recent study in previously untreated patients.

HUNTINGTON'S CHOREA

This is an hereditary disease which presents in adult life with progressively impaired motor co-ordination and bizarre limb movements. The pathology is a loss of GABA neurones within the neostriatum which connect with the substantia nigra (Fig. 25.1). There is a consequent reduction of inhibitory activity on dopaminergic cells in the substantia nigra and cells in the thalamus. These cells generate uncoordinated discharges, producing bursts of excess motor activity. Treatment aims to reduce the excessive dopaminergic activity.

TETRABENAZINE

Mechanism of action

Tetrabenazine produces selective monoamine depletion from neurones in the CNS. Storage vesicles become leaky and the released contents are degraded by monoamine oxidase. It is more effective for choreiform movements than the antipsychotic drugs which block dopamine receptors.

Unwanted effects

- Drowsiness.
- Postural hypotension.
- Dysphagia, which may be due to extrapyramidal dysfunction.

SPASTICITY

Spasticity is a state of sustained muscle tone or tension which is often associated with an increase in stretch reflexes. The increase in muscle tone may arise from continued spinal reflex activity in the absence of input from the primary motor cortex such as may result from a stroke. Spasticity in skeletal muscles often results in a partial or complete loss of voluntary movement.

Neuromuscular junction blocking drugs are not used to treat spasticity, since their main effect would probably be the further loss of voluntary movement. The primary sites of action of drugs for spasticity are the spinal reflexes and the release of calcium in the muscle fibre. Muscular hypotonia is a common problem in the drug therapy of spasticity.

DIAZEPAM

Diazepam enhances inhibitory pathways by facilitating GABA-mediated opening of chloride channels (see Chapter 21). In spasticity, diazepam acts via presynaptic inhibitory GABA receptors to decrease the activity of excitatory pathways in the spinal cord. The main disadvantage is sedation due to inhibitory activity in higher centres at the doses necessary for a spasmolytic action.

BACLOFEN

Mechanism of action

Baclofen inhibits excitatory activity at mono- and polysynaptic reflexes at the spinal level. It binds stereoselectively to and is an agonist at $GABA_B$ receptors. It probably acts via an increase in presynaptic inhibition with a possible action to inhibit presynaptic calcium influx. It also has an analgesic action, probably by inhibition of the release of substance P.

Pharmacokinetics

Baclofen is absorbed rapidly from the gastrointestinal tract. It has a short half-life and is eliminated largely in the urine in the unchanged form.

Unwanted effects

- Sedation and drowsiness.
- Nausea.
- Various CNS effects, e.g. lightheadedness, confusion, dizziness and headache.
- Sudden withdrawal may cause hallucinations.

DANTROLENE

Mechanism of action

Acts on the muscle fibres to inhibit the release of calcium from the sarcoplasmic reticulum. It reduces excitation–contraction coupling, but does not abolish contraction of skeletal muscle.

Pharmacokinetics

Dantrolene is absorbed slowly and incompletely (about 80%) from the gastrointestinal tract. It is eliminated by hepatic metabolism and the metabolites, which are also active, are eliminated in urine and bile. The half-life is intermediate/long with wide interpatient variability.

Unwanted effects

- Liver dysfunction and hepatotoxicity (sometimes fatal).
- Diarrhoea (which may necessitate discontinuation of treatment).

26

Migraine

Migraine is characteristically a unilateral throbbing headache often associated with nausea and occasionally with vomiting. In a few patients ("classical" migraine) this is preceded by an aura which often consists of visual disturbances but occasionally more severe focal neurological episodes.

The pathogenesis of migraine is believed to involve neuronal, vascular and biochemical influences. The initiation of pain may have a neural origin, but its development is probably due to the release of 5-hydroxytryptamine (5HT) from tissue stores. Receptors for 5HT are distributed widely in cerebral blood vessels and many receptor subtypes have been identified (see Table 17.1). Receptors on cerebral arteries are mainly $5HT_1$, while those on temporal arteries are $5HT_2$ and both are present on meningeal arteries. Dilation of cranial blood vessels is believed to contribute to the pain of migraine, augmented by a neurogenic inflammatory process with extravasation of plasma protein from dural vessels. This is probably provoked by release of transmitters such as substance P or neurokinin A.

SPECIFIC DRUGS FOR THE ACUTE MIGRAINE ATTACK

ERGOTAMINE

Mechanism of action

Ergotamine is a potent vasoconstrictor as a consequence of partial agonist activity (Chapter 1) at the $5HT_{1A}$ vascular receptor and at α_1-adrenoceptors.

Pharmacokinetics

Absorption from the gut is often accompanied by nausea. It is better tolerated when given sublingually, as a rectal suppository or by inhalation from a pressurized aerosol. Absorption is unreliable whichever route is chosen. Ergotamine undergoes extensive metabolism in the liver and has a short half-life. However, tight receptor binding produces a long duration of action.

Unwanted effects

- Nausea and vomiting, possibly due to dopaminergic stimulation of the chemoreceptor trigger zone (Chapter 34).
- Severe vasoconstriction which can lead to peripheral gangrene (acute ergotism). Ergotamine should be avoided in patients with known vascular disease or those concurrently receiving β-adrenoceptor antagonists (Chapter 6).
- Chronic intoxication with dependence. Withdrawal produces nausea and headache similar to an acute migraine attack.

SUMATRIPTAN

Mechanism of action and effects

Sumatriptan is a selective $5HT_{1D}$ agonist and produces constriction in cranial arteries believed to be involved in migraine attacks. This brings rapid pain relief for the majority of patients.

Pharmacokinetics

Absorption from the gut is rapid but erratic, although effective plasma concentrations are usually reached within 30 min. It is also available for subcutaneous injection. It is extensively metabolized in the liver and has a short half-life.

Unwanted effects

- Pain or irritation at the injection site.
- Tingling or sensation of warmth.
- Dizziness or vertigo.

PROPHYLACTIC DRUGS FOR MIGRAINE

β-ADRENOCEPTOR ANTAGONISTS

Examples: propranolol, atenolol.

Mechanism of action in migraine

Full details of these drugs are found in Chapter 6. In migraine, drugs with partial agonist activity (e.g. pindolol) are ineffective suggesting that vasoconstriction may contribute to their action. Some (e.g. propranolol) are also weak 5HT receptor antagonists.

PIZOTIFEN

Mechanism of action

Pizotifen is a non-selective antagonist at $5HT_1$ and $5HT_2$ receptors and may have central actions which prevent the onset of the inflammatory response associated with established migraine attacks.

Pharmacokinetics

Oral absorption is almost complete and extensive metabolism occurs in the liver. The half-life of pizotifen is long.

Unwanted effects

- Appetite stimulation with weight gain, which may be due to enhanced insulin release.
- Drowsiness.

METHYSERGIDE

Mechanism of action

This is similar to pizotifen, with some additional partial agonist activity at $5HT_{1D}$ receptors (cf. sumatriptan).

Pharmacokinetics

Oral absorption is complete and liver metabolism extensive. Methysergide has a very short half-life.

Unwanted effects

- Drowsiness.
- Retroperitoneal fibrosis with long-term use, producing ureteric compression, hydronephrosis and renal failure. It is reversible, but methysergide should only be given for a maximum of 6 months, followed by a 1 month drug-free interval.

MANAGEMENT OF MIGRAINE

THE ACUTE ATTACK

Withdrawal of possible triggers such as cheese, chocolate, citrus fruits or alcoholic drinks may reduce the frequency of attacks by up to 50%. The oral contraceptive pill is a potential exacerbating factor.

For relief of an acute attack, simple analgesia, for example aspirin, paracetamol or a non-steroidal anti-inflammatory drug (NSAID) (Chapter 31) may be sufficient. Nausea frequently accompanies a migraine attack; absorption of the drug will be more rapid if gastric emptying is enhanced by metoclopramide (Chapter 34). If vomiting is prominent, rectal or intramuscular analgesia, for example the NSAID diclofenac, may be needed. Ergotamine can be given occasionally (by tablet, suppository or metered dose inhaler) but the potential for vasospasm and habituation means that it should be avoided in older patients and those with frequent attacks. If attacks are poorly controlled by standard therapies, sumatriptan is often highly effective.

PROPHYLAXIS

Prophylaxis is usually recommended for patients experiencing at least two attacks of migraine each month. β-Adrenoceptor antagonists are widely held to be the best choice if there are no contraindications. Pizotifen is an alternative, but weight gain limits its acceptability, especially in young women. Methysergide can be given intermittently.

Small doses of tricyclic antidepressants, for example amitriptyline, can be helpful, either alone or in combination with a β-adrenoceptor antagonist. Clonidine (Chapter 7), although once recommended for the prophylaxis of migraine, is ineffective.

The Musculoskeletal System

27

The Neuromuscular Junction

NEUROMUSCULAR TRANSMISSION

Acetycholine (ACh) is the neurotransmitter at the N_2 nicotinic receptor of the neuromuscular junction. The processes of synthesis and release of ACh have been described briefly in Chapter 4, in relation to the general properties of neuro-transmitters in the autonomic nervous system.

The neuromuscular junction represents a specialized part of the sarcolemma of skeletal muscle, the motor-end plate (Fig. 27.1). In mammals depolarization of the postsynaptic membrane at the motor-end plate causes contraction of the whole muscle. The presynaptic nerve terminal contains 300 000 or more vesicles, each of which may contain up to 5000 molecules of ACh. In the presence of an action potential, up to 500 vesicles are discharged over a very short period (0.5 ms). This produces rapid depolarization of the motor-end plate due to the binding of ACh to the N_2 receptors, which opens the associated Na^+ channel (Chapter 1) allowing an influx of Na^+ ions. The extent of channel opening is dependent on the amount of ACh released and binding to N_2 receptors; a minimum amount of depolarization is necessary in order to reach the firing threshold at which full depolarization is triggered (Fig. 27.1). The action of ACh on N_2 receptors is very short lived (about 0.5 ms) since the motor-end plate has large amounts of acetyl-choline esterase (AChE) associated with it (mouse diaphragm end-plate has 12 000 AChE molecules per square micrometre).

Although ACh is the neurotransmitter causing contraction of both skeletal muscle and most smooth muscles, the basic organization and functioning of these neuroeffector systems are very different as shown in Table 27.1.

AGONISTS AT THE NEUROMUSCULAR JUNCTION

There are no clinical indications for the use of specific direct agonists at the skeletal neuromuscular junction. Administration of a long-acting direct N_2-receptor agonist would *not* be of clinical value because the necessary *voluntary* control would not be possible. In addition, prolonged occupancy of nicotonic receptors (both N_1 and N_2) by an agonist leads to a depolarizing blockade (see Chapter 28).

ANTAGONISTS/BLOCKERS AT THE NEUROMUSCULAR JUNCTION

Relaxation of skeletal muscles is an essential prerequisite for many surgical operations. To avoid the need for deep anaesthesia, this is achieved by drugs which specifically block the neuromuscular junction without affecting autonomic functioning, that is the actions of ACh on muscarinic and N_1 receptors. Drugs which block the neuromuscular junction almost all resemble ACh to the extent that they contain a quaternary amino group which produces strong binding to the

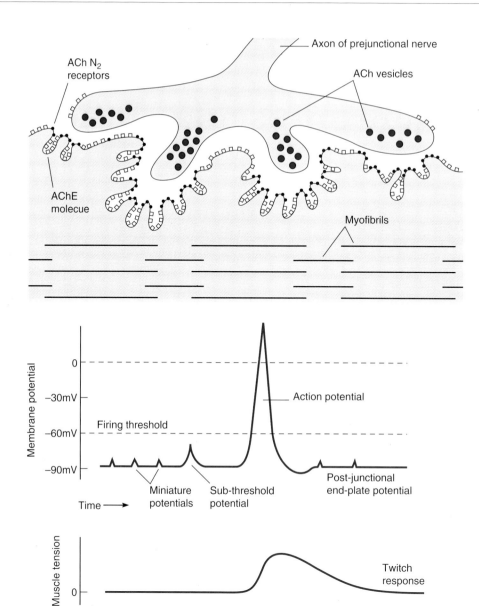

Figure 27.1 Neuromuscular junction and action potential.

Table 27.1 Comparison of skeletal and smooth muscle innervation

Property	Skeletal muscle	Smooth muscle
Innervation	Single	Multiple
Junction	Highly organized motor-end plate	Simple
Neurotransmitter	ACh	ACh
Receptor subtype	Nicotinic — N_2	Muscarinic — M
Receptor distribution	Only at motor-end plate	Widely on the muscle surface
Effects of stimulation	Single nerve contracts the whole muscle fibre (all or none response)	Each nerve contracts part of muscle fibre (graded response)
Inhibition of AChE	Flaccid paralysis	Spasticity

anionic site of the N_2 receptor. Antagonists/ blockers at the neuromuscular junction are presented in Chapter 28.

ACETYLCHOLINE ESTERASE (AChE) INHIBITORS

AChE inhibitors block the breakdown of ACh following its release in synapses and neuro-effector junctions. The mechanisms of action of different types of AChE inhibitor have been described under autonomic nervous system (Chapter 4) but it should be appreciated that they are non-selective and affect the actions of ACh at N_1, N_2 and muscarinic sites. A major clinical use for these drugs is in the treatment of myasthenia gravis and details are presented in that section (Chapter 29).

Neuromuscular Blockade

There are two major classes of antagonists/blockers at the neuromuscular junction (Chapter 27).

COMPETITIVE ANTAGONISTS

Examples: tubocurarine, vecuronium, atracurium, pancuronium.

Mechanism of action and effects

These drugs bind to the N_2 ACh receptor without causing depolarization of the postsynaptic membrane. There is simple concentration-dependent competition between the blocker and ACh. Prevention of ACh breakdown by an AChE inhibitor (usually neostigmine, see Chapter 29) will therefore reverse the blockade. A period of continuous nerve stimulation (tetanic stimulation) decreases neuronal ACh stores and increases ACh synthesis. If tetanic stimulation occurs during partial blockade, the release of ACh decreases, the blockade increases and the tetanic contraction fades. However, after cessation of tetanic stimulation there is an enhanced response to a subsequent single stimulation which is known as post-tetanic potentiation (Fig. 28.1).

Pharmacokinetics

Because of their high polarity (quaternary N atom) these drugs are not absorbed from the gastrointestinal tract (hence the successful use of curare as a native arrow tip poison in hunting) and they are given by intravenous injection. They have a low volume of distribution and do not cross the blood–brain barrier or placenta; they are eliminated in urine and/or bile, largely as the unmetabolized compound but there is limited metabolism (up to about 30%). The terminal half-lives are short. Atracurium undergoes non-enzymatic spontaneous degradation, which is an advantage in patients with hepatic or renal impairment.

There is a rapid onset of action as the motor-end plate equilibrates readily with the high plasma concentrations following the intravenous dose. With the exception of atracurium the duration of action (from about 15 min for vecuronium up to 30 min for tubocurarine) is limited by redistribution of the drug into the body tissues which lowers the plasma concentration (see Chapter 2) and therefore the concentration at the motor-end plate.

Unwanted effects

- The blockade of ganglionic N_1 receptors (tubocurarine) and cardiac muscarinic receptors (pancuronium) indicating limited selectivity.
- Tubocurarine and atracurium can cause the release of histamine from mast cells, which can result in flushing, bronchospasm and a rash.
- Vecuronium appears to have the fewest unwanted effects, and does not produce these problems.

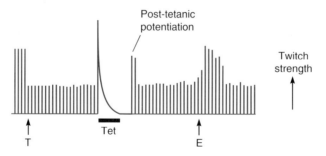

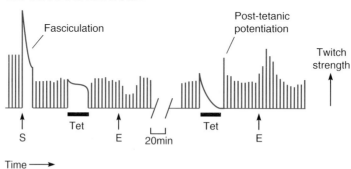

Figure 28.1 The effects of tetanic stimulation and an AChE inhibitor during a partial neuromuscular blockade. T, Start of tubocurarine infusion to maintain a consistent partial block; S, start of suxamethonium infusion to maintain a consistent partial block; Tet, period of tetanic stimulation; E, bolus administration of edrophonium (an AChE inhibitor).

DEPOLARIZING BLOCKERS

Example: succinylcholine (suxamethonium).

Mechanism of action and effects

Suxamethonium binds to the N_2 receptors and acts as an agonist to cause both depolarization of the end-plate and muscle contractions.

Suxamethonium

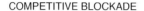

$$CH_3-N^{(+)}-CH_2CH_2O.CCH_2-CH_2C.OCH_2CH_2-N^{(+)}-CH_3$$

Acetylcholine

$$CH_3-N^{(+)}-CH_2CH_2O.CCH_3$$

Suxamethonium is not hydrolysed by AChE and causes prolonged depolarization of the motor-end plate. Prolonged occupancy of N_2 receptors leads to a conformational change which allows the Na^+ channel to close despite the continued presence of an agonist. Thus, the muscle repolarizes and can respond to direct electrical stimulation but can no longer be stimulated via the neuronal release of ACh. Indeed enhanced amounts of ACh, due to the use of an AChE inhibitor, would add to the depolarizing blockade not reverse it. Suxamethonium is described as producing a "dual block" because after about 20 min of blockade the nature of the effect resembles that of a non-depolarizing antagonist, that is tetanic stimulation no longer produces a sustained contraction and is accompanied by post-tetanic potentiation, and in addition the blockade may be partially reversed by an AChE inhibitor (Fig. 28.1).

Pharmacokinetics

Suxamethonium contains two quaternary amino groups and because of its very high polarity it is given intravenously. It has a low volume of distribution and does not cross the blood–brain barrier or placenta. It is rapidly hydrolysed by plasma pseudocholinesterase and this results in a very short duration of action (about 5 min); therefore an infusion is necessary to give a prolonged effect. A very prolonged paralysis occurs in those rare patients (about 1 in 3000) who have a genetically determined deficiency in plasma pseudocholinesterase. In these patients, the action of suxamethonium is terminated after some 2–3 h by renal excretion.

Unwanted effects

- There is an initial depolarization of the motor-end plates prior to blockade; this results in muscle fasciculations and postoperative muscle pain.
- Prolonged apnoea occurs when low circulating levels of pseudocholinesterase arise from either a genetic deficiency or a decreased synthesis of the enzyme due to severe liver disease.
- The use of suxamethonium during anaesthesia has been linked with the development of rare but potentially fatal malignant hyperthermia.
- Other effects include some stimulation of ACh receptors at ganglia (N_1) and muscarinic sites (such as salivation); these are mostly observed with high doses.
- Profound bradycardia or cardiac arrest with repeated doses especially in the presence of hyperkalaemia.

The Treatment of Myasthenia Gravis

Myasthenia gravis is an autoimmune disease in which there is an antibody to the acetylcholine nicotinic N_2 receptor system which impairs the responsiveness of the neuromuscular junction. In effect there is a reduced number of functional N_2 receptors on the motor-end plate. Therefore, in order to depolarize enough receptors to reach the firing potential, it is necessary to have a higher percentage receptor occupancy compared with normal. Thus, myasthenic patients experience muscle weakness. Even in a healthy neuromuscular junction, the availability of receptors declines rapidly after initiation of a series of nerve impulses. In the myasthenic patient, the smaller receptor pool leads to a rapid progressive reduction in receptor availability with repeated release of ACh so that increasing numbers of muscle fibres fail to fire. This produces the characteristic muscle fatiguability. Patients with myasthenia gravis show altered sensitivity to muscle relaxant drugs: they are more sensitive to competitive non-depolarizing receptor antagonists but are resistant to depolarizing blockers (Chapter 28).

ACETYLCHOLINE ESTERASE (AChE) INHIBITORS

Examples: neostigmine, pyridostigmine, edrophonium; physostigmine.

Mechanism of action and effects

AChE inhibitors block the breakdown of released ACh (Chapter 4); they are non-selective and produce beneficial effects at N_2 receptors (Chapter 27) while unwanted effects arise from the actions of ACh at N_1 and muscarinic sites.

Pharmacokinetics and clinical uses

Neostigmine and pyridostigmine are quaternary amines and are slowly and incompletely absorbed from the gut so that oral doses are about 10 times greater than parenteral doses; they have short half-lives and are eliminated by a combination of metabolism and renal excretion. Both are used to treat myasthenia gravis and neostigmine is also used to reverse the effect of competitive neuromuscular blockers (Chapter 28).

Edrophonium is given as an intravenous bolus dose to test therapeutic response in myasthenia gravis (see below); it has a very short duration of action (2–5 min) largely due to tissue redistribution of the bolus dose.

Physostigmine is a tertiary amine isolated from the Calabar-bean which is readily absorbed from the gut. It is sufficiently lipid soluble to cross the blood–brain barrier and has a short half-life due to its rapid metabolism. It is therefore reserved for topical use in the eye (Chapter 53).

Organophosphate compounds could *theoretically* be used to enhance the actions of ACh at N_2 receptors because they inactivate AChE; however they have a "hit-and-run" effect and therefore they would not allow reversibility or the fine control of symptoms.

Unwanted effects

- These arise from the non-specific inhibition of AChE and the actions of ACh on the autonomic nervous system (particularly neostigmine) and include effects on the gastrointestinal tract (diarrhoea), heart (bradycardia), eye (miosis) and airways (bronchoconstriction) (see Chapter 4). The peripheral parasympathetic effects can be blocked by administration of atropine or propantheline.

- The more lipid soluble drug physostigmine, produces CNS effects including convulsions if given systemically.

- Excessive dosage will lead to a depolarizing neuromuscular blockade by ACh, and weakness (see below).

THE TREATMENT OF MYASTHENIA GRAVIS

Myasthenia gravis can be treated with an AChE inhibitor (Chapter 4), which reduces the normal rapid breakdown of ACh and thereby enhances the activity of any ACh released by normal nerve stimulation. Pyridostigmine is usually given since its action is more consistent and constant than neostigmine and the dosing frequency less. An antimuscarinic agent may be necessary to block the effects of ACh on the parasympathetic nervous system, especially if large doses of AChE inhibitor are given.

Excessive dosage of an AChE inhibitor can lead to prolonged stimulation of the N_2 receptors by ACh resulting in a depolarizing blockade of the neuromuscular junction similar to that produced by suxamethonium (Chapter 28). Therefore, muscle weakness in myasthenia gravis can be the result of either inadequate or excessive dosage of AChE inhibitor. The clinical problem of deciding whether to increase or lower the dose is overcome by observing the response (i.e. an improvement or deterioration) following a small dose of a very short-acting AChE inhibitor such as edrophonium.

Patients who do not respond adequately to an AChE inhibitor are usually treated by immunosuppression with prednisolone (Chapter 47) alone or with azathioprine (Chapter 42). Some patients with myasthenia have a tumour of the thymus gland (thymoma); removal of this can produce lasting remission in younger patients. Plasma exchange to remove circulating anti-ACh receptor antibodies can be used to gain a short-term response.

30

Joint Disorders and the Inflammatory Process

PROSTAGLANDINS, LEUKOTRIENES AND INFLAMMATION

Tissue inflammation is produced by the interaction of many inflammatory mediators. However, most anti-inflammatory drugs interfere principally with the generation of one class of mediator, the prostaglandins (PGs). Prostaglandins are members of a family of related polyunsaturated fatty acids (known as "eicosanoids" because they contain 20 carbon atoms) which also includes thromboxanes and leukotrienes. All are formed from essential fatty acid precursors. Arachidonic acid, the major precursor, is formed in the liver from dietary constituents containing linoleic acid such as vegetable oils, for example sunflower oil. A related series of eicosanoids is formed from eicosapentaenoic acid which can be obtained from oily fish; the platelet thromboxane in this series is less pro-aggregatory than that produced from linoleic acid (Chapter 10).

Prostaglandins are synthesized by oxygenation and ring closure of arachidonic acid, controlled by a rate-limiting enzyme, cyclooxygenase, which is associated with the cell membrane. The products are unstable intermediates known as cyclic endoperoxides. Specific enzymes, which differ from cell to cell, convert these intermediates to "classical" prostaglandins, prostacyclin (PGI_2) or thromboxane A_2 (Fig. 30.1). The products of the cyclooxygenase pathway therefore differ among various tissues, reflecting the diverse nature of their actions. PGE_2 is the principal inflammatory prostaglandin, which produces vasodilation, increased vascular permeability and sensitizes pain fibre nerve endings to the stimulant action of bradykinin. A comparison of the major actions of prostaglandins is shown in Table 30.1.

The second route for arachidonic acid metabolism is via the lipoxygenase pathway to produce leukotrienes (Fig. 30.1). These are also involved in the inflammatory process by enhancing vascular permeability (LTB_4 and LTC_4) and through chemotaxis of neutrophil leucocytes (particularly LTB_4).

(a)

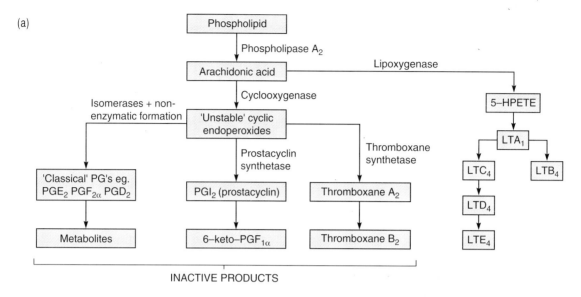

Key:

PG: Prostaglandin
LT : Leukotriene
The subscript numeral denotes the number of unsaturated carbon bonds
The subscript α or β denotes the orientation of the –OH group at C9

(b)

'Core' structure of a typical prostaglandin

Figure 30.1 (a) Biosynthetic pathways for prostaglandins and leukotrienes. (b) 'Core' structure of a typical prostaglandin. Each carbon atom is identified by a number.

Table 30.1 Actions of major prostaglandins and leukotrienes

Tissue	Effect	Eicosanoid
Platelets	↑ aggregation ↓ aggregation	TXA_2 PGI_2
Vascular smooth muscle	Vasodilation Vasoconstriction	PGI_2, PGE_2, PGD_2 TXA_2, LTC_4
Other smooth muscle	Bronchodilation Bronchoconstriction GI tract (contraction/relaxation depends on muscle orientation) Uterine contraction	PGE_2 PGD_2, $PGF_{2\alpha}$, TXA_2, LTC_4, LTD_4, LTE_4 $PGF_{2\alpha}$, PGE_2, PGI_2 PGE_2, $PGF_{2\alpha}$
Vascular endothelium	Increased permeability	LTC_4, LTB_4
Neutrophils	Chemotaxis	LTB_4
Gastrointestinal mucosa	Reduced acid secretion Increased mucus secretion	PGE_2, PGI_2 PGE_2
Nervous system	Inhibition of noradrenaline release Endogenous pyrogen in hypothalamus Sedation, sleep	PGD_2, PGE_2, PGI_2 PGE_2 PGD_2
Endocrine/metabolic	Secretion of ACTH, GH, prolactin, gonadotrophins Inhibition of lipolysis	PGE_2 PGE_2
Kidney	Increased renal blood flow Antagonism of ADH Renin release	PGE_2, PGI_2 PGE_2 PGI_2, PGE_2, PGD_2

Key:
PG: Prostaglandin
LT: Leukotriene
TX: Thromboxane

31

Non-steroidal Anti-inflammatory Drugs (NSAIDs)

CLASSIFICATION OF NSAIDs

Most NSAIDs have common structural origins. A simplified "family tree" is shown in Fig. 31.1. They differ in the extent of cyclooxygenase inhibition *in vitro* which is one determinant of their efficacy, and in elimination half-life which determines the duration of action (Table 31.1).

Examples: aspirin, ibuprofen, indomethacin, naproxen, piroxicam.

Mechanism of action and effects

All NSAIDs share the ability to inhibit the enzyme cyclooxygenase and reduce the formation of prostaglandins. Although they may have actions on other chemical mediators of inflammation, such as reducing superoxide production and inhibition of leucocyte migration, they do not inhibit the lipoxygenase pathway, and leukotriene production is unimpaired. The effect on prostaglandin synthesis is not selective for inflamed tissues, and widespread inhibition of cyclooxygenase is responsible for several of the unwanted effects of this group of drugs. With most of the drugs, enzyme inhibition is reversible; aspirin, however, produces irreversible acetylation of cyclooxygenase.

Inhibition of prostaglandin synthesis produces several potentially therapeutic effects:

- Analgesia is largely a peripheral action at the site of pain, and is most effective when the

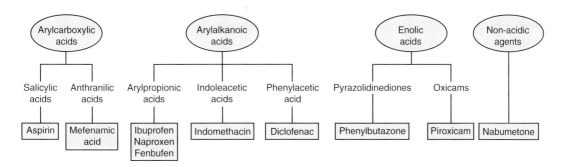

Figure 31.1 Classification of non-steroidal anti-inflammatory drugs with selected drug examples.

Table 31.1 Comparisons among some non-steroidal anti-inflammatory drugs

	Anti-inflammatory activity	Half-life
Aspirin	Moderate	Short/intermediate
Propionic acid derivatives		
Ibuprofen	Weak	Short
Naproxen	Moderate	Intermediate
Fenamates		
Mefenamic acid	Moderate	Short
Acetic acids		
Diclofenac	Strong	Short
Indomethacin	Strong	Short
Enolic acids		
Phenylbutazone	Strong	Long
Oxicams		
Piroxicam	Moderate	Long
Others		
Nabumetone	Moderate	Intermediate/long

pain has an inflammatory origin. A small component of the analgesic action is due to a central effect by reduction of prostaglandin production in the CNS; this is the main site of action of paracetamol (see below).

- An anti-inflammatory effect which is related to reduced peripheral prostaglandin synthesis; paracetamol has no anti-inflammatory action.
- An antipyretic effect which is a consequence of central prostaglandin inhibition. Circulating pyrogens enhance prostaglandin production in the hypothalamus which depresses the response of temperature-sensitive neurones. NSAIDs do not affect normal body temperature.
- Impaired platelet aggregation due to reduced thromboxane synthesis. This action can be used to prevent vascular occlusion (Chapter 10).

There are additional minor actions which can have useful therapeutic consequences:

- Closure of a patent ductus arteriosus in the neonate. Patency may be inappropriately maintained by prostaglandin production.
- Inhibition of uterine contraction. Stimulation of the uterus by prostaglandins can produce the painful symptoms of primary dysmenorrhoea.

Pharmacokinetics

Most NSAIDs are weak acids which undergo some gastric absorption by pH partitioning (Chapter 2). This explains the relatively high concentration in gastric mucosal cells. However, most absorption occurs from the larger surface area of the small bowel. Enteric-coated formulations can be used to reduce release of drug in the stomach and limit exposure of the gastric mucosa. Absorption is usually fairly rapid from conventional formulations, but the compounds differ widely in their elimination half-lives (Table 31.1). Short-acting drugs require frequent dosing for continuous effect, but the dose interval can be extended by using modified-release formulations to prolong absorption time.

Alternative routes of administration are intramuscular for rapid onset of analgesia or rectally to achieve a prolonged action. The transcutaneous route has recently been used to provide high local drug concentrations while attempting to minimize systemic actions. However, widespread distribution probably occurs throughout the body once the drug has penetrated the skin.

In plasma, most NSAIDs are extensively bound to albumin where competition with other acidic protein-bound drugs, such as warfarin (Chapter 10), can occur. Many NSAIDs undergo hepatic metabolism to inactive compounds. However, some compounds are given as prodrugs (Chapter 2), for example nabumetone. Prodrugs are absorbed as an inactive molecule and undergo conversion (usually in the liver) to an active metabolite.

Aspirin (acetylsalicylic acid) is also initially converted to an active metabolite, salicylic acid, and finally inactivated by conjugation. The latter process is saturable at higher doses and the metabolism of salicylate then changes from first-order to zero-order elimination kinetics (Chapter 2). This has important implications for aspirin overdose (Chapter 57).

Some NSAIDs, for example piroxicam, undergo enterohepatic cycling which contributes to a long half-life.

Unwanted effects

Most unwanted effects arise from the non-selective inhibition of prostaglandin synthesis throughout the body.

- Gastric irritation is due to inhibition of production of prostaglandin E_2. PGE_2 has several actions which confer cytoprotection in the stomach (Chapter 35). Inhibition within the mucosal cells occurs by direct absorption of the drug from the gastric lumen; there is also systemic delivery of the drug to the gastric mucosa and consequently rectal administration or use of a prodrug will reduce but not eliminate the risk of gastric damage. Superficial gastric erosions or occasionally ulceration can occur. Occult blood loss is increased and the risk of overt bleeding is greater during regular treatment with NSAIDs. Clinical sequelae include heartburn, nausea and epigastric discomfort.

    Treatment of gastric damage involves withdrawal of the NSAID if this is practicable, combined with standard ulcer-healing therapy. If NSAID treatment must be continued then prophylactic treatment with ulcer-healing agents or a cytoprotective agent should be considered (Chapter 35).

- Renal impairment. Prostaglandins are involved in the maintenance of renal blood flow and probably have additional effects on the renal tubule to promote natriuresis. NSAIDs can produce a reversible decline in renal function with a rise in serum creatinine and salt and water retention leading to oedema. The problem is more frequent if renal function is already impaired, as is often the case in the elderly. Salt retention can exacerbate heart failure or further raise blood pressure in the hypertensive patient. The efficacy of treatments for these conditions (e.g. diuretics, ACE inhibitors, β-adrenoceptor antagonists) can be blunted by NSAIDs.

- Hypersensitivity reactions occur occasionally producing asthma, urticaria, angioedema and rhinitis. These are most common with aspirin and may be due to inhibition of prostaglandin E_2 production in the lung, with diversion of arachidonic acid towards leukotriene synthesis. Patients with nasal polyps and known allergic disorders appear to be more susceptible.

Other unwanted effects appear to be relatively specific for individual compounds:

- Aspirin produces tinnitus in toxic doses. Overdose of aspirin can be particularly hazardous (Chapter 57).

- Indomethacin causes CNS unwanted effects such as dizziness and confusion, particularly in the elderly.

- Phenylbutazone can produce bone marrow aplasia. Its use is now restricted to patients with ankylosing spondylitis for which it is particularly effective.

PARACETAMOL

Mechanism of action and effects

Paracetamol is believed to inhibit prostaglandin production, but unlike most NSAIDs it shows tissue specificity for the CNS. Consequently it has antipyretic and analgesic effects but little anti-inflammatory action (Table 31.2).

Pharmacokinetics

Absorption from the gut is almost complete, including drug administered rectally. Elimination occurs by hepatic metabolism (see also Chapter 57) and the half-life is short.

Unwanted effects

- Hepatic damage in overdose (Chapters 56 and 57).

Table 31.2 Differences between peripherally acting analgesic drugs

	Aspirin (moderate doses)	Paracetamol	Indomethacin
Analgesic	++	++	+
Anti-inflammatory	+	−	+++
Antipyretic	+	+	+
Metabolic effects‡	+	−	−
GI bleeding	+	−	+

‡See Chapter 57.

32

"Second-line" or "Disease-modifying" Drugs for Rheumatoid Arthritis

Non-steroidal anti-inflammatory drugs do not alter the long-term progression of joint destruction in rheumatoid arthritis. However, a diverse group of compounds may reduce the rate of progression of joint erosion and destruction leading to improvement both in symptoms and in the clinical and serological markers of rheumatoid arthritis activity. The mechanisms by which they achieve this are poorly understood but long-term depression of the inflammatory response is probably important, although they have little or no direct anti-inflammatory effect. They all have a slow onset of action, with most producing little improvement until about 3 months after starting treatment. It is unclear whether they modify the long-term outcome of the disease.

GOLD

Examples: sodium aurothiomalate, auranofin.

Mechanism of action

The precise mechanism by which gold acts is unknown, and it has been suggested that the oral and parenteral forms could act differently. A popular concept is that gold is taken up by mononuclear cells and inhibits their phagocytic function. This will reduce the release of inflammatory mediators and inhibit cell proliferation. Other factors involved in inflammation may also be modified, such as complement and the production of free radicals.

Oral gold (auranofin) has a rather slower onset of action than intramuscular gold, and is less efficacious but much better tolerated.

Pharmacokinetics

Gold binds readily to albumin and accumulates in many tissues such as the liver, kidney, bone marrow, lymph nodes and spleen. Accumulation also occurs in the synovium of inflamed joints. The parenteral form is given by deep intramuscular injection (sodium aurothiomalate). An initial test dose is given to screen for acute toxicity (see below) followed by injections at weekly intervals to gradually achieve a therapeutic concentration in the tissues. Subsequently a smaller dose is used to maintain remission. Elimination is largely by the kidney, and to a lesser extent by biliary excretion. Gold has a half-life of several weeks, probably largely due to its extensive tissue binding.

Oral gold (auranofin) is taken daily.

Unwanted effects

These can be serious and all but the most minor effects should lead to immediate cessation of treatment.

- Oral ulceration.
- Proteinuria due to membranous glomerulonephritis. Proteinuria can develop after several weeks of treatment sometimes progressing to nephrotic syndrome. Recovery may take up to 2 years following drug withdrawal.
- Blood disorders, especially thrombocytopenia but also agranulocytosis and aplastic anaemia.
- Skin rashes.
- Diarrhoea is common with oral gold.

Prevention and management of unwanted effects

Urine should be checked for protein and a blood count obtained before each injection of gold, and regularly during oral therapy. Major complications may require chelation of gold with dimercaprol or penicillamine (Chapter 57) to increase its elimination. Corticosteroids can be helpful for blood dyscrasias. Gold should not be used if there is a history of renal or hepatic disease, blood dyscrasias or severe skin rashes. If stomatitis, a pruritic rash, leucopaenia, thrombocytopenia or significant proteinuria (>1 g/24 h) develop, gold should be stopped.

PENICILLAMINE

Mechanism of action

Modulation of the immune system is believed to underlie the action of penicillamine. The precise details are uncertain but may include reduced production of immunoglobulins, formation of mixed disulphide bonds with macromolecules, reduction in the number of activated lymphocytes, and stabilization of lysosomal membranes in inflammatory cells. It has not, however, been shown to slow the progression of joint erosions.

Penicillamine can chelate many metals. This is probably of little relevance to its use in arthritis, but has given the drug a role in the management of poisonings (Chapter 57) and in Wilson's disease, a genetically determined illness which is associated with copper overload.

Pharmacokinetics

Pencillamine is well absorbed from the gut, although oral iron supplements substantially reduce this. The half-life is very long (about 1 week) due to tight binding of drug to plasma protein and tissues. Penicillamine is partially metabolized but also excreted unchanged in the urine. Doses should be increased gradually to reduce the incidence of unwanted effects.

Unwanted effects

These are not infrequent and lead about 30% of patients to stop treatment. Many unwanted effects resemble those of gold.

- Nausea, vomiting, abdominal discomfort and rashes (often with fever), especially early in treatment.
- Loss of taste is common but may resolve despite continued treatment.
- Oral ulceration.
- Proteinuria which is due to immune complex glomerulonephritis and is dose-related. Nephrotic syndrome can occur.
- Blood disorders, especially thrombocytopenia but also neutropenia or rarely aplastic anaemia.

Regular monitoring of urine protein and blood counts should be carried out during treatment.

ANTIMALARIALS

Examples: chloroquine, hydroxychloroquine.

These drugs (Chapter 54) are believed to reduce lymphocyte transformation and chemotaxis, stabilize lysosomal membranes in phagocytic cells and trap free radicals that cause tissue damage. Their major toxic effect is on the retina. However, at the low doses that are now recommended they are relatively safe. Annual specialist monitoring of the eyes is still recommended by some rheumatologists.

SULPHASALAZINE

Sulphasalazine (Chapter 36) has a poorly understood action. It is hydrolysed in the colon to 5-aminosalicylic acid (which is believed to contribute little to the antirheumatic action) and to sulphapyridine. The latter moiety probably acts by reducing absorption of antigens from the colon.

High doses are required, which often produce gastrointestinal upset. This can be minimized by increasing the dose slowly and using an enteric-coated formulation. Other problems include oligospermia (therefore avoid in males who have not completed their family) and blood dyscrasias.

IMMUNOMODULATING DRUGS

Several **drugs** with **immuno**modulating actions have been shown to be effective in rheumatoid arthritis. These include:

- Antimetabolites: methotrexate, azathioprine (Chapter 55).
- Alkylating agents: cyclophosphamide, chlorambucil (Chapter 55).
- Cyclosporin A (Chapter 42).
- Immunostimulants: gamma interferon (Chapter 42).

The success of both immunosuppressant and immunostimulant drugs in rheumatoid arthritis is a paradox which is unexplained. Inhibition of the production of immunologically active cells such as lymphocytes may be important for the clinical effectiveness of immunosuppressants.

MANAGEMENT OF ARTHRITIS

OSTEOARTHRITIS

Osteoarthritis is the clinical manifestation of joint degeneration which results from loss of articular cartilage. Most osteoarthritis is primary or idiopathic but a small proportion is secondary to other conditions such as joint injury or chondrocalcinosis. The integrity of cartilage depends on the balance of production and resorption of the cartilage matrix by embedded chondrocytes. Osteoarthritis may result from reduced secretion by chondrocytes of the proteoglycan which forms the majority of the matrix. Loss of matrix leads to disruption of the cartilage with swelling and fissuring of the surface. Subchondral bone becomes increas-

ingly vascular and new bone is laid down in response to the changes in the cartilage.

The cardinal symptom of osteoarthritis is pain during physical activity which is most pronounced later in the day. Pain also occurs at rest with advanced disease. Stiffness may be troublesome for short periods after rest. Various joints can be involved, particularly the distal interphalangeal joints of the fingers and the carpometacarpal joint of the thumb. Large joints such as the knee, hip, elbow and shoulder are often asymmetrically affected.

Simple analgesics should usually be considered as first-line treatment. Non-steroidal anti-inflammatory drugs (NSAIDs) may be helpful for inflammatory episodes that accompany advanced osteoarthritis. Concern has recently been expressed that some NSAIDs may accelerate the loss of articular cartilage in osteoarthritis. Clinical studies are inconclusive, but provide some support for the avoidance of strong NSAIDs when possible. Much of the long-term management of osteoarthritis is non-pharmacological and includes weight loss, physiotherapy and ultimately surgical joint replacement. Compounds under development may in future offer the possibility of prevention of cartilage degeneration or even promote regeneration.

RHEUMATOID ARTHRITIS AND OTHER INFLAMMATORY ARTHRITIDES

Rheumatoid arthritis is an inflammatory condition of unknown cause. Autoimmune processes contribute to the maintenance of the condition, but it is uncertain whether autoimmunity plays a part in the initiation. The primary process is a proliferative inflammation of the synovial membrane around the joint. The synovium subsequently invades and destroys cartilage. This process appears to result in the formation of antibodies to the collagen exposed in the damaged cartilage. Complexes of collagen antibody along with other immune complexes such as rheumatoid factor-IgG in the cartilage probably act as chemoattractants to the inflammatory cells in invasive synovial tissue.

Rheumatoid factor is present in the majority of cases of rheumatoid arthritis and appears to amplify the inflammation of rheumatoid disease. The inflammatory reaction is further enhanced by lymphocytic infiltration and the release of cytokines by activated T-lymphocytes and macrophages (Chapter 40). New vessel formation occurs in the synovium with local proliferation of B-lymphocytes and the production of antibodies. Neutrophils are attracted to the joint cavity. The end result is irreversible destruction of cartilage and erosion of peri-articular bone. The symptoms of rheumatoid arthritis appear gradually in most patients and usually involve the proximal interphalangeal joints of the fingers, metacarpophalangeal joints and wrists. Other joints such as the ankles and hips may be involved later. The affected joints are warm, swollen and painful. Stiffness is troublesome, particularly in the morning, due to an increase in extracellular fluid in and around the joint. Systemic disturbance is common, including general fatigue and malaise, while extra-articular manifestations such as vasculitis and neuropathy can occur.

Non-steroidal anti-inflammatory drugs are the mainstay of drug treatment which is given in conjunction with physical aids such as splinting and bed rest for acute episodes. The choice of NSAID is arbitrary with considerable variation in individual responses to different drugs. Propionic acid derivatives are often used first; they are somewhat weaker than other classes but generally have fewer unwanted effects. More powerful drugs such as indomethacin are used when others fail to control symptoms. About 60% of patients can be expected to respond to the first-choice agent and most can be controlled by one of the NSAIDs. Morning stiffness is often disabling in inflammatory arthritis: this is helped by late evening dosing with a long half-life NSAID, a modified-release formulation of a short half-life compound or an NSAID suppository. The value of topical NSAIDs applied over the affected joint(s) is controversial but some patients find them helpful for acutely inflamed joints.

Many inflammatory arthritides (the sero-negative spondylarthritides) do not usually progress to extensive erosive arthritis with joint destruction. By contrast, progressive joint damage is common in rheumatoid arthritis. "Second-line" drugs are often used early in rheumatoid arthritis. Indications for these agents include the prevention of erosive damage, the suppression of persistent inflammation that fails to respond to 6 months' treatment with NSAIDs and patient intolerance to NSAIDs. A high titre of rheumatoid factor or extra-articular manifestations of rheumatoid disease should also encourage their early use. Second-line drugs are almost always used with NSAIDs, particularly in the first few weeks of treatment since they do not have significant anti-inflammatory action. There is no consensus for choice among second-line drugs. Sulphasalazine is often chosen for its low toxicity but methotrexate is probably the most effective single agent. Gold (despite being associated with increased mortality) and penicillamine are also widely accepted as second-line drugs while immunomodulators other than methotrexate are generally reserved as third-line agents. Cytotoxic drugs, especially cyclophosphamide, appear to be particularly useful for the management of extra-articular manifestations of rheumatoid disease, such as vasculitis, pericarditis or pleurisy.

The role of corticosteroids in rheumatoid arthritis is controversial. Intra-articular injections are used for individual inflamed joints (especially knee and shoulder). Due to their unwanted effects, oral corticosteroids should be avoided unless all other options are unsuccessful; an exception to this general rule is the treatment of extra-articular disease.

33

Drugs Specifically Used for Gout

Uric acid is a relatively insoluble derivative of the nucleic acid purine bases, guanine and adenine (Fig. 33.1). If the plasma concentration is high it can crystallize as monosodium urate in tissues, which initiates an inflammatory response. Phagocytic cells internalize the crystals and subsequent enzyme release enhances tissue inflammation. Deposition of uric acid crystals in joints produces an extremely painful acute arthritis. In some patients, chronic urate deposits (tophi) are found in tendon sheaths and soft tissues.

Uric acid is normally eliminated by the kidney. Its renal handling is complex but involves glomerular filtration with initial proximal tubular reabsorption. Subsequently, there is considerable distal tubular secretion with a small amount of reabsorption at the same site. Excess uric acid can be deposited in the interstitium of the kidney or filtered uric acid can form stones in the calyces. Both will produce progressive renal damage.

Hyperuricaemia results from either:

- Over-production of uric acid: excessive cell destruction (e.g. lymphoproliferative or myeloproliferative disorders, especially during treatment; Chapter 55), inherited defects increasing purine synthesis and alcohol.
- Reduced renal excretion: renal failure and drugs that reduce tubular secretion of uric acid (e.g. most diuretics, low dose aspirin and lactate formed from alcohol).

There are two approaches to drug treatment:

- Treatment of an acute attack.
- Reduction of plasma uric acid concentration for prophylaxis against recurrent attacks. This is achieved either by inhibition of uric acid production or by increasing its urinary excretion.

SPECIFIC TREATMENT FOR ACUTE GOUT

COLCHICINE

Mechanism of action

Colchicine was originally used as an antimitotic agent. It is believed to act in gout by inhibiting

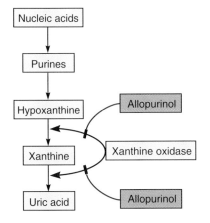

Figure 33.1 The pathway of uric acid production.

leucocyte migration into inflamed tissue. Colchicine depolymerizes proteins of the neutrophil microtubules which are involved in cell movement. It produces a specific response in the gouty joint, not seen in other forms of inflammatory arthritis, with symptom relief beginning after about 2 h.

Pharmacokinetics

Colchicine is poorly absorbed from the gut and partially excreted unchanged in the urine and bile. Some hepatic metabolism also occurs. The initial half-life of colchicine is very short but enterohepatic circulation prolongs its action. It is usually given every 2 h until symptomatic relief or the onset of unwanted effects. Intravenous colchicine can be used if there is intolerance to oral administration.

Unwanted effects

- Gut toxicity, due to inhibition of mucosal cell division, is common producing abdominal pain, vomiting and diarrhoea. These effects often limit dosing.

DRUGS FOR REDUCING PLASMA URIC ACID CONCENTRATION

ALLOPURINOL

Mechanism of action

Allopurinol inhibits the enzyme xanthine oxidase, thereby reducing uric acid formation (Fig. 33.1). The increases in xanthine and hypoxanthine concentrations in blood do not lead to crystallization due to their greater water solubility. These compounds are also available for reincorporation into the purine metabolic cycle which by a feedback mechanism decreases *de novo* purine formation.

Pharmacokinetics

Allopurinol is well absorbed from the gut and converted in the liver to an active metabolite, oxypurinol. Both compounds are excreted by the kidney. The half-life of oxypurinol is long.

Unwanted effects

- An increased risk of acute gout during the first few weeks of treatment. This may be due to fluctuations in plasma uric acid perhaps due to reabsorption from tissue deposits.
- Allergic reactions, especially rashes.

URICOSURICS

Examples: probenecid, sulphinpyrazone.

Mechanism of action

These drugs compete with uric acid for reabsorption from the distal renal tubule. Low doses inhibit tubular secretion of uric acid which can raise plasma levels. There is a risk of precipitation of uric acid crystals in the kidney, particularly during the early stages of treatment, which can be prevented by maintaining a high fluid intake and an alkaline urine (using potassium citrate or sodium bicarbonate). Aspirin and other salicylates should not be given with uricosurics since small doses inhibit tubular uric acid secretion.

Pharmacokinetics

Both probenecid and sulphinpyrazone are well absorbed from the gut and eliminated partly by metabolism and partly by renal excretion. The half-lives are intermediate.

Unwanted effects

- Renal uric acid deposition. Deterioration of renal function can occur if there is pre-existing impairment.
- Gastrointestinal upset.
- Probenecid reduces urinary elimination of several drugs, for example penicillins, cephalosporins, NSAIDs, sulphonylureas.

TREATMENT OF GOUT

For acute attacks, NSAIDs (Chapter 31) are the treatment of choice, especially indomethacin. Colchicine is usually reserved for patients intolerant of NSAIDs. Corticosteroids, for example prednisolone (Chapter 47), can be used for resistant episodes.

Allopurinol is given for recurrent attacks or chronic deposition of urate in the tissues (tophi) or for uric acid-induced renal damage. It should not be used during an acute attack and cover with an NSAID should be provided during the first 2 months. Uricosuric drugs are reserved for patients who do not tolerate allopurinol, but should be avoided if there is renal damage.

The Gastrointestinal System

Nausea and Vomiting

NAUSEA AND VOMITING

Vomiting is initiated by the vomiting centre in the brain stem. Efferent connections activate the vasomotor, respiratory and salivary centres in the brain stem and inhibit gastric motility, which provokes vomiting. The afferent trigger to the vomiting centre comes from several sources (Fig. 34.1). An important input is from the chemoreceptor trigger zone (CTZ) in the 4th ventricle which lies outside the blood–brain barrier. Many drugs produce

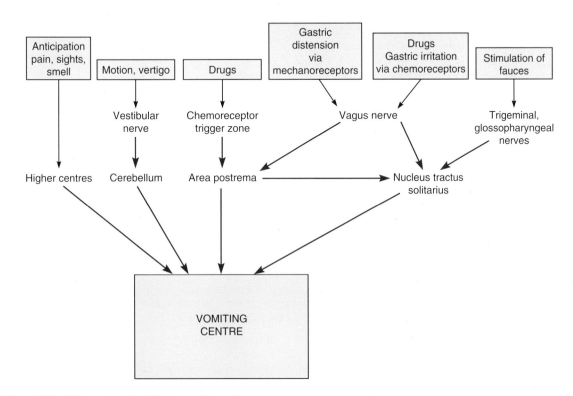

Figure 34.1 Pathways involved in the vomiting reflex.

Table 34.1 Drugs which produce a high incidence of nausea and vomiting

Allopurinol
Antibiotics (oral use)
Bromocriptine
Cytotoxic agents (especially cisplatin, cyclophosphamide, doxorubicin, nitrosoureas)
Digoxin
Gold
Iron (oral use)
Levodopa
Non-steroidal anti-inflammatory drugs
Oestrogens (oral use)
Opiate analgesics
Penicillamine
Sulphasalazine
Theophylline

vomiting by an action on the CTZ (Table 34.1) although stimulation of chemoreceptors in the gut may also be important. In many situations, vomiting can involve several inputs. For example, postoperative nausea and vomiting frequently occurs in the first 24 h after anaesthesia and surgery. It is provoked by inhalational rather than intravenous anaesthesia, more often by abdominal, ophthalmic or ear, nose and throat procedures, by opiate analgesics and by postoperative pain, hypotension and gastric stasis. In this situation several sub-emetic stimuli may summate to trigger vomiting.

Several receptors are involved in activation of the vomiting centre including those for dopamine (D_2), 5HT ($5HT_3$), acetylcholine muscarinic (M_1 and M_2) and histamine (H_1). Clinical applications of the various drugs are summarized in Table 34.2.

ANTIEMETIC AGENTS

ANTIMUSCARINIC AGENTS

Examples: hyoscine, promethazine, cyclizine.

Mechanism of action and clinical use

Hyoscine has antimuscarinic activity (Chapter 4) and some antiemetic drugs classed as antihistamines such as promethazine and cyclizine (Chapter 41) or phenothiazines, for example prochlorperazine (Chapter 22) also have antimuscarinic activity. Promethazine and cyclizine are most useful for motion sickness or vomiting due to vestibular disease. Promethazine is also used for vomiting in pregnancy, since it appears to be free from teratogenic effects. Hyoscine, which is used for the treatment of motion sickness and postoperative vomiting, acts on visceral afferents in the gut and the vestibular nuclei.

Pharmacokinetics

Hyoscine is available for parenteral or transdermal use. Oral absorption is poor. It is partially metabolized in the liver and has an intermediate half-life.

Unwanted effects

- Typical antimuscarinic actions (Chapter 4).
- Sedation.

ANTIDOPAMINERGIC AGENTS

Examples: metoclopramide, domperidone, prochlorperazine.

Table 34.2 Common indications for various antiemetic agents

Motion sickness	Hyoscine, cyclizine, promethazine
Postoperative vomiting	Hyoscine, metoclopramide, domperidone, prochlorperazine, ondansetron (reserved for resistant vomiting)
Drug-induced vomiting	Prochlorperazine, metoclopramide, cyclizine (particularly for opiate-induced vomiting)
Cytotoxic drug-induced vomiting	Prochlorperazine, metoclopramide (especially high doses), nabilone, ondansetron Adjunctive treatments, e.g. corticosteroids, benzodiazepines
Pregnancy-induced vomiting	Promethazine, metoclopramide, pyridoxine

Mechanism of action and clinical use

Several agents including the phenothiazines and metoclopramide block central dopamine D_2 receptors and inhibit dopaminergic stimulation of the chemoreceptor trigger zone (CTZ). They are used to reduce vomiting induced by drugs (e.g. cytotoxics, opiate analgesics) and post-operatively. Metoclopramide is sometimes used for severe vomiting in pregnancy (hyperemesis gravidarum), but promethazine (see above) is the drug of first choice in this situation. Phenothiazines, for example prochlorperazine (Chapter 22) are useful for labyrinthine disorders. All antidopaminergic agents are ineffective in motion sickness.

The pharmacology of the phenothiazines is discussed in Chapter 22: both dopamine and muscarinic receptor blockade contribute to their effects. Antiemetic doses of phenothiazines are generally less than one-third of those used to treat psychoses. Domperidone acts solely by dopamine receptor blockade. This is also an important mechanism for metoclopramide at usual oral doses. However, metoclopramide is most effective at high doses given intravenously (e.g. for the vomiting induced by the cytotoxic agent cisplatin) when it acts via blockade of $5HT_3$ receptors. It also has antiemetic actions on the gut, increasing the tone of the gastro-oesophageal sphincter and enhancing both gastric emptying and small intestinal motility, actions which may be due to cholinergic stimulation.

Pharmacokinetics

Metoclopramide is well absorbed orally and is also available for parenteral use. It is eliminated mainly by metabolism in the liver and has a short half-life. Domperidone is also well absorbed orally but undergoes extensive first-pass metabolism in the gut wall and liver. A rectal formulation of domperidone is available. Domperidone has an intermediate half-life and penetrates poorly into the brain, which reduces CNS unwanted effects, but it still reaches the CTZ which lies outside the blood–brain barrier.

Unwanted effects

Centrally mediated effects are produced by metoclopramide and to a lesser extent domperidone (as a result of lower CNS penetration):

- Acute or chronic effects of dopamine receptor blockade in the basal ganglia (cf. phenothiazines, Chapter 22). Extrapyramidal responses include acute dystonias (especially in children and young adults), akathisia and a Parkinsonian-like syndrome in the elderly.
- Galactorrhoea due to hyperprolactinaemia from pituitary dopamine receptor blockade.
- Drowsiness, mainly with high doses of metoclopramide.

$5HT_3$-RECEPTOR ANTAGONISTS

Example: ondansetron.

Mechanism of action and clinical use

Ondansetron blocks the $5HT_3$ receptors in the CTZ and in the gut where they stimulate the vagal reflex to the vomiting centre (Fig. 34.1). It is effective in emesis induced by cisplatin and other highly emetogenic chemotherapeutic agents for treating malignancy (Chapter 55), and for postoperative vomiting. It is often used in combination with corticosteroids (see below) for vomiting produced by cancer chemotherapy.

Pharmacokinetics

Oral absorption is rapid and an intravenous formulation is also available. It is extensively metabolized in the liver and has a short-half life.

Unwanted effects

- Headache is common, but there is little sedation, unlike high-dose metoclopramide.
- Constipation, probably due to $5HT_3$ receptor blockade in the gut.

CANNABINOIDS

Example: nabilone.

Mechanism of action and clinical use

Nabilone, a synthetic derivative of tetrahydro-cannabinol (an active substance in marihuana), is effective in combating sickness induced by cytotoxic drugs; but it must be given before chemotherapy is started. The mechanism is uncertain, but may involve inhibition of cortical activity and anxiolysis; cannabinoid receptors are found in several areas of the CNS.

Pharmacokinetics

Nabilone is absorbed from the gut and has an intermediate half-life.

Unwanted effects

- Dysphoric reactions, most disturbing to older patients. This may be reduced by concurrent use of prochlorperazine (see antidopaminergic drugs).
- Sedation, dry mouth and dizziness are common.

CORTICOSTEROIDS

These drugs, for example dexamethasone or methylprednisolone, are weak antiemetics. However, they produce additive results when given with high dose metoclopramide or with ondansetron. High doses of dexamethasone are given intravenously before chemotherapy, with subsequent oral doses to prevent delayed emesis. They are discussed in Chapter 47.

BENZODIAZEPINES

These drugs have no intrinsic antiemetic activity. They are given orally or intravenously to sedate and produce amnesia before cancer chemotherapy. They are especially useful if the patient has previously experienced vomiting with a course of treatment since anticipatory nausea and vomiting are then common with subsequent courses. Benzodiazepines are discussed in Chapter 21.

OTHER ANTIEMETIC AGENTS FOR USE IN PREGNANCY

Vomiting in pregnancy can be troublesome and there is a natural desire to avoid drugs whenever possible. Some clinicians advocate a trial of the vitamin pyridoxine or ground ginger in this situation. Psychotherapeutic counselling or hypnotism may also be considered, since psychological abnormalities are a frequent trigger.

35

Dyspepsia and Peptic Ulcer Disease

Dyspepsia is the term used for a group of symptoms that arise from the upper gastrointestinal tract. They include heartburn, abdominal pain or discomfort, belching and nausea.

GASTRO-OESOPHAGEAL REFLUX

This can produce heartburn, pain or difficulty on swallowing and regurgitation of gastric contents into the mouth. If associated with oesophagitis, there may be additional chest pain, and chronic bleeding can also occur. Reflux is produced by relaxation of the lower oesophageal sphincter in the absence of swallowing which allows gastric acid, pepsin and bile to come into contact with the vulnerable epithelium of the oesophagus. Poor oesophageal peristalsis can reduce clearance of refluxed material.

PEPTIC ULCER DISEASE

Characteristic features include epigastric pain (relieved by antacids or by food), nocturnal pain and vomiting. It is more common in males and in smokers, and there is often a family history of the disorder. Women more commonly have gastric rather than duodenal ulceration. Symptoms are a poor guide to the location of an ulcer, although patients with gastric ulcer may have pain that is made worse by food and they are more likely than those with duodenal ulcer to have weight loss, anorexia and nausea. Ulcers only occur in the presence of both acid and peptic activity (Fig. 35.1). Gastric ulcers are often associated with breakdown of the "protective" functions of gastric mucosa, while duodenal ulceration is usually accompanied by excess acid secretion. Duodenal ulceration is characteristically a relapsing disorder even after successful healing with drugs. Peptic ulceration is more common in patients who use non-steroidal anti-inflammatory drugs (Chapter 31) or who have a heavy alcohol intake. A proportion of patients who present with ulcer symptoms, especially over the age of 45 years will have a gastric cancer. Investigation above this age is important since drug treatment can produce symptomatic improvement in patients with early gastric cancer.

HELICOBACTER PYLORI AND DYSPEPSIA

Helicobacter pylori is a bacterium that is frequently present in the stomach of healthy individuals most of whom do not develop peptic ulceration. However, it is found in most patients with chronic active (Type B) antral gastritis and is an independent risk factor for active peptic ulceration. Its presence is particularly associated with relapse of duodenal ulcer disease. *Helicobacter pylori* is believed to stimulate acid secretion by creating a relatively alkaline environment in the gastric antrum through release of urease. Figure 35.1 illustrates the interaction of the various factors associated with peptic ulceration.

CONTROL OF GASTRIC ACID SECRETION AND MUCOSAL PROTECTION

Acid secretion into the cannaliculi of gastric parietal cells is due to the activity of a membrane-bound proton pump which exchanges potassium and hydrogen ions (H^+/K^+-ATPase). The activity of the pump is controlled by several mediators including histamine, gastrin and acetylcholine. Stimulation of histamine H_2 receptors appears to be important for facilitating the action of gastrin and acetylcholine (Fig. 35.2).

Gastric mucosal cells are protected against acid digestion by several mechanisms. These include:

- Secretion of a barrier of mucus from the cells.
- Secretion of bicarbonate into the mucus layer.
- Intrinsic resistance of the cell membranes to hydrogen ion back-diffusion.

- High mucosal blood flow which removes hydrogen ions from the mucosa.

Many of these protective functions are dependent on the synthesis of prostaglandins (especially PGE_2 and PGI_2; see Chapter 30) by gastric mucosa.

DRUGS FOR TREATING DYSPEPSIA AND PEPTIC ULCER

ANTACIDS

Examples: aluminium hydroxide, magnesium trisilicate.

Mechanism of action

Antacids neutralize gastric acidity. They have a more prolonged effect if taken after food; if used without food the effect lasts no more than an hour due to gastric emptying. Magnesium salts neutralize acid much more rapidly than aluminium salts. Antacids quickly produce symptom relief in ulcer disease, but large doses are required to heal ulcers. Most are relatively poorly absorbed from the gut. Liquids work more rapidly, but tablets are more convenient to use.

Unwanted effects

- Constipation with aluminium salts, diarrhoea with magnesium salts.
- Systemic alkalosis can occur with very large doses.
- Retention of absorbed aluminium in advanced renal failure requiring dialysis may contribute to metabolic bone disease and encephalopathy.
- Drug interactions: aluminium salts can bind other drugs and reduce their absorption, for example non-steroidal anti-inflammatory drugs. This effect is reversed if aluminium and magnesium salts are mixed.

ALGINIC ACID

Alginic acid is an inert substance. It is claimed to form a raft of high pH foam which floats on the gastric contents and it is suggested that

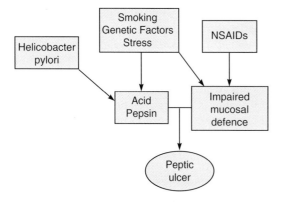

Figure 35.1 Factors predisposing to peptic ulceration.

alginic acid will protect the oesophageal mucosa during reflux but objective evidence for this mechanism is lacking. All proprietary preparations combine alginic acid with an antacid which is probably responsible for much of the clinical effect.

ANTISECRETORY AGENTS

It is only necessary to raise intragastric pH above 3 for a few hours in the day to promote healing of most ulcers. The duration of acid suppression will then determine the rate of healing but not the eventual proportion of healed ulcers. Rapid healing requires acid suppression for a minimum of 18–20 h per day. Several classes of drug have antisecretory actions, including histamine H_2 receptor antagonists, anticholinergic drugs and proton pump inhibitors (Fig. 35.2).

HISTAMINE H_2-RECEPTOR ANTAGONISTS

Examples: cimetidine, ranitidine.

Mechanism of action

These are competitive antagonists of the histamine H_2 receptor on gastric parietal cells. They reduce basal acid secretion and pepsin production and prevent the increase that occurs in response to a number of secretory stimuli, but they do not produce complete suppression of acid secretion.

Pharmacokinetics

Absorption of cimetidine and ranitidine from the gut is almost complete but both undergo first-pass metabolism. Elimination is mainly by renal excretion for cimetidine, and partially by metabolism. The half-lives are short.

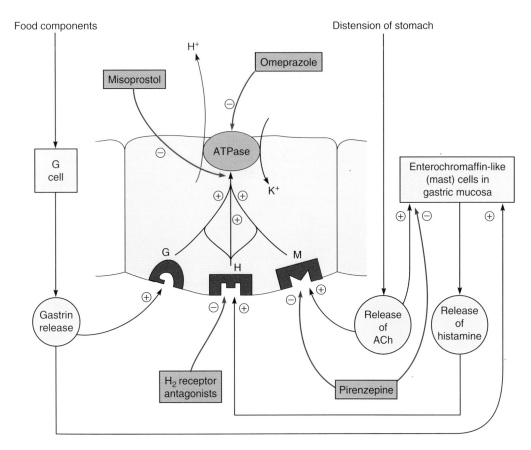

Figure 35.2 Control of gastric acid secretion. G, Gastrin receptor; H, histamine receptor; M, muscarinic acetylcholine receptor. ⊖, Inhibition. ⊕, Augmentation.

Unwanted effects

- Diarrhoea.
- Headache.
- Confusion in the elderly.
- Gynaecomastia with cimetidine.
- Therapeutic doses of cimetidine, but not ranitidine, inhibit the hepatic cytochrome P450 enzyme complex. This creates the potential for important drug interactions with compounds such as warfarin, phenytoin, tolbutamide and theophylline (Chapter 2).

ANTICHOLINERGIC DRUGS

Example: pirenzepine.

Mechanism of action

Pirenzepine is a competitive antagonist at muscarinic M_1 receptors in autonomic ganglia, and to a lesser extent gastric parietal cell muscarinic M_3 receptors (Chapter 4) and reduces the acid and pepsin secretion induced by vagal stimulation. The volume of gastric juice is reduced but not the acid concentration.

Pharmacokinetics

Absorption of pirenzepine from the gut is poor. It does not cross the blood–brain barrier. Pirenzepine has a long half-life and is eliminated unchanged by the kidney.

Unwanted effects

These are less common than with less selective anticholinergic agents such as atropine (Chapter 4).

- Dry mouth.
- Blurred vision.

PROTON PUMP INHIBITORS

Example: omeprazole.

Mechanism of action

Since the proton pump is the final common pathway for acid secretion in gastric parietal cells, inhibition can completely block acid secretion (Fig. 35.2). Omeprazole is an irreversible inhibitor of H^+/K^+-ATPase, and the return of acid secretion is dependent on the synthesis of new enzyme.

Pharmacokinetics

Omeprazole is a prodrug which is unstable in acid. It is therefore given as an enteric-coated formulation. The parent drug is a weak base and is concentrated in the acid environment of the secretory canaliculi of the gastric parietal cell. Activation then occurs by protonation. Absorption is variable and incomplete, improving with repeated dosing. Elimination is by hepatic metabolism, with a short plasma half-life; due to its irreversible mechanism of action the half-life of the drug bears no relationship to the duration of action.

Unwanted effects

- Gastrointestinal upset, for example epigastric discomfort, nausea and vomiting, diarrhoea.
- Headache.
- Skin rashes.
- Inhibition of the cytochrome P450 system in the liver occurs. Important drug interactions are few, but may occur with warfarin or phenytoin (Chapter 2).

Concern that substantial reduction of gastric acid, associated with a rise in gastrin secretion, may predispose to an increased incidence of gastric cancer (cf. the risk in pernicious anaemia) appears to be unfounded. Omeprazole does not completely abolish acid secretion and intragastric pH can still fall below 4 during part of the day.

CYTOPROTECTIVE AGENTS

SUCRALFATE

Mechanism of action

Sucralfate is an aluminium salt of sucrose octasulphate. It dissociates to leave negative ions in an acid environment which bind to the ulcer base and create a protective barrier to pepsin and bile and inhibit the diffusion of gastric acid. Sucralfate also stimulates the gastric secretion of bicarbonate and prostaglandins. It is not absorbed from the gut.

Unwanted effects

- Constipation.

BISMUTH SALTS

Example: tripotassium dicitratobismuthate.

Mechanism of action

Bismuth salts precipitate in the acid environment of the stomach and then bind to glycoprotein on the base of an ulcer. The resulting complex adheres to the ulcer and has similar local effects to sucralfate. An additional action which may make a major contribution to ulcer healing is suppression of *Helicobacter pylori* in most patients, and long-term eradication in 20%.

Unwanted effects

- Blackens stools.
- Absorption of bismuth chelates from the gut is minimal but in severe renal failure, the inability to excrete the small amounts of absorbed bismuth could produce encephalopathy.

Because of the risk of accumulation of bismuth, courses are usually limited to a maximum of 6 weeks.

PROSTAGLANDIN ANALOGUES

Example: misoprostol.

Mechanism of action

Misoprostol is an analogue of prostaglandin E (Chapter 30) and has several potentially useful actions including:

- Increased gastric mucus production.
- Enhanced duodenal bicarbonate secretion.
- Increased mucosal blood flow which aids buffering of hydrogen ions that diffuse back across the mucosa.
- Inhibition of gastric acid secretion. Misoprostol has both a direct effect, and also reduces endogenous histamine release.

The overall effect is to limit the damage caused by agents such as acid and alcohol to superficial mucosal cells.

Pharmacokinetics

Misoprostol is well absorbed from the gut but undergoes extensive first-pass metabolism. The half-life is very short (20 min) and elimination is mainly by hepatic metabolism.

Unwanted effects

- Diarrhoea and abdominal cramps, caused by a local effect on gut motility, are fairly common.
- Uterine contractions, therefore avoid in pregnancy.
- Menorrhagia and postmenopausal bleeding.

CARBENOXOLONE

Mechanism of action

This is a synthetic derivative of a liquorice constituent. It has a steroid structure and enhances the synthesis of gastric mucus perhaps by stimulating prostaglandin secretion. This increases the protective barrier in the stomach against acid and peptic digestion. It is rarely used since the advent of newer ulcer-healing agents.

Pharmacokinetics

Absorption from the gut is almost complete. The major route of elimination is conjugation in the liver and the half-life is long.

Unwanted effects

- Aldosterone-like actions on the kidney produce salt and water retention and hypokalaemia. Hypertension or heart failure can result from the fluid retention.

PROKINETIC DRUGS

Examples: cisapride, metoclopramide.

Mechanism of action

Metoclopramide is fully discussed in Chapter 34. Cisapride stimulates the release of acetylcholine in the myenteric plexus of the oesophagus. This increases the pressure of the lower oesophageal sphincter and reduces oesophageal reflux. It also increases motility throughout the gut. Cisapride has no dopamine receptor blocking activity, unlike metoclopramide, and therefore has no central antiemetic effect. It may, however, have effects on gastrointestinal $5HT_3$ or $5HT_4$ receptors (Chapter 17).

Pharmacokinetics

Oral absorption of cisapride is good but it undergoes extensive first-pass metabolism. It does not cross the blood–brain barrier and is eliminated by hepatic metabolism. The half-life is long.

Unwanted effects

- Abdominal cramps, borborygmi, diarrhoea.

MANAGEMENT OF DYSPEPSIA AND PEPTIC ULCER DISEASE

Most patients with dyspepsia do not have significant underlying disease and investigations should not be necessary. In all cases, efforts should be made to remove causative agents, for example smoking, excess alcohol or non-steroidal anti-inflammatory drugs.

For persistent symptoms, antacids provide symptomatic relief. Many physicians treat younger patients who fail to respond to simple measures, and who do not have associated features such as weight loss or persistent vomiting, without initial investigation. A histamine H_2-receptor antagonist is usually the first choice drug but should not be given for more than about 6 weeks in the absence of a confirmed diagnosis.

Accurate diagnosis requires investigation, usually by gastroduodenoscopy although more specialized tests may be required in some patients.

CONFIRMED PEPTIC ULCERATION

Histamine H_2-receptor antagonists usually give symptomatic relief for both gastric and duodenal ulcers within a week, but healing of the ulcer is much slower (Table 35.1). Other agents such as colloidal bismuth, pirenzepine and sucralfate will heal ulcers in a similar proportion of patients but do not improve symptoms as quickly. Omeprazole produces the fastest rate of healing

Table 35.1 Healing and relapse rates during treatment of peptic ulceration

(a) Duodenal ulcer

Drug	Percentage healed		
	2 weeks	4 weeks	8 weeks
H_2 antagonist	40	80	95
Colloidal bismuth	40	80	95
Proton pump inhibitor	>60	95	95

Healing drug	Maintenance drug	% relapse at 1 year
H_2 antagonist	None	80
H_2 antagonist	H_2 antagonist	20–40
Bismuth salt	None	40–60
"Triple therapy"	None	20

(b) Gastric ulcer

Drug	Percentage healed	
	4 weeks	8 weeks
H_2 antagonist	60	85
Proton pump inhibitor	80	95

but is usually reserved for patients who are resistant to H_2-receptor antagonists.

RELAPSING DUODENAL ULCER DISEASE

Long-term maintenance therapy with a low dose of one of the healing agents can reduce recurrence rates. However, eradication of *Helicobacter pylori* with "triple therapy" of metronidazole, amoxicillin or tetracycline and colloidal bismuth has been shown to produce a much lower relapse rate (Table 35.1). Similar results may be obtained using "dual therapy" of omeprazole with amoxycillin.

PEPTIC ULCERATION ASSOCIATED WITH NON-STEROIDAL ANTI-INFLAMMATORY DRUGS

If the provoking agent cannot be withdrawn, then ulcers will often heal if a standard healing agent is co-prescribed. Prophylaxis against *gastric* ulceration or its recurrence is probably most successful with the prostaglandin analogue misoprostol, while antisecretory agents protect equally well against recurrent *duodenal* ulceration. Careful patient selection is recommended before prophylaxis is given. Those at higher risk are the elderly, smokers, alcohol users and patients with a history of previous ulceration.

GASTRO-OESOPHAGEAL REFLUX DISEASE

Initial measures include avoidance of tight clothing, smoking, alcohol and caffeine and encouraging weight loss. Raising the head of the bed at night can be helpful. There are three approaches to drug treatment. First, reduction of gastric acid with antacids can relieve mild symptoms with or without the addition of an alginate to provide a mechanical barrier. Antisecretory agents are helpful but H_2-receptor antagonists often relieve symptoms without producing mucosal healing. Better response rates can often be achieved by using these drugs at high dosages. Standard treatment with an antacid/alginate and an H_2-receptor antagonist will provide relief in about 40% of patients. For severe, resistant or relapsing disease, a proton pump inhibitor is more effective. A second approach is to enhance oesophageal motility with metoclopramide or cisapride. These encourage normal peristalsis in the upper gastrointestinal tract and produce similar symptomatic relief to H_2-receptor antagonists. The third form of treatment is stimulation of mucosal defence with sucralfate or carbenoxolone. Both offer similar efficacy to H_2-receptor antagonists but are less widely used.

36

Inflammatory Bowel Disease

Crohn's disease and ulcerative colitis are chronic inflammatory disorders of the gastrointestinal tract, together termed inflammatory bowel disease. Their aetiology is unknown. Patients experience periods of relapse and remission over many years.

CHRONIC INFLAMMATORY BOWEL DISEASE

- Ulcerative colitis is a mucosal and submucosal disorder which produces continuous inflammation confined to the large bowel. Symptoms include bloody diarrhoea, fever and weight loss; the extent of colonic disease varies but the rectum is always involved. Ulcerative colitis can be associated with extra-colonic manifestations such as uveitis and sacroileitis. The cause is unknown.

- Crohn's disease is a transmural granulomatous condition which can involve any part of the gut. The bowel involvement is discontinuous, often sparing the rectum. Fistula formation, small bowel strictures and perianal disease such as abscesses and fissures are common. Clinical features of colonic involvement include diarrhoea, abdominal pain and fatigue. Involvement of more proximal parts of the gut produces various symptoms depending on the site of the disease.

Treatment is intended to induce and maintain remissions and the drugs used for these two conditions are broadly similar.

DRUGS FOR INFLAMMATORY BOWEL DISEASE

AMINO SALICYLATES

Examples: sulphasalazine, mesalazine, olsalazine.

Mechanism of action and effects

Sulphasalazine was the first amino salicylate shown to be effective in treating inflammatory bowel disease. Colonic flora cleave sulphasalazine into its constituent parts, 5-aminosalicylic acid (5-ASA) and sulphapyridine. The active anti-inflammatory component is 5-ASA while sulphapyridine is thought to be responsible for many unwanted effects. 5-ASA (mesalazine) can be given *per se* without the sulphapyridine component, or alternatively as olsalazine which is two molecules of 5-ASA joined by an azo bond. The mechanisms of action of aminosalicylates are not clear but may be via their ability to inhibit leucocyte chemotaxis, free radical generation and leukotriene synthesis. Amino salicylates are all effective in achieving remission and reducing the relapse rate in ulcerative colitis and Crohn's colitis. Sulphasalazine is still considered to be the drug of first choice.

Pharmacokinetics

Sulphasalazine is partially absorbed from the gut intact, but most reaches the colon where it undergoes reduction by gut bacteria. Sulphapyridine and about 20% of the 5-ASA are absorbed from the colon, and then metabolized in the liver. Both have intermediate half-lives in the circulation. Olsalazine is not absorbed from the upper gut; 5-ASA is released after splitting of the azo bond by the colonic flora. Mesalazine is given as an enteric-coated or modified-release formulation to avoid absorption from the small bowel.

Unwanted effects

Those due to sulphapyridine are:

- Headache, nausea, vomiting.
- Blood dyscrasias, especially agranulocytosis.
- Oligospermia.
- Rashes.

Those due to 5-ASA are:

- Nausea, diarrhoea, abdominal pain.
- Skin rashes including urticaria.
- Nephrotoxicity: this is unusual but may result from the structural relationship to phenacetin, an analgesic that produces chronic interstitial nephritis.

CORTICOSTEROIDS

Prednisolone or hydrocortisone (Chapter 47) are used to induce remission in patients with active inflammatory bowel disease but there is little evidence that corticosteroids prevent relapse. Following remission, the dose is gradually tapered to minimize the well-known unwanted effects. Topical treatment with liquid or foam enemas or suppositories is used for localized rectal disease but systemic administration is used for more severe or extensive disease.

IMMUNOSUPPRESSIVES

Azathioprine and 6-mercaptopurine are both useful in some cases of active inflammatory bowel disease and may enable reduced steroid doses. They are slow acting, requiring months of treatment for full effectiveness. Cyclosporin A and methotrexate are also being evaluated. Details of these drugs are found in Chapters 42 and 55.

ANTIBIOTICS

Metronidazole (Chapter 54) is moderately effective in some cases of Crohn's disease, although the mechanism of action is uncertain.

37

Constipation and Diarrhoea

CONSTIPATION

Humans normally defecate with a frequency from once every 2 days (sometimes less in women) to three times a day. Maintenance of "regular" bowel habits is a western preoccupation best controlled by increasing dietary fibre. Drugs are widely prescribed or taken without prescription and are frequently abused.

Constipation is the infrequent passage of hard, small stools. There are many causes including:

- Disease, for example colonic cancer, myxoedema.
- Iatrogenic (drug induced) for example opiate analgesics, anticholinergic agents, antacids.
- Slow gut transit, especially in young women.
- Immobility.

Underlying organic disease should be excluded in cases where there is persistent constipation or if there has been a recent change in bowel habit. Symptoms of constipation include mild abdominal discomfort and distension, similar to those of irritable bowel syndrome (see below).

LAXATIVES

BULKING AGENTS

These include various polysaccharides: wheat bran, ispaghula husk, sterculia or the synthetic alternative, methylcellulose. They are not broken down by digestive processes. As they are hydrophilic compounds, their action is retention of water in the gut lumen, and stimulation of colonic mucosal receptors to promote peristalsis. Increased numbers of colonic bacteria also increase faecal bulk. Bulking agents are given orally and generally take at least 24 h to work. A liberal fluid intake should accompany bulking agents to lubricate the colon and minimize the risk of obstruction. They are useful for establishing a regular bowel habit in patients with chronic constipation, diverticular disease and irritable bowel syndrome. They increase faecal bulk by "natural" means, but can produce a sensation of bloating, flatulence or griping abdominal pain.

OSMOTIC LAXATIVES

Examples of these are magnesium salts and lactulose. These are poorly absorbed, osmotically active solutes, which increase the small and large bowel luminal fluid volume. Magnesium salts may also stimulate cholecystokinin release from the small intestinal mucosa which enhances intestinal secretion and motility. These actions result in more rapid transit of gut contents into the large bowel, while large bowel distension promotes evacuation after about 3 h. About 20% of magnesium is absorbed and has CNS and neuromuscular blocking activity if it is retained in the circulation in large enough amounts, for example in renal failure. Lactulose is a semisynthetic disaccharide of fructose and galactose. In the bowel, bacteria release fructose and galactose. Fermentation yields lactic and acetic acids which are osmotically active and at the same time lower intestinal pH which favours overgrowth of selected colonic flora. Sodium acid phosphate is an osmotic preparation that is given as an enema or suppository.

IRRITANT AND STIMULANT LAXATIVES

Important examples are senna, bisacodyl, danthron and sodium picosulphate. They act by largely unknown mechanisms, probably stimulating local reflexes through intramural plexuses, thereby reducing net reabsorption of water and electrolytes and enhancing gut motility. They are useful for more severe forms of constipation, but tolerance is often seen with regular use and they can produce abdominal cramps. Senna has the most gentle purgative action of this group. It is hydrolysed by colonic bacteria to release irritant anthracene glycoside derivatives, sennosides A and B, which stimulate the myenteric plexus; the onset of action is after 6–12 h. Bisacodyl can be given orally, or rectally for a more rapid action in 15–30 min; it undergoes enterohepatic recirculation. Sodium picosulphate is a powerful irritant and is used to prepare the bowel for surgery or colonoscopy. Danthron is an effective alternative to the drugs already discussed but is carcinogenic at high doses in animals and it is advised that its use in man should be limited to the elderly or terminally ill. Chronic use of any of these compounds may lead to progressive deterioration of normal colonic function (cathartic colon) possibly by damaging the myenteric plexus.

LUBRICANTS AND STOOL SOFTENERS (EMOLLIENTS)

Docusate sodium has detergent properties which may soften stools by increasing intestinal fluid secretion; it also has stimulant activity but overall is a relatively ineffective compound. Arachis oil or glycerol can be given rectally or liquid paraffin orally. Glycerol, used as a suppository, is a gentle method for stimulating colonic activity and provoking evacuation. Liquid paraffin is not recommended since it impairs the absorption of fat soluble vitamins, can cause anal seepage and accidental inhalation produces lipoid pneumonia.

DIARRHOEA

Severe acute diarrhoea can be the consequence of both reduced absorption of fluid and an increase in intestinal secretions. Viral gastroenteritis is a common cause in children, but bacteria are more often responsible in adults. Diarrhoea may result from local release of toxins (e.g. bacterial enterotoxins) which have a variety of actions on gut mucosal cells, including stimulation of intracellular cyclic AMP which causes chloride secretion into the bowel. Drugs can also produce diarrhoea, most often magnesium salts (see above), cytotoxic agents (Chapter 55) and α and β-adrenoceptor blocking drugs (Chapters 4 and 7).

It is essential to maintain electrolyte and fluid balance which can be achieved by rehydration therapy using intravenous or oral fluid, glucose, sodium, potassium and chloride replacement; the route depending upon the severity of the diarrhoea. Appropriate antimicrobial therapy should be given in severe diarrhoea caused by specific organisms, for example amoebic dysentery, shigella dysentery, typhoid, cholera.

Broad-spectrum antibiotics can produce diarrhoea by altering colonic flora. Occasionally this is associated with Pseudomembranous colitis due to overgrowth of *Clostridium difficile* in the bowel. The organism can be eradicated with oral metronidazole or vancomycin (Chapter 54). Antimicrobial prophylaxis, for example with trimethoprim, can protect against organisms that produce travellers' diarrhoea. Specific antidiarrhoeal agents such as antimotility and adsorbent drugs, can also be helpful for acute diarrhoea.

Chronic diarrhoea requires full investigation for non-infectious causes such as carcinoma of the colon, inflammatory bowel disease or coeliac disease.

DRUG TREATMENT FOR DIARRHOEA

ANTIMOTILITY AGENTS

Antimotility drugs allow greater time for fluid absorption from gut contents. Two classes of drug are used:

- Opiate drugs: for example codeine, loperamide, diphenoxylate. The antimotility action of opiates is probably due to an action on μ and possibly κ receptors in the myenteric plexus of the intestinal wall (Chapter 20). Receptor binding inhibits smooth muscle contractions and propulsive movements of the gut, enhancing segmental contractions and prolonging transit time of intestinal contents. Loperamide has an intermediate half-life, the others have short half-lives. Loperamide, in addition to a longer duration of action, has a more rapid onset of action and is more selective for the gut, partly due to a high first-pass metabolism which limits systemic absorption. Unwanted effects of opiate drugs are discussed in Chapter 20.
- Anticholinergic agents: loperamide has anticholinergic activity which also inhibits peristalsis in addition to its opioid receptor stimulation. Other anticholinergic drugs (Chapter 4) have too many unwanted effects to be clinically useful for this indication.

ADSORBENT AGENTS

Kaolin, chalk, ispaghula and methylcellulose are adsorbents which have a minor role in the treatment of diarrhoea. They may act by adsorbing toxins from microorganisms.

IRRITABLE BOWEL SYNDROME

Irritable bowel syndrome is characterized by abdominal pain and alterations in bowel habit, varying from diarrhoea to constipation, for which no cause can be identified. It is said to occur in 15% of the population. Abdominal pain can often be relieved by defecation, but there is a sensation of incomplete evacuation and mucus is passed per rectum. Altered, but ill-defined, patterns of motility throughout the gut have been reported. A strong psychological component is also evident.

Drug therapy should form only part of the treatment, supplemented by counselling and psychological support. Constipation or diarrhoea should be treated with agents previously described. Some patients will also respond favourably to alterations in diet, antispasmodic agents or short courses of benzodiazepines (Chapter 21) or antidepressants (Chapter 23).

ANTISPASMODIC AGENTS

Examples: mebeverine, dicyclomine, propantheline.

Mechanism of action

These compounds have both antimuscarinic and, in the case of mebeverine and dicyclomine, direct antispasmodic properties (possibly by phosphodiesterase inhibition). They can relieve gut spasm and the associated pain. Propantheline also inhibits gastric emptying.

Pharmacokinetics

Oral absorption of mebeverine and dicyclomine is good and the compounds are metabolized in the liver. The half-lives are short. Propantheline is a poorly absorbed quaternary amine; most is hydrolysed in the bowel.

Unwanted effects

- Mainly anticholinergic actions (Chapter 4).

38

Biliary Disease

Bile is secreted by the liver cells and stored in the gall bladder. The presence of food in the duodenum stimulates the release of cholecystokinin from the intestinal mucosa which causes the gall bladder to contract. Bile enters the duodenum to aid in the breakdown and digestion of fats. When bile is excluded from the intestine there is severe malabsorption of fat and fat soluble vitamins. Bile is concentrated in the gall bladder as water is absorbed. Bile consists of conjugated bile salts (derived from bile acids which are themselves formed from cholesterol), bile pigments, phospholipids and small amounts of cholesterol. The bile salts undergo enterohepatic recycling.

The formation of gallstones (cholelithiasis) is a common condition and it is estimated that 20% of women and 5% of men between the ages of 50 and 65 years have them. Gallstones arise from bile stasis and its concentration in the gall bladder, so that cholesterol becomes saturated in the bile. The solubility of cholesterol in bile is dependent upon the content of bile acids and phospholipids. About 10% of gallstones are predominantly formed from cholesterol and are small enough to be amenable to drug treatment. Mixed gallstones containing calcium, protein and bile pigments, and pure pigment stones cannot be dispersed by drug treatment.

GALLSTONE DISSOLUTION

SEMISYNTHETIC BILE ACIDS

Examples: chenodeoxycholic acid, ursodeoxycholic acid.

Mechanism of action and effects

Bile acids reduce biliary secretion of cholesterol and increase the bile acid pool. Cholesterol synthesis is reduced by inhibition of the rate-limiting enzyme HMG Co-A reductase (Chapter 51). Dissolution of small stones is most effective, beginning after about 6 months and completed in 2–3 years. Treatment is successful in up to 60% of cases, but gallstones recur in about 50% during the 5 years following dissolution. There is some evidence that a combination of the two semisynthetic bile acids may be more effective than either alone. A small dose of ursodeoxycholic acid given regularly after complete dissolution may reduce the risk of gallstone recurrence. Dissolution of large stones can be enhanced by fragmentation using external shock-wave lithotripsy.

Pharmacokinetics

Oral absorption is complete, mainly from the terminal ileum, and about 60% is secreted into the bile after conjugation in the liver. Enterohepatic circulation of ursodeoxycholic acid occurs rather less readily than with natural bile acids. Intestinal bacteria degrade the compounds to lithocholic acid.

Unwanted effects

- Diarrhoea is the only significant effect, occurring with chenodeoxycholic acid but not ursodeoxycholic acid.

39

Obesity

Obesity (body weight greater than 30% above ideal) reduces life expectancy and is associated with the development of hypertension, diabetes, gout, osteoarthrosis, hiatus hernia and hyperlipidaemia. Most excess weight is stored as fat, but about one-quarter is in other tissues. Weight loss depends mainly on generating a negative energy balance by appropriate dietary restriction and increasing energy expenditure, but dietary compliance is often poor. Drugs are sometimes of use under close supervision to reduce hunger and appetite, but have a limited application since tolerance often occurs with long-term use.

ANORETIC AGENTS

AMPHETAMINE DERIVATIVES

Example: diethylpropion.

The amphetamine derivatives produce central stimulation and cardiovascular actions which limit their usefulness. There is also a risk of dependency with long-term use and these drugs are not recommended. Amphetamine is discussed in Chapter 58.

5HT RECEPTOR AGONISTS

Example: dexfenfluramine.

Mechanism of action

Dexfenfluramine (the *d*-optical isomer of fenfluramine) is a 5HT reuptake inhibitor which reduces appetite without producing central stimulation or dependence.

Pharmacokinetics

Oral absorption of fenfluramine is good, and most is metabolized in the liver. It has a long half-life.

Unwanted effects

- Dryness of the mouth.
- Drowsiness.

The Immune System

40

The Immune Response

The body has both innate and adaptive immune response systems. Phagocytic macrophages and natural killer cells comprise the first line of defence against invading organisms. If this innate system is breached, the adaptive system is triggered. This comprises two elements: humoral and cellular immunity.

HUMORAL IMMUNITY

The production of antibodies specific for an invading organism requires initial presentation of the antigenic organism to the B lymphocyte. Antigen presentation is followed by B-cell differentiation into clones capable of producing an antibody directed against the initial antigen. Several cells are able to initiate this process of differentiation and are collectively known as antigen presenting cells (APCs). APCs are found principally in the skin, lymph nodes, spleen and thymus and include macrophages, Langerhan's cells in the skin and interdigitating cells in the lymph nodes. Antigen on the surface of the APC triggers T helper lymphocytes (T_H cells) to produce cytokine mediators known as lymphokines. Several lymphokines have been characterized, including various interleukins, gamma interferon and tumour necrosis factor. Recognition of the antigen by B lymphocytes makes them responsive to the lymphokines released by both APCs and T_H lymphocytes. This leads to expression of receptors for additional cytokines on the B-cell surface and their subsequent differentiation into antibody producing cells (Fig. 40.1). The nature of the lymphokine stimulation will help to determine which immunoglobulin class is produced.

IMMUNOGLOBULINS

Five classes of immunoglobulin (Ig) are recognized, known as IgA, IgD, IgE, IgG and IgM. IgG is the major immunoglobulin in the blood, with IgM forming most of the rest. IgA is predominantly found in seromucous secretions. IgD is present in the membrane of circulating B lymphocytes while IgE is mainly attached to the surface of basophils and mast cells. Antibodies, in addition to their defensive role, can become involved in various different types of hypersensitivity reaction (see Chapter 56).

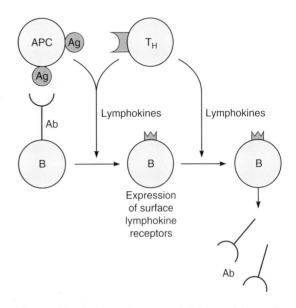

Figure 40.1 Pathways for expressing humoral immunity. APC, Antigen presenting cells; T_H, T-helper lymphocyte; B, B lymphocyte; Ag, antigen; Ab, antibody.

IgE is most commonly associated with immediate (type I) hypersensitivity disease such as hay fever and asthma. IgE responses to antigen are localized to the site of the challenge and will initially sensitize mast cells. This is followed by IgE spill-over into the circulation with binding to basophils and mast cells in other tissues. Subsequent exposure to antigen results in release from these cells of preformed mediators, including histamine and newly generated mediators including PGD_2 and LTC_4 (Chapter 30).

IgM and IgG are involved in type II hypersensitivity reactions, when antibody is directed against cell surface or tissue antigens. Interactions with complement or mononuclear cells leads to damage of the target tissue.

Immune complexes are responsible for type III hypersensitivity reactions. These are formed by combination of antibody and antigen and lead to tissue damage by complement activation or by release of mediators from mast cells and basophils.

CELL-MEDIATED IMMUNITY

When APCs interact with T_H cells, the lymphokines produced by the T_H cells stimulate cytotoxic T lymphocytes (T_C cells) as well as B lymphocytes. Other mononuclear cells such as natural killer cells, macrophages and granulocytes also respond. T lymphocytes are responsible for cell-mediated immune responses and

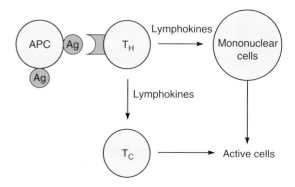

Figure 40.2   Expression of cellular immunity. APC, Antigen presenting cell; T_H, T-helper cell; T_C, cytotoxic T lymphocytes.

can be involved in type IV or delayed hypersensitivity reactions. Release of lymphokines from sensitized T cells activates local macrophages which are particularly important in the development of such reactions and the consequent tissue damage (Fig. 40.2).

T SUPPRESSOR CELLS

These are also stimulated by the presentation of antigen and regulate both T_H and B cells. This regulation is achieved by release of humoral factors which interact with target cell membranes and diminish their responses.

41

Antihistamines and Allergic Disease

HISTAMINE AS AN AUTACOID

Histamine is a heterocyclic amine (Chapter 1) which functions as a local hormone. It is found in mast cells, particularly in tissues which come into contact with the outside world, for example skin, lungs and gut, where it forms part of the tissue defence mechanisms. It is also present in circulating basophils where it may have a similar role. Histamine is found also in the stomach where it participates in acid secretion (Chapter 35) and in the brain where it may act as a neurotransmitter (Chapter 17).

Histamine is synthesized from dietary histadine by decarboxylation. After release from cells it is rapidly metabolized. Its effects are mediated by three distinct types of receptor known as H_1, H_2 and H_3. In general, the H_1-receptors are involved in the "defensive" actions of histamine while gastric acid secretion is mediated by H_2-receptors and H_3-receptors are involved in neurotransmission, possibly in the autonomic nervous system and in itch and pain perception.

Histamine released from mast cells is one of the chemical mediators of type 1 or immediate hypersensitivity reactions, that is, anaphylaxis, urticaria and allergic rhino-conjunctivitis. Other mediators include prostaglandins and leukotrienes (Chapter 30). The major effects of H_1-receptor stimulation are:

- Capillary and venous dilation which can produce marked hypotension. In its most dramatic form, this can present as anaphylactic shock. In the skin it produces the histamine wheal and flare response, an axon reflex via H_1-receptors being responsible for the spread of vasodilation or flare.
- Increased capillary permeability producing oedema.
- Smooth muscle contraction, especially bronchiolar and intestinal.
- Skin itching: but in combination with kinins and prostaglandins, histamine produces pain.

H_2-receptor stimulation inhibits further release of inflammatory mediators including histamines from mast cells and activates suppressor T lymphocytes.

H_1-RECEPTOR ANTAGONISTS: "ANTIHISTAMINES"

Examples: chlorpheniramine, promethazine, terfenadine, astemizole.

Mechanisms of action and effects

The classical antihistamines are selective for H_1-receptors (H_2-receptor antagonists are not usually called antihistamines). Most are competitive antagonists, except astemizole, which binds tightly to the receptor and produces non-competitive inhibition. Antihistamines suppress many of the vascular effects of histamine. Some compounds have other actions which can be used therapeutically, for example the sedative effect of older compounds (e.g. chlorphenira-mine, promethazine) or the suppression of nausea in motion sickness (e.g. promethazine), which is believed to be an anticholinergic effect (Chapter 34). Newer antihistamines such as terfenadine and astemizole do not have these additional actions.

Pharmacokinetics

Antihistamines are well absorbed from the gut and metabolized in the liver. Most have a long half-life. Astemizole has a very long half-life of 10 days, with a very long duration of action which is largely due to an active metabolite. Like most drugs with very long half-lives its onset of effect is slow unless a loading dose is given (Chapter 2). Intravenous chlorphenira-mine is available for medical emergencies. Several topical formulations of antihistamines exist, including a nasal spray for allergic rhinitis, skin preparations for insect stings (but see unwanted effects) and eyedrops for allergic rhinitis.

Unwanted effects

- Sedation or fatigue (not with astemizole or terfenadine).
- Appetite stimulation (astemizole).
- Dry mouth (older drugs with anticholinergic effects).
- Topical antihistamines for use on the skin should be avoided because hypersensitivity reactions are common.
- Ventricular arrhythmias can occur with high doses of terfenadine or astemizole, particu-larly if used in combination with imidazole antifungal agents or macrolide antimicrobials (Chapter 54).

MANAGEMENT OF ALLERGIC DISORDERS

Allergic rhinitis (both seasonal and perennial), urticaria and immediate hypersensitivity reactions share certain principles for management. Precipitating factors should be avoided when possible, but symptomatic relief is often necessary.

Antihistamines are the mainstay of treatment, the initial choice being governed mainly by the degree of sedation required. More sedative drugs can be useful to control nocturnal itching. Less sedative compounds are an advan-tage if the patient wishes to drive or operate machinery. Responses to individual drugs vary and it can be helpful to try an alternative drug if the initial choice is unsuccessful. Topical anti-histamines for the nose or eye can be effective.

Oral or depot injections of corticosteroids (Chapter 47) are valuable for severe or resistant allergic reactions. Topical corticosteroids should be used in preference to systemic treat-ment where possible, for example to treat rhinitis. However, responses to topical corticos-teroid may be incomplete, for example if the nose is severely obstructed. Corticosteroid eye drops should only be given under specialist supervision because of the risk of exacerbating local infection or accelerating cataracts. Other useful topical formulations include sodium cromoglycate (Chapter 11) for rhinitis or conjuctivitis, while an anticholinergic spray (e.g. ipratropium; Chapter 11) can be especially effec-tive for persistent rhinorrhoea.

Anaphylactic shock or angioedema of the mouth, tongue, pharynx and larynx are medical emergencies. Severe hypotension or respiratory obstruction can occur for which adrenaline (Chapter 4) is given intramuscularly. An antihis-tamine should be given intravenously by slow injection. Intravenous hydrocortisone (Chapter 47) is given when the initial measures do not produce a rapid response. Patients who are known to have severe reactions to wasp or bee venom can be given a prefilled adrenaline syringe or an inhaler to reduce the risk of anaphylaxis if they are stung.

42

Immunomodulator Drugs

IMMUNOMODULATOR DRUGS

CYCLOSPORIN A

Mechanism of action

Cyclosporin A is a cyclic peptide, formed as a fungal metabolite which inhibits the production of lymphokines by T-helper cells. It has a particular suppressive effect on interleukin-2 production and inhibits the maturation of cytotoxic T cells (Fig. 40.2). There is a lesser effect on γ-interferon production, which suppresses the expression of major histocompatibility antigens on macrophages. Cyclosporin A is believed to act in the cell nucleus preventing transcription of the genes for lymphokine production.

Pharmacokinetics

Oral absorption is variable and incomplete. After absorption there is selective concentration in some tissues including liver, kidney, several endocrine glands, lymph nodes, spleen and bone marrow. Extensive metabolism by cytochrome P450 occurs in the liver and the half-life is long. Plasma drug concentration monitoring is important to guide dosage for optimal effectiveness and to minimize toxicity.

Unwanted effects

- Nephrotoxicity almost always occurs and includes interstitial fibrosis and tubular atrophy. The decline in renal glomerular func-

tion is usually reversible but permanent renal impairment can result.
- Hypertension, often associated with fluid retention, occurs in up to 50% of patients. It usually responds to standard antihypertensive drug treatment.
- Convulsions can occur, most frequently if corticosteroids are given concurrently. They often occur in association with hypertension and are more common in children.
- Hypertrichosis and gum hypertrophy are common.
- Gastrointestinal disturbance including anorexia, nausea and vomiting.
- Drug interactions: caution should be taken when cyclosporin A is used with other nephrotoxic drugs such as aminoglycoside antimicrobials (Chapter 54). Drugs which induce liver cytochrome P450 can reduce the plasma concentration of cyclosporin to subtherapeutic levels (Chapter 2).

AZATHIOPRINE

Mechanism of action

Most of the effects of azathioprine result from cleavage to the active derivative 6-mercaptopurine (Chapter 55). Effects on the immune response include impaired synthesis of immunoglobulins by B lymphocytes, and inhibition of the infiltration of mononuclear cells into inflamed tissue. These arise from the antimetabolite action of 6-mercaptopurine, which interferes with purine biosynthesis, thus impairing DNA synthesis in the S-phase of the cell cycle.

Pharmacokinetics

Oral absorption is almost complete. Azathioprine is a prodrug, and metabolism in the liver produces active compounds. The half-life is short.

Unwanted effects

- Bone marrow suppression with dose-dependent leucopenia. Regular monitoring of the white cell count is essential.
- Carcinogenicity, especially lymphomas, although the risk is small.
- Increased susceptibility to infection, often with "opportunistic" organisms.
- Gastrointestinal disturbances, especially nausea and vomiting.
- Alopecia.
- Drug interactions: the most important interaction is with allopurinol (Chapter 33), which inhibits the enzyme xanthine oxidase that is involved in the metabolism of azathioprine. The dose of azathioprine should be reduced by 75% if the drugs are used together.

IMMUNOSUPPRESION IN ORGAN TRANSPLANTATION

Effective immunosuppression has improved the early survival of kidney, liver, heart and lung transplants. However, suppression of acute rejection is more effective than prevention of chronic rejection. Most transplant units use "triple therapy" with oral corticosteroids (usually prednisolone) (Chapter 47), azathioprine and cyclosporin. After renal transplantation, cyclosporin is withheld until an adequate urine output is established. Maintenance immunosuppression is often continued with triple therapy. Cyclosporin doses are adjusted by monitoring blood concentrations, while the dose of prednisolone is gradually reduced to minimize chronic unwanted effects. Rejection episodes are usually treated with large doses of corticosteroids, supplemented by biological agents such as antilymphocyte globulin or a specific monoclonal antibody against CD_3 lymphocytes.

IMMUNOSUPPRESSION IN OTHER DISORDERS

Immunosuppression therapy is used in several diseases in which an "autoimmune" component may contribute to the pathogenesis. These include various connective tissue diseases such as vasculitis or systemic lupus erythematosus, certain types of glomerulonephritis, chronic active hepatitis, Crohn's disease and some haematological disorders. Drugs may be given alone or in combination. Those most widely used include corticosteroids, azathioprine and cyclophosphamide (Chapter 55).

The Endocrine System
and Metabolic Disorders

Blood Glucose Regulation and Diabetes Mellitus

CONTROL OF BLOOD GLUCOSE

Glucose occupies a central positon in metabolism as the predominant substrate for energy production. Cells receive their supply of glucose from blood, where control mechanisms ensure concentrations remain within certain limits. Glucose enters the blood by absorption from the gut and from breakdown of stored glycogen in tissues such as liver. At physiological concentrations it leaves the blood almost entirely by active transfer into the cells, which is dependent in most tissues on the polypeptide hormone insulin.

Insulin is a protein which is secreted from the β-cells of the islets of Langerhans in the pancreas in response to a rise in blood glucose, and inhibited by a fall. Occupation of specific cell surface receptors by insulin leads to active transport of glucose into the cell, accompanied by potassium. Insulin also provides a powerful anabolic stimulus not only to metabolism of carbohydrate but also to that of amino acids and fatty acids which enter cells more readily in the presence of insulin.

Several hormones antagonize the anabolic action of insulin, particularly on carbohydrate metabolism. These include glucagon, growth hormone, cortisol and catecholamines. Most of these are released in stressful situations requiring the breakdown of glycogen reserves for energy.

DIABETES MELLITUS

Failure to secrete sufficient insulin to maintain a normal level of blood glucose results in diabetes mellitus. Two patterns are recognized.

TYPE I (OR INSULIN-DEPENDENT) DIABETES MELLITUS; IDDM

Type I diabetes represents a severe deficiency of insulin, usually presenting in youth. The clinical picture reflects failure of glucose to enter the cells in sufficient quantities to maintain energy production and anabolic metabolism. Patients are tired and unwell, lose weight and become keto-acidotic. Replacement of insulin is almost always necessary, in addition to control of carbohydrate intake. Close control of blood sugar concentrations has been shown to reduce the development of diabetic retinopathy, nephropathy and neuropathy. Excess saturated fat should also be avoided to protect against premature atheroma.

TYPE II (OR NON-INSULIN-DEPENDENT) DIABETES MELLITUS; NIDDM

Type II diabetes presenting later in life, represents a relative deficiency of insulin. Sufficient glucose enters cells to permit adequate energy production for most situations, and the main problem is excess glucose outside the cells rather than a shortfall inside. Such patients are often overweight (which increases cellular resistance to insulin) and do not usually become ketotic. They can often be treated successfully with a diet which avoids immediate hyperglycaemia by limiting intake of low molecular weight carbohydrate, and by shedding of excess weight. If satisfactory control of blood sugar is not achieved by diet alone, insulin secretion and action in these patients can be enhanced by oral hypoglycaemic drugs, supplemented if control is poor by the α-glucosidase inhibitor acarbose. However, a proportion of patients presenting with typical Type II diabetes will eventually require treatment with insulin.

ORAL HYPOGLYCAEMIC DRUGS

SULPHONYLUREAS

Examples: tolbutamide, chlorpropamide, glibenclamide, gliclazide.

Mechanism of action

Sulphonylureas act mainly by increasing the release of insulin from the β-cells in response to stimulation by glucose. They also increase the effect of insulin on target tissues by up-regulation of receptors.

Pharmacokinetics

Sulphonylureas are structurally related to sulphonamides. They are absorbed rapidly (although the rate of absorption is reduced when taken with food), they are highly protein bound, and are metabolized by the liver. Chlorpropamide depends partly on the kidney for its elimination. The very long half-life of chlorpropamide (about 3 days) may lead to accumulation and its use in the elderly is dangerous. Tolbutamide and gliclazide have short half-lives; glibenclamide has a longer duration of action than would be predicted from its short plasma half-life due to selective concentration in islet cells.

Compounds with a short duration of action are usually preferred when starting treatment with a sulphonylurea to minimize the risk of hypoglycaemia.

Unwanted effects

- Excessive (and particularly nocturnal) hypoglycaemia is most frequent with the longer acting drugs.
- Weight gain is almost inevitable unless dietary restrictions are observed.
- Skin rashes and, rarely, blood dyscrasias (in common with most sulphonamides; see Chapter 54).
- Chlorpropamide increases renal sensitivity to antidiuretic hormone and can produce water retention with dilutional hyponatraemia.
- Chlorpropamide can produce flushing if alcohol is taken.

BIGUANIDES

Example: metformin.

Mechanism of action and effects

Metformin does not affect insulin secretion; it reduces hepatic gluconeogenesis and may also limit glucose absorption or facilitate its peripheral uptake. Metformin can also suppress appetite which is useful in overweight patients, and when used alone it does not cause hypoglycaemia. An additional benefit is improvement in the adverse plasma lipid profile found in diabetes; it raises high density lipoprotein cholesterol and reduces triglycerides (Chapter 51). The action of metformin is complementary to that of sulphonylureas.

Pharmacokinetics

Metformin is well absorbed from the gut and excreted unchanged by the kidney. It has a short half-life.

Unwanted effects

Gastrointestinal upset, including anorexia, abdominal discomfort and diarrhoea which are usually short-lived.

- Inhibition of pyruvate metabolism encourages lactate accumulation. In situations which lead to an increase in anaerobic metabolism, severe lactic acidosis can result. This is also more common in the presence of cardiac, renal or hepatic impairment.

α-GLUCOSIDASE INHIBITORS

Example: acarbose.

Mechanism of action and effects

Carbohydrate digestion in the bowel involves several enzymes which sequentially degrade complex polysaccharides such as starch into monosaccharides such as glucose. Initial digestion in the gut lumen is carried out by amylases from the saliva and pancreas. The final digestion of oligosaccharides is carried out by β-galactosidase (including lactase) and various α-glucosidases (such as maltase, isomaltase, glucoamylase and sucrase which hydrolyses the disaccharide, sucrose) in the small intestinal brush border. Acarbose competes with dietary oligosaccharides for α-glucosidase, and has a higher affinity for the enzymes. Binding is reversible so that digestion and absorption of glucose after a meal is slower than usual but not prevented. As a result, the postprandial peak of blood glucose is reduced and blood glucose concentrations are more stable through the day. Acarbose has no effect on insulin secretion or its tissue action.

Pharmacokinetics

Oral absorption of acarbose is very poor. Only about 2% of the active parent drug reaches the circulation. Inactive metabolites are formed in the gut lumen by enzymic degradation. About one-third of the oral dose is absorbed as inactive metabolite and most metabolite is excreted in the faeces.

Unwanted effects

- Gastrointestinal effects include flatulence, abdominal distension and diarrhoea due to fermentation of unabsorbed carbohydrate in the bowel.

INSULIN

The half-life of insulin in plasma is very short (about 8–16 min), and to avoid the need for frequent injections, the absorption of insulin from injection sites must be prolonged. Insulin solutions are either "soluble" and clear or are complexed with a substance to delay absorption from the injection site and appear cloudy. The main chemical modifications to insulin are shown in Table 43.1.

Insulins for therapeutic administration used to be extracted either from cattle or pig pancreas. Bovine insulin differs chemically from human insulin in three amino acid residues, and porcine in one, but their action is very similar to human insulin. More recently, recombinant DNA technology has allowed *in vitro* manufacture of insulin with the same structure as human insulin and increasingly these preparations are superceding those of animal origin. All current insulin preparations have a low content of impurities, which has been a cause of problems in the past.

Insulin is initially purified by protein extraction to form a crystalline product. It may then undergo either gel filtration to produce a single peak (SP) insulin or gel filtration and ion exchange chromatography which generates monocomponent (MC), single component (SC) or rarely immunogenic (RI) insulin.

Pharmacokinetics

Insulin must be given parenterally as it is digested in the gut. Subcutaneous injection is

Table 43.1 Comparisons among insulins

Type	Onset of action (h)	Peak activity (h)	Duration (h)	
Neutral	0.5	1–3	7	Short-acting
Isophane	1	2–6	20 ⎫	Intermediate-acting
Lente	2	6–14	22 ⎬	
Protamine-zinc	4	12–24	30	Long-acting

used for routine treatment, and intravenous infusion for emergency situations. Normal insulin secretion from the pancreas is into the portal circulation, and strictly related to metabolic needs. Sixty per cent of insulin released from the pancreas is extracted by the liver before reaching the systemic circulation. Therapeutic delivery of insulin is to the systemic circulation, and the relationship to metabolic needs can only be approximated by the dosages used and their timing in relation to meals. Up to 60% of insulin in the systemic circulation is degraded by the kidney.

There is substantial evidence that close control of plasma glucose concentrations throughout the day can reduce the risk of complications associated with diabetes, making the choice of an appropriate regimen of considerable importance. To generate intermediate or long-acting insulin, it is complexed with:

- *Protamine*: to create the intermediate-acting isophane insulin.
- *Zinc*: to create the intermediate/long acting lente insulin.
- *Protamine and zinc*: to create the long-acting protamine zinc insulin.

These complexes act as modified-release formulations for subcutaneous administration (Table 43.1).

THERAPEUTIC REGIMENS

- *Single daily injections:* used mainly for elderly patients in whom long-term complications of diabetes are less relevant. An intermediate or long-acting insulin is used which can be combined with a short-acting one to optimize control.
- *Twice daily injections:* suitable for patients who have a reasonably stable pattern of activity and eating habits. Short and intermediate-acting insulins are combined, either in fixed ratios provided by the manufacturers, or in varying ratios according to individual requirements. Fixed ratios vary from 10% short with 90% intermediate acting to a 50% mixture of each component.
- *Multiple injections:* increasingly used in younger, active patients who require more flexibility in their lifestyle. Short-acting insulin is given before each main meal and the amount related

to the size of the meal. Administration can be facilitated by the use of portable "pen-injectors". An additional daily injection of a longer-acting insulin is given, usually in the evening, to ensure a "background" effect of insulin throughout the 24 h. This is also known as the "basal-bolus" regimen.

- *Infusion pump:* used for patients in diabetic crises, in labour, during and after surgery or at other times when the patient's usual routine cannot be adhered to. Short-acting insulin is infused in 5% dextrose solution.
- *Intraperitoneal:* patients being treated for chronic renal failure by continuous ambulatory peritoneal dialysis can add their insulin to the dialysis fluid. This is the only therapeutic regimen in which insulin has direct access to the portal circulation.

Unwanted effects

- The main problem is an excessive action producing hypoglycaemia. Neuroglycopaenia with confusion and coma can occur. It can usually be avoided by careful matching of meals, exercise and insulin. All patients taking insulin should carry a card with details of their treatment. Although most diabetics get warning symptoms of hypoglycaemia, some do not and are prone to sudden and severe hypoglycaemic coma. This has been reported to develop after transfer from animal to human insulin. The cause and extent of this problem is currently under investigation.
- Animal insulins, particularly older impure preparations, produced circulating antibodies. These could diminish the activity of the insulin (insulin resistance) or produce local reactions (lipo-atrophy) at injection sites. Modern insulins can cause fat hypertrophy or local fibrosis if given repeatedly at the same site.

GLUCAGON

Use and mechanism of action

Glucagon is used to counter severe hypoglycaemia. It is a peptide, synthesized in man by the A cells of the pancreatic islets of Langerhans, which binds to specific hepatocyte receptors activating adenylate cyclase. The increase in intracellular cyclic AMP leads to inhibition of glycogen synthetase, which blocks the effect of insulin and mobilizes stored liver glycogen.

Pharmacokinetics

Glucagon must be given by intramuscular or intravenous injection, and acts in 10–20 min. It is degraded by enzymes in the bloodstream, liver and kidney.

Unwanted effects

- Nausea and vomiting.
- Very occasionally allergic reactions.

44

The Thyroid and Control of Metabolic Rate

The term "basal metabolism" refers to the energy-utilizing chemical processes of the body at rest. Its rate is controlled by the thyroid hormones, L-thyroxine (T4) and tri-iodothyronine (T3), which stimulate oxygen consumption. This creates a drain on energy reserves such as glycogen and fat, but thyroid hormones also promote gluconeogenesis with consequent wasting of tissues such as muscle and bone. The hormones interact with the sympathetic nervous system, in particular enhancing the effects of β-adrenoceptor stimulation (Chapter 4).

T3 and T4 are synthesized in the thyroid gland. Inorganic iodine is trapped with great avidity by the gland, oxidized and attached to tyrosine. Combination of mono- and/or di-iodinated tyrosine forms T3 and T4. The enzyme thyroxine peroxidase is important both in the initial oxidation and the final combination steps (Fig. 44.1).

Synthesis and release of thyroid hormones are controlled by the anterior pituitary hormone, thyrotrophin or thyroid-stimulating hormone (TSH). This in turn is controlled by the hypothalamus which secretes thyrotrophin-releasing hormone (TRH). Circulating T3 and T4 exert a negative feedback on both the hypothalamic and pituitary hormones.

Circulating thyroid hormones are highly protein-bound (particularly T4 of which less than 0.1% is free), mostly to thyroxine-binding globulin (TBG). Only the free fraction can bind to specific cell receptors. The thyroid secretes both T3 and T4, but most T3 is derived from peripheral de-iodination of T4.

T3 is much more biologically active than T4, but its half-life in the circulation is about 1.5 days compared to about 7 days for T4. Elimination of T3 and T4 is by conjugation, mainly in the liver.

HYPERTHYROIDISM

The commonest form of hyperthyroidism is Graves disease, an autoimmune condition in which thyroid-stimulating immunoglobulins act at TSH receptors on thyroid cells. In many patients there is also an immunologically mediated inflammatory reaction in the extrinsic muscles of the eyes causing swelling and the characteristic exophthalmos. Single or multiple autonomous thyroid adenomata ("hot nodules") are also fairly common. Symptoms of hyperthyroidism, which include weight loss, palpitation and tremor, are in part mediated by excess β-adrenoceptor stimulation.

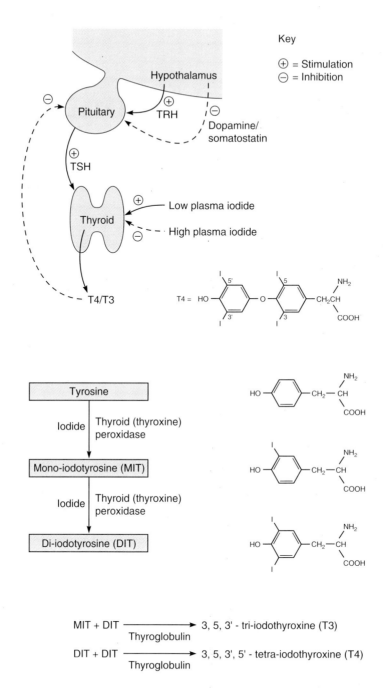

Figure 44.1 Synthesis and regulation of thyroid hormones.

DRUGS FOR TREATMENT OF HYPERTHYROIDISM

THIOUREAS

Examples: carbimazole, propylthiouracil.

Mechanism of action

Thioureas inhibit thyroxine peroxidase, and therefore synthesis of thyroid hormone. Because of the long half-lives of thyroid hormones, particularly T4, changes in the rate of synthesis take several weeks to lower circulating concentrations to normal. In patients with autoimmune thyroid disease these drugs also appear to have an immunosuppressive effect, reducing the levels of TSH receptor-stimulating antibody. This may explain their ability to produce long-term remissions.

Pharmacokinetics

Carbimazole is the drug of choice and is almost completely absorbed from the gut and rapidly converted by first-pass metabolism to the active derivative methimazole. Methimazole has a short half-life and is excreted mainly in the urine. Propylthiouracil has only about one-tenth of the activity of methimazole and has a short half-life due to rapid liver metabolism. It is usually reserved for patients intolerant of carbimazole. Although the antithyroid drugs have short half-lives, they accumulate in the thyroid and have a longer duration of action.

Unwanted effects

- Gastrointestinal upset, especially nausea and taste disturbance.
- Allergic rashes. There is incomplete cross-sensitivity between carbimazole and propylthiouracil.
- Bone marrow suppression, especially agranulocytosis. A severe sore throat with fever is often the presenting complaint, and should be immediately reported by the patient. The onset is sudden and routine blood counts are unhelpful.
- Placental transfer and secretion in breast milk can produce neonatal hypothyroidism, but small doses are probably safe.

β-ADRENOCEPTOR ANTAGONISTS (β-BLOCKERS)

These are fully described in Chapter 6. β-Blockers act on the target tissues to modulate the additive effects of thyroid hormones and β-adrenoceptor stimulation. They have immediate effects on symptoms such as palpitation and tremor but do not alter the rate of thyroid hormone synthesis.

MANAGEMENT OF THYROTOXICOSIS

Carbimazole is the drug of choice, and initially treatment should be continued for 12–18 months, using the lowest possible dose to control symptoms and normalize circulating thyroid hormone concentrations. Carbimazole is occasionally given in high doses for resistant patients with thyroxine replacement to prevent hypothyroidism. Exophthalmos associated with Graves disease responds poorly to treatment. β-Blockers are particularly useful for symptomatic relief during the early period of treatment with carbimazole.

Approximately 40% of patients with Graves disease have a single episode which is cured by drug treatment. Those who relapse will usually do so repeatedly and most are offered definitive treatment by either a subtotal thyroidectomy (for a large goitre) or a therapeutic dose of radioactive iodine (^{131}I). Both may produce hypothyroidism delayed by several months or years.

Before surgery, patients are usually given oral potassium iodide for up to 2 weeks. Iodides inhibit thyroxine synthesis and release, and importantly reduce the vascularity of the hyperplastic thyroid gland.

Before radioactive iodine treatment, patients should be stabilized with carbimazole to reduce the risk of a thyroid crisis immediately after isotope treatment. However, drug treatment must be stopped before radioactive iodine is given or it will prevent uptake of the iodine by the thyroid cells. β-Blockers can be useful in this period to prevent symptomatic relapse.

A toxic nodule can be removed surgically but radioactive iodine is extremely effective since the isotope is taken up only by the abnormal tissue (the remainder is suppressed by the absence of TSH in the circulation). Multinodular toxic goitres are often treated by radio-iodine.

HYPOTHYROIDISM

Hypothyroidism is usually due to thyroid failure and the low circulating T4 concentration is accompanied by a raised TSH. Autoimmune thyroiditis is the commonest cause, but it is occasionally congenital or can follow treatment for hyperthyroidism by surgery or radio-iodine. Rarely, hypothyroidism can be secondary to pituitary or hypothalamic failure, when the circulating TSH will be low. Typical symptoms of hypothyroidism are non-specific and include lethargy, cold intolerance, weight gain, constipation or menorrhagia. Severe hypothyroidism (myxoedema) produces marked changes in facial appearance and may ultimately lead to a hypothermic, comatose state.

MANAGEMENT OF HYPOTHYROIDISM

Standard treatment is with oral thyroxine (T4) although absorption is incomplete and variable. Some T3 will be formed by peripheral de-iodination of T4, but the proportion of circulating T3 is usually lower than normal. Therefore, circulating levels of T4 will often need to be higher than those in healthy subjects to obtain a satisfactory response and a normal serum TSH

is a better guide to the adequacy of therapy. In some patients, particularly those with ischaemic heart disease, a rapid increase in metabolic activity can cause excessive cardiac stimulation. Thyroxine should, therefore, be introduced gradually. After initiation of a fixed dose, steady-state plasma concentrations will not be achieved for about 5 weeks due to the long half-life.

Tri-iodothyronine (T3) is usually reserved for patients with severe hypothyroidism (myxoedema coma) when its potency and shorter half-life allows more rapid attainment of a therapeutic blood concentration. It can be given orally or intravenously.

45

Calcium Metabolism and Metabolic Bone Disease

REGULATION OF CALCIUM METABOLISM

Calcium ions play a part in a large number of cellular activities, including stimulus–response coupling in striated and smooth muscle, endocrine and exocrine glands. Calcium modulates the action of intracellular cyclic AMP and is a co-factor for numerous intracellular enzymes and for blood clotting. In addition, calcium in the form of hydroxyapatite crystals deposited on the protein matrix of bone gives it mechanical strength.

Calcium circulates in plasma partly bound to protein and partly in the free ionized (and therefore "active") form. The free fraction is maintained within narrow limits principally by parathyroid hormone (PTH) and vitamin D. Calcitonin also reacts to changing calcium levels but its effect in overall control is less important. Calcium in plasma is in constant flux with calcium in the gut, renal tubules and bone. This is illustrated, with the main controlling variables in Fig. 45.1.

PTH is a polypeptide hormone which is the main physiological regulator of calcium in blood. Its secretion is stimulated by a reduction of ionized calcium. PTH binds to receptors on renal tubular cells and various cells in bone, where cyclic AMP generation triggers an influx of calcium. The main renal action is to inhibit tubular phosphate reabsorption and to promote calcium retention. The principal action in bone is stimulation of resorption by osteoclasts, which increases bone turnover although enhanced osteoblastic activity results in some bone repair.

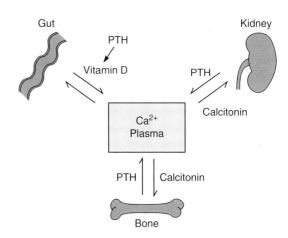

Figure 45.1 Major influences of hormones on calcium metabolism. PTH, Parathyroid hormone.

Vitamin D has a steroid nucleus. A precursor of active vitamin D, ergocalciferol (vitamin D_2), is absorbed from the gut but given adequate sunlight the major source is conversion of 7-dehydro-cholecalciferol in the skin to cholecalciferol (vitamin D_3). This is further metabolized to 25-hydroxy D_3 in the liver and then in the kidney to 1,25-dihydroxy D_3 (calcitriol). PTH promotes the hydroxylation in the kidney. Cholecalciferol is really a skin-derived hormone rather than a vitamin, but this source was discovered after the dietary origins. The main effect of vitamin D is to increase the plasma concentration of calcium by stimulating its absorption from the gut. It acts via typical steroid receptors (Chapter 47), which trigger synthesis of an intracellular calcium-binding protein. In the kidney, vitamin D enhances phosphate retention in contrast to the action of PTH. Actions of vitamin D on bone are poorly understood, but it may stimulate bone formation.

Calcitonin is a peptide secreted by the parafollicular, or C, cells of the thyroid when plasma calcium rises. The main target cell is the osteoclast which it inhibits by stimulation of adenylate cyclase, thus reducing bone turnover. It also enhances the excretion of calcium and phosphate by the kidney.

HYPERCALCAEMIA

The main causes of hypercalcaemia are:

- Increased resorption from bone, for example primary hyperparathyroidism, bony metastases.
- Increased absorption from gut, for example excessive use of vitamin D.
- Reduced renal excretion, for example thiazide diuretics.

Chronic moderate hypercalcaemia is associated with a decline in renal function, formation of renal stones and ectopic calcification (e.g. cornea, blood vessels). Severe hypercalcaemia causes nausea, vomiting, drowsiness and confusion leading to coma. Renal failure can occur, particularly if hypercalcaemia-related impairment of urinary concentrating ability and vomiting have led to dehydration. Sudden death may occur from cardiac arrest.

ANTIRESORPTIVE DRUGS FOR HYPERCALCAEMIA

CALCITONIN

Mechanism of action and effects

The actions of calcitonin on bone and kidney have been discussed above. Calcitonin acts within a few hours of administration and the effect lasts up to 10 h. The hypocalcaemic effect of repeated administrations lasts between 2 and 3 days. Downregulation of calcitonin receptors on the osteoclast then results in a rebound increase in bone resorption, and loss of the clinical response.

Pharmacokinetics

Salmon calcitonin is most commonly used. It is given by intramuscular or subcutaneous injection. The half-life is very short at 15 min, and it is broken down to inactive fragments by enzymic degradation in plasma and in the kidney.

Unwanted effects

- Facial flushing occurs in most patients.
- Nausea is common.

BISPHOSPHONATES

Examples: etidronate, pamidronate.

Mechanisms of action and effects

Bisphosphonates are pyrophosphate analogues with a high binding affinity for receptors on osteoclasts. They inhibit bone reabsorption by preventing osteoclast attachment to bone matrix. Pamidronate also inhibits osteoclast development and recruitment. The fall in serum calcium following a single intravenous infusion is maximal after about a week, and can persist for up to 4 weeks after treatment. Bisphosphonates can also reduce osteolysis in bone malignancy.

Pharmacokinetics

Bisphosphonates are poorly absorbed by mouth (less than 10% of the ingested dose). They are best taken with the stomach empty, to avoid binding by calcium in food. A more reliable route is by intravenous infusion (pamidronate is only available for intravenous use). Removal from blood is rapid via the kidney, but their effect persists as they remain bound to calcium salts in bone.

Unwanted effects

- Oral etidronate causes gastrointestinal disturbance, particularly nausea and diarrhoea.
- Taste disturbance and transient pyrexia with infusion.
- Prolonged use impairs mineralization of newly formed bone with consequent risk of osteomalacia.

PLICAMYCIN (formerly called mithramycin)

This is a cytotoxic agent which inhibits osteoclastic bone resorption. It is given by intravenous infusion. Its action is slower in onset than calcitonin and maximal after about 3 days. The most common unwanted effects are nausea and vomiting. It is rarely used now because of its propensity to cause thrombocytopenia and liver and kidney damage.

TREATMENT OF HYPERCALCAEMIA

When possible the primary cause should be corrected, for example removal of parathyroid adenomata or treatment of myeloma. Specific measures to lower the plasma calcium must be taken in acute, severe hypercalcaemia of any cause, and chronic moderate hypercalcaemia where there is no curative treatment.

Most patients with severe hypercalcaemia are fluid depleted at presentation and rehydration with intravenous saline is essential, which also promotes a sodium-linked calcium diuresis in the proximal renal tubule. Loop diuretics (Chapter 15) are sometimes advocated to increase calcium elimination but require very high volumes of saline and intensive monitoring of fluid balance for safe use.

Bisphosphonates, especially pamidronate by intravenous infusion, are now the drug treatment of first choice. If this is unsuccessful or only partially effective, calcitonin can be substituted or added. Glucocorticoids, such as prednisolone (Chapter 47), are effective in lowering calcium when vitamin D excess is an important factor, for example in sarcoidosis and acute treatment of vitamin D overdose. They probably act by reducing the effect of 1,25-dihydroxycholecalciferol on intestinal calcium transport.

HYPOCALCAEMIA

There are two major underlying causes for hypocalcaemia:

- Deficiency of parathyroid hormone, for example idiopathic hypoparathyroidism, after surgical parathyroid removal.
- Deficiency of vitamin D, for example dietary deficiency, limited exposure to sunlight, renal failure (failure of 1α-hydroxylation).

Hypocalcaemia increases neuromuscular excitability, causing tetany. When severe it may produce fits. Chronic hypocalcaemia, especially in congenital hypoparathyroidism, is associated with mental deficiency, fits, intracranial calcification (e.g. choroid plexus) and ocular cataracts.

DRUGS FOR HYPOCALCAEMIA

VITAMIN D

Examples: ergocalciferol (vitamin D_2) 1α-hydroxy-cholecalciferol (alfacalcidol), 1,25-dihydroxy cholecalciferol (calcitriol).

Mechanism of action

This is discussed above. A dose-related increase in calcium and phosphate absorption from the gut occurs at lower concentrations than those which stimulate bone resorption.

Pharmacokinetics

The fat-soluble D vitamins are well absorbed orally in the presence of bile. Conversion of ergocalciferol to active derivatives has been discussed above. Both alfacalcidol and calcitriol have short half-lives and are excreted mainly in the bile.

Unwanted effects

- Excessive dosing will produce hypercalcaemia.
- Excretion of vitamin D supplements in breast milk can cause hypercalcaemia in an infant.

TREATMENT OF HYPOCALCAEMIA

In the absence of reversible pathology such as coeliac disease, the mainstay of treatment for hypocalcaemia is vitamin D. With the exception of patients who have vitamin D deficiency from inadequate diet or sunlight exposure, much larger doses of vitamin D (usually given as ergocalciferol, vitamin D_2) are required to maintain normocalcaemia than those derived from the diet. Oral calcium supplements are also used for some patients. For patients with severe renal impairment, 1α-hydroxy-cholecalciferol (alfacalcidol) should be used.

Parathyroid hormone is not available for replacement therapy and alfacalcidol is given for hypoparathyroidism. 1,25-dihydroxy cholecalciferol (calcitriol) is rarely required unless a very rapid onset of action is required.

METABOLIC BONE DISEASE

OSTEOMALACIA

This is the bone disease resulting from failure of adequate bone mineralization due to lack of vitamin D. Bone pain is prominent and low plasma calcium and phosphate concentrations produce muscle weakness. In developing children the bones become distorted (rickets). Treatment is with vitamin D (ergocalciferol) supplements.

OSTEOPOROSIS

Osteoporosis is the loss of bone mass due to reduced organic matrix, and consequently mineral content, which reduces the mechanical strength of bone. To some extent it is a natural and inevitable part of the ageing process. In females, however, a marked increase in bone loss occurs after the menopause. Osteoporosis in younger patients is associated with trabecular bone loss predisposing to spontaneous vertebral fractures. In older patients cortical bone is also lost, increasing the risk of traumatic fracture, particularly of the neck of the femur. Sometimes osteoporosis is secondary to other conditions such as corticosteroid therapy (Chapter 47), myeloma, alcoholism or thyrotoxicosis. Once established it is extremely difficult to reverse and emphasis should be placed on prevention where possible:

- The major opportunity for preventing osteoporosis is the use of hormone replacement therapy with oestrogens (Chapter 48) in peri- and postmenopausal women. Unless a hysterectomy has been performed progestogens must be given as well to prevent endometrial hyperplasia and an increased risk of carcinoma. The duration of treatment remains controversial, due to slight concern during long-term use of provoking breast cancer. However, 5–10 years of oestrogen therapy may be required.
- Oral calcium supplements probably reduce the risk of vertebral fractures in postmenopausal women.

Treatments for established osteoporosis include:

- Salmon calcitonin given subcutaneously which produces a modest increase in bone mass. Introduction of an intranasal formulation may make this a more attractive treatment in the future.
- Oral bisphosphonates which produce an increase in bone mass although most studies are confined to postmenopausal women. Oral etidronate, given for 2 weeks at 3-monthly intervals usually with continuous calcium supplements, increases vertebral bone mineral content, and may reduce fractures.
- Oral fluoride supplements increase bone formation in osteoporotic bone, but also produce a defect in mineralization of cortical bone. This can be minimized by giving calcium supplements but the ability of fluoride to prevent fractures is unproven.

PAGET'S DISEASE OF BONE

Paget's disease of bone is characterized by excessive bone reabsorption by osteoclasts with a compensatory increase in bone formation. This produces new bone matrix and non-lamellar woven bone which is often structurally weakened. The aetiology is unknown but a slow virus infection has been implicated.

Clinical features include bone pain and deformity and pathological fractures. Active treatment should be given if symptoms or complications are identified. Apart from symptomatic measures, two main treatments are used:

- Calcitonin, by reducing osteoclastic bone resorption can reduce pain and then improve the structural abnormalities in Pagetic bone.

Response to treatment may be delayed by up to 6 weeks, and therapy may be necessary for several months. About 50% of patients will relapse on stopping treatment.

- Bisphosphonates also inhibit bone resorption but long-term use can also impair bone mineralization. With intermittment treatment (e.g. 6 months out of every 12 months) prolonged remission of symptoms and complications can be achieved.

46

Pituitary and Hypothalamic Hormones

ANTERIOR PITUITARY AND HYPOTHALAMIC HORMONES

GROWTH HORMONE

Growth hormone (GH) or somatotrophin, is a 191-amino acid peptide which is synthesized in specific cells in the anterior pituitary. Its secretion is controlled by both a releasing hormone (GHRH) and a release-inhibiting hormone (GHRIH or somatostatin) from the hypothalamus. Like other peptides GH binds to cell surface receptors and activates adenylate cyclase. It has direct metabolic effects which can be summarized as anabolic in relation to protein metabolism and catabolic in relation to fat and carbohydrate metabolism. It also has tissue differentiating and proliferating effects particularly on cartilage and therefore bone growth, which are indirectly mediated by "insulin-like" growth factors (IGFs). IGF-1C appears to be most closely associated with growth hormone action; it is released from the liver and other tissues and bound to proteins in plasma. GH release has a circadian variation, highest levels being found soon after onset of sleep.

Sources of GH for therapeutic use

GH from human cadaveric pituitary origin (which could transmit slow-virus infection) has been replaced since 1985 by biosynthetic GH (somatropin) developed using genetic engineering techniques. Treatment has been extended to patients other than severe GH-deficient children (who usually lack GHRH: pituitary dwarfism). In particular, patients with "partial" GH deficiency who are of short stature and Turner's syndrome are now receiving GH. To be effective the hormone must be given before the closure of the epiphyses.

Pharmacokinetics

GH has a very short half-life of approximately 25 min so plasma concentrations fluctuate widely whereas, due to its protein binding, those of IGF-1 are much more constant. As a consequence three doses of GH per week give good clinical results, although daily dosing is often used. It must be given by subcutaneous or intramuscular injection. Antibody production is frequent, but few patients need higher doses as a result of this; it may also be less of a problem with the purer preparations now available. Patients with a genetically determined complete absence of GH do not recognize GH as "self" and have the greatest tendency to produce antibodies.

Unwanted effects

- There is a transient insulin-like action which occasionally produces hypoglycaemia.
- If excessive doses are used (as may happen during illicit use by athletes) there is a risk of diabetes mellitus in predisposed individuals.
- Pain or lipoatrophy at the injection site.

ACROMEGALY

This results from excessive production of GH, almost always by an adenoma in the anterior pituitary. The clinical features arise from excessive growth of bone and soft tissue. Complex metabolic changes occur including insulin resistance with diabetes, and hypertension is common.

Production of other pituitary hormones may be abnormal, due to compression of normal pituitary tissue by the adenoma. Occasionally, the tumour will extend above the sella turcica causing compression of the optic chiasm. This usually results in a bi-temporal hemianopia progressing eventually to complete loss of vision.

The morbidity and mortality of acromegaly vary according to its severity but untreated acromegalic patients have a life expectancy approximately half that of individuals without acromegaly. It is therefore usually treated actively. Surgery by the trans-sphenoidal route is the usual treatment of choice, sometimes followed by external radiotherapy. Three groups of patients may be suitable for drug treatment:

- Those in whom an excess of growth hormone persists despite surgery and radiotherapy.
- Those with mild acromegaly.
- The elderly.

DRUGS FOR ACROMEGALY

BROMOCRIPTINE

Full details about bromocriptine can be found in Chapter 25. In normal subjects dopaminergic receptor stimulation increases secretion of growth hormone, but acromegalic patients have a paradoxical response. The long-acting dopamine agonist, bromocriptine, reduces GH secretion but the clinical response is unpredictable.

OCTREOTIDE

This synthetic derivative of somatostatin (GHRIH) is both more potent and longer-acting than the native compound. Like somatostatin, it also inhibits the release of gastro-entero-pancreatic peptide hormones, for example insulin, glucagon and gastrin via specific intestinal receptors with generation of intracellular cyclic AMP and calcium influx into the cell. It is used preoperatively and for persistent acromegaly after surgery and radiotherapy. Given by subcutaneous injection it reduces GH release and pituitary tumour size.

Additional uses of octreotide are in the management of other endocrine tumours, for example carcinoid tumours (to reduce flushing and diarrhoea), VIPoma (to reduce diarrhoea) and glucagonoma (to improve the characteristic necrolytic rash).

Unwanted effects

- Gallstones, due to suppression of cholecystokinin secretion with decreased gall bladder motility.
- Gastrointestinal upset, which usually resolves with continued treatment.

ADRENOCORTICOTROPHIC HORMONE (ACTH)

ACTH is a straight-chain polypeptide with 39 amino acids; the first 24 which form the N-terminal are essential for full biological acitivity. It is one of a family of peptides cleaved from a glycoprotein, called pro-opio-melanocortin (POMC). ACTH promotes steroidogenesis in adrenocortical cells by occupying cell surface receptors and stimulating adenylate cyclase.

Release of ACTH is triggered by the hypothalamic peptide corticotrophin releasing factor (CRF), which reaches the anterior pituitary via the portal capillary venous plexus: CRF stimulates secretion of ACTH and other POMC-derived peptides. CRF secretion is pulsatile and has a circadian rhythm which is influenced by several chemical, physical and psychological stimuli.

The main inhibitory influence on ACTH release is feedback control by circulating cortisol. This occurs at both hypothalamic and pituitary levels. Adrenal androgens, although stimulated by ACTH, play no part in feedback control.

THERAPEUTIC USES OF ACTH

ACTH preparations of animal origin have been replaced by a less allergenic synthetic peptide, tetracosactrin, which consists of the active N1-24 part of the ACTH molecule. It is given by injection and there are two formulations:

- A rapid-acting form which increases steroidogenesis for about an hour and is suitable for tests of adrenocortical function. In patients with suspected adrenal insufficiency, there is a subnormal or absent rise of plasma cortisol after intramuscular or intravenous injection.

- A depot form which is absorbed slowly into the circulation over several hours and is used as an alternative to exogenous corticosteroid therapy. In children production of a mixture of anabolic and catabolic steroids by ACTH means less risk of growth inhibition than with oral glucocorticoids alone.

Once absorbed into the circulation tetracosactrin is metabolized rapidly with a half-life of about 10 min.

Unwanted effects

- Prolonged use will produce all the features of corticosteroid excess (Chapter 47).

- Tetracosactrin has been advocated in preference to glucocorticoid administration to avoid adrenal atrophy during long-term treatment (Chapter 47). However, hypothalamic suppression still limits responsiveness of the hypothalamic pituitary–adrenal axis when ACTH is withdrawn.

PROLACTIN

Prolactin is a glycoprotein similar in structure to growth hormone but secreted by distinct cells in the anterior pituitary. The major hypothalamic control mechanism is inhibition by dopamine which stimulates specific D_2 receptors (Chapter 17). Interference with this mechanism, either by hypothalamic dysfunction, or by interruption of blood flow between hypothalamus and pituitary — the "stalk compression syndrome" — results in an increase in secretion of prolactin.

The main target tissue for prolactin is the breast, which secretes milk if primed by ovarian hormones. High levels of prolactin interfere with hypothalamic–pituitary control of gonadotrophin secretion (Chapter 48) resulting in low plasma concentrations of luteinizing hormone and to a lesser extent follicle-stimulating hormone. This leads to a failure of Graafian follicle growth and a low oestrogen state in the female. High concentrations of circulating prolactin are physiological during pregnancy and lactation, and release is stimulated by stress.

HYPERPROLACTINAEMIA

Persistent hyperprolactinaemia is usually due to a micro-adenoma of the anterior pituitary. Dopamine receptor antagonist drugs such as phenothiazines (Chapter 22) can also be responsible. In a younger woman hyperprolactinaemia can produce amenorrhoea, infertility and symptoms of oestrogen deficiency (e.g. vaginal dryness and dyspareunia, galactorrhoea and osteoporosis). In men it may cause hypogonadism. The long-acting dopamine receptor agonist bromocriptine (Chapter 25) can be used to suppress prolactin secretion.

GONADOTROPHIN-RELEASING HORMONE (GnRH)

Also known as luteinizing hormone-releasing hormone (LHRH), this decapeptide is synthesized in the hypothalamus and controls release of both luteinizing hormone (LH) and follicle-stimulating hormone (FSH). Surface receptors on the secretory cells are induced by repeated stimulation with GnRH, but pulsatile exposure is essential to maintain responsiveness. (Tolerance to constant-rate infusions of GnRH is rapid due to downregulation of receptors.)

CLINICAL USE OF SYNTHETIC GnRH (GONADORELIN)

In patients with hypogonadotrophic hypogonadism, particularly when there is a lack of endogenous GnRH, repeated pulses of exogenous GnRH will often lead to normal pituitary–gonadal function, including a regular menstrual cycle in females. The hormone is usually infused subcutaneously from a portable syringe-driving pump.

GnRH ANALOGUES

Examples: buserelin, goserelin.

Structurally similar to the natural hormone, these analogues initially stimulate GnRH receptors but subsequently inhibit them by promoting receptor downregulation. Buserelin can be given either by subcutaneous injection or by nasal spray. It has a short half-life. Goserelin must be given by subcutaneous injection and is available as an oily depot preparation. Depot formulations maintain gonadotrophic receptor blockade for up to 4 weeks after a single injection.

Clinical uses of GnRH analogues

- The main use is to reduce testosterone secretion in men with prostatic cancer. Reduction to castrate levels can be maintained but an initial rise in testosterone from receptor stimulation is undesirable. An anti-androgen (Chapter 49) is usually given to counteract this effect.
- Treatment of endometriosis and advanced breast cancer in women by reducing oestrogen secretion.
- Buserelin is also used in female patients undergoing preparation for assisted conception by methods such as *in vitro* fertilization (IVF) or gamete intrafallopian transfer (GIFT). In these patients ovulation is targeted on a particular date. Buserelin inhalation will "switch off" their natural cyclical menstrual activity. Ovarian stimulation treatment (see gonadotrophins) is then begun to achieve maturation of oocytes at the time chosen for the procedure of IVF or GIFT.

Unwanted effects

- Hypogonadism, for example loss of libido, gynaecomastia, vasomotor instability.

GONADOTROPHINS

Luteinizing hormones (LH) and follicle-stimulating hormone (FSH) are glycoproteins. Release of both hormones from the anterior pituitary is stimulated by pulsatile exposure to gonadotrophin-releasing hormone (GnRH), A negative feedback by inhibin, a hormone of gonadal origin, selectively inhibits FSH secretion. In addition, both gonadotrophins are subject to negative feedback from gonadal steroids, including progesterone.

In the male, LH acts on specific receptors on the surface of the Leydig cells in the testes and stimulates adenylate cyclase, leading mainly to the production of testosterone. FSH acts in a similar way on the Sertoli cells of the seminiferous tubules, stimulating the formation of a specific androgen-binding protein.

In the female, receptors for FSH and LH are found in granulosa cells of ovarian follicles. FSH is responsible for follicular development. The rising oestradiol concentration in the late follicular phase has a positive feedback effect on secretion of LH, and produces a short-lived surge of LH release. This triggers rupture of the follicle, release of the ovum, and formation of the corpus luteum (Chapter 48).

SOURCE OF GONADOTROPHIN FOR THERAPEUTIC USE

FSH is extracted from urine obtained from postmenopausal women (human menopausal gonadotrophin: HMG). It is administered by intramuscular injection in either a relatively unpurified form, menotrophin, which contains some LH or as a more purified preparation, urofollitrophin, containing very little LH. A third preparation, human chorionic gonadotrophin (HCG) is secreted by the placenta and extracted from the urine of pregnant women. It contains large quantities of LH.

Clinical uses of gonadotrophins

- Treatment of infertility when deficiency of gonadal stimulation by gonadotrophin is the limiting factor. Intramuscular menotrophin encourages the development of a single mature Graafian follicle. Release of the ovum is then stimulated by a single large intramuscular injection of HCG.

- Preparation for assisted conception (IVF or GIFT) involves giving large doses of menotrophin to stimulate the development of several follicles. These ova are then "harvested" by aspiration of the follicles.

- Male patients with gonadotrophin deficiency require long courses of gonadotrophin injections initially to achieve external sexual maturation and then to maintain satisfactory sperm production. Spermatozoa take 70–80 days to mature, and a year or more of treatment may be needed to achieve optimal response. A combination of menotrophin and HCG is usually given.

Unwanted effects

- The main risk in the female is hyper-stimulation of the ovaries which can become grossly enlarged as a result of multiple follicle stimulation leading to considerable abdominal pain, ascites and even pleural effusions.

- In the male the commonest problem is gynaecomastia.

POSTERIOR PITUITARY HORMONES

VASOPRESSIN

Vasopressin is a nonapeptide, often referred to as arginine vasopressin (AVP) because human vasopressin has an arginine residue in position 8. It is released from neurosecretory cells of the hypothalamus and transported down the axons of the nerve cells which form the pituitary stalk. AVP is stored in the nerve endings in the posterior pituitary and released in response to stimulation of the hypothalamus via osmoreceptors, sodium receptors and volume receptors.

AVP has two main target tissues: vascular smooth muscle (V_1-receptors) and distal tubules of the kidney nephron (V_2-receptors). In the latter it facilitates water reabsorption to produce a more concentrated urine. Vasoconstriction sufficient to raise blood pressure only occurs at high blood AVP concentrations. The renal effect is associated with the intracellular production of cyclic AMP, whereas the effect on vascular smooth muscle is mediated by calcium influx. Vasopressin is metabolized in many tissues including the liver and kidney, and has a very short half-life of about 10 min. It is given therapeutically by subcutaneous or intramuscular injection or by intravenous infusion.

Clinical uses of vasopressin

- Treatment of cranial diabetes insipidus (see below), although the long-acting derivative desmopressin is usually used for maintenance treatment.

- To control bleeding from oesophageal varices in portal hypertension. Aqueous vasopressin is infused intravenously to produce vasoconstriction.

DESMOPRESSIN

AVP has a short duration of action. By deamination of residue 1 and substitution of D-arginine for L-arginine in position 8 the diuretic effect is increased, the pressor effect is reduced and the action is prolonged. The resulting compound, known as des-amino-D-arginine vasopressin (DDAVP or desmopressin), is absorbed through the nasal mucosa and is most conveniently administered by a metered-dose nasal spray. It can also be given parenterally. An additional action of parenteral DDAVP is to increase clotting factor VIII concentration in blood; it is sometimes given to patients with haemophilia.

Like the native hormone, DDAVP is metabolized in the liver and kidney, but has a longer half-life of around 75 min.

Unwanted effects

- Potentiation by drugs which mimic AVP (see treatment of nephrogenic diabetes insipidus) producing dilutional hyponatraemia as a result of excess water retention.

DIABETES INSIPIDUS

Diabetes insipidus (DI) is usually caused by a failure of secretion of AVP in the hypothalamus ("cranial" DI). Tumours, inflammatory and granulomatous conditions such as sarcoidosis, and trauma to the hypothalamus are the main causes. A distinct condition known as nephrogenic DI occurs when the kidney is unresponsive to vasopressin. It results from a hereditary deficiency of renal AVP receptors or arises as a consequence of drug therapy, particularly with lithium (Chapter 23) or the tetracycline demeclocycline. DI presents clinically with thirst, polyuria and a tendency to high plasma osmolality with an inappropriately low urine osmolality. Vasopressin produces concentrated urine in patients with cranial DI but the response in nephrogenic DI is impaired. Treatment of cranial DI is by nasal administration of desmopressin.

Treatment of nephrogenic diabetes insipidus

To a greater extent than in cranial DI the patient is dependent on taking an adequate fluid intake. Paradoxically, thiazide diuretics (Chapter 15) can reduce the polyuria as can carbamazepine (Chapter 24). Chlorpropamide (Chapter 43) is also used but acceptability is limited by hypoglycaemia. The latter two compounds are believed to sensitize the renal tubule to the effect of AVP.

OXYTOCIN

This is discussed in Chapter 48.

47

Corticosteroid (Glucocorticoid and Mineralocorticoid) Hormones

STRUCTURE OF STEROID HORMONES

Steroid hormones constitute a range of compounds synthesized mainly in the adrenal cortex and the gonads. They are derived from cholesterol and share a common nucleus (Fig. 47.1). In addition to the 17-carbon ring structure, methyl groups can be present at positions 10 and 13, the extra carbon atoms being numbered 19 and 18 respectively. In addition, a further two carbon atoms (numbered 20 and 21) can be attached at position 17 to form a side-chain.

The steroid hormones produced principally in the adrenal cortex (adrenal corticosteroids) are classified according to their effects into glucocorticoid and mineralocorticoid hormones (see below and Table 47.1). The other major group of steroid hormones, the sex hormones are considered in Chapters 48 and 49. There is some overlap in activity of individual molecules particularly when their structures are similar,

for example hydrocortisone has mainly glucocorticoid but also some mineralocorticoid activity. Synthetic analogues of these hormones do not necessarily conform to these chemical types and indeed may not even be steroids (e.g.

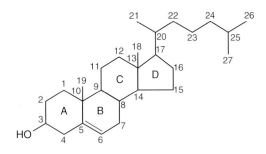

Figure 47.1 The "core" structure of steroid hormones is derived from the cholesterol molecule shown. Note: the four rings are each identified by a letter and each carbon atom by a number.

Table 47.1 Relative glucocorticoid and mineralocorticoid activities of some natural and synthetic steroid hormones

	Glucocorticoid	Mineralocorticoid
Cortisol (hydrocortisone)	1	1
Prednisolone	4	0.8
Dexamethasone	30	Negligible
Aldosterone	0	80
Fludrocortisone	10	125

diethylstilboestrol, a synthetic oestrogen). Most synthetic progestogens are 19-carbon steroids which tend to have androgenic actions as well. Synthetic androgens may be methylated giving a 20-carbon structure or demethylated (at position 18, e.g. nandrolone) giving an 18-carbon structure.

SYNTHESIS OF STEROID HORMONES

The pathways of steroid hormone synthesis are shown in Fig. 47.2.

MODE OF ACTION OF STEROID HORMONES

All steroid hormones share a common receptor mechanism. The distribution of the various receptors in different tissues gives specificity to each type of steroid hormone and defines its activity. Cytoplasmic receptors initially bind the steroid and the resulting complex is transported into the nucleus, where it binds to "hormone responsive elements" on DNA. This stimulates mRNA transcription and initiates specific intracellular protein synthesis. These proteins mediate the action of the hormone.

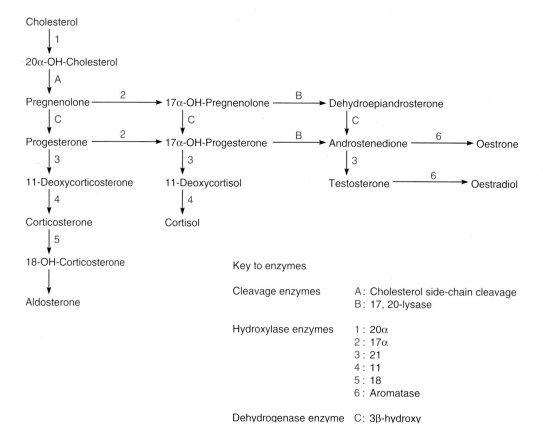

Figure 47.2 Pathways of steroid biosynthesis.

GLUCOCORTICOIDS

Cortisol (also known as hydrocortisone) is the main glucocorticoid in humans. It is synthesized in the adrenal cortex in response to ACTH from the anterior pituitary (Chapter 46). Receptors are found in many tissues giving cortisol a wide variety of actions.

ACTIONS OF GLUCOCORTICOIDS

Therapeutic doses of glucocorticoids produce a wide range of effects.

Metabolic effects

These are catabolic in nature:

- Carbohydrate: gluconeogenesis is increased and leads to increased storage of glycogen in the liver and to a lesser extent in muscle. Tissue uptake of glucose is impaired.
- Fat: redistribution of fat from the steroid-sensitive fat stores in the limbs to the steroid-resistant stores in the face, neck and trunk.
- Protein: protein is degraded to enable synthesis of glucose and to increase the available pool of amino acids, while protein synthesis is inhibited. As a result there is breakdown of tissues such as skin, muscle and bone, and an overall negative nitrogen balance.

Cardiovascular effects

Capillary permeability is decreased, which has a protective effect on blood volume and raises blood pressure. The sensitivity of vascular walls to the vasoconstrictor actions of catecholamines is also enhanced.

Immunological effects

The main effect is involution of lymphoid tissue (especially T-lymphocytes), but there is also reduced responsiveness of lymphocytes to lymphokines (Chapter 40).

Anti-inflammatory effects

The immunological and vascular actions of glucocorticoids confer anti-inflammatory activity. In addition, they inhibit mononuclear and neutrophil cell migration and their adhesion to inflamed capillary endothelium. Production of prostaglandins and leukotrienes is reduced by inhibition of the enzyme phospholipase A_2 (Chapter 30). These anti-inflammatory actions of glucocorticoids result from the production of several intracellular proteins known collectively as lipocortins.

Central nervous system effects

Plasma cortisol concentrations rise to a peak at the time of awakening and are lowest during sleep. In general, high circulating concentrations of cortisol are associated with alertness, but severe disturbances of mood may occur with abnormally high levels. Low concentrations produce a feeling of lethargy.

Mineralocorticoid effects

Natural glucocorticoids also have mineralocorticoid activity (see below). Synthetic glucocorticoid compounds are altered structurally to change the relationship between the amount of mineralocorticoid and glucocorticoid activity (Table 47.1).

PHARMACOKINETICS OF GLUCOCORTICOIDS

Both natural and synthetic glucocorticoids are used in clinical practice. They are readily absorbed from the gut. The natural glucocorticoid hydrocortisone is extensively metabolized in the gut wall and liver. Prednisone is a synthetic glucocorticoid which is effectively a prodrug because most of its activity is due to conversion in the liver to prednisolone which is preferred in clinical practice. Synthetic glucocorticoids are more potent than hydrocortisone and more slowly metabolized in the liver, giving them a longer duration of action. Substantial amounts are excreted via the kidney.

Most glucocorticoids are available in formulations for parenteral use. This does not appreciably shorten the time to onset of action which is delayed by up to 8 h while protein synthesis is stimulated intracellularly.

Plasma half-lives of all glucocorticoids are short, but their biological (i.e. effective) half-lives are long (varying from 12 h for hydrocortisone to 2 days for dexamethasone), due to their intracellular effects.

Table 47.2 Examples of diseases for which systemic glucocorticoid therapy is useful

Acute inflammatory disease
  Bronchial asthma
  Anaphylaxis and angioneurotic oedema
  Acute fibrosing alveolitis

Chronic inflammatory disease
  Connective tissue disorders, e.g. systemic lupus erythematosus, polymyositis, vasculitides
  Renal disorders, e.g. glomerulonephritis
  Hepatic disorders, e.g. chronic active hepatitis
  Bowel disorders, e.g. inflammatory bowel disease
  Eye disorders, e.g. posterior uveitis

Neoplastic disease
  Myeloma
  Lymphomas
  Lymphocytic leukaemias

Miscellaneous disorders
  Bell's palsy
  Sarcoidosis
  Organ transplantation

CLINICAL USES OF SYSTEMICALLY ADMINISTERED GLUCOCORTICOIDS

Physiological replacement therapy

Cortisol deficiency can result from:

- Primary adrenocortical destruction (Addison's disease).
- Secondary adrenocortical failure (deficient ACTH from the anterior pituitary).
- Suppression of the hypothalamic–pituitary–adrenal axis by prolonged glucocorticoid treatment at pharmacological doses (see below).
- Various enzyme defects in cortisol synthesis (congenital adrenal hyperplasia).

Hydrocortisone or an equivalent synthetic glucocorticoid is given in doses as close as possible to the amount normally secreted by the adrenal cortex. In stressful situations, for example intercurrent infection, the dose must be increased.

Pharmacological actions

The anti-inflammatory and immunosuppressive effects of glucocorticoids are used for various inflammatory diseases (especially those which are immunologically mediated) and neoplastic conditions particularly when they involve lymphoid tissue (Table 47.2). Powerful gluco-corticoids such as prednisolone with little miner-alocorticoid activity are usually chosen.

TOPICAL ADMINISTRATION OF GLUCOCORTICOIDS

Topical use of glucocorticoids can deliver high concentrations to a target site but at higher doses significant absorption into the blood can occur. Examples of the clinical uses of topical corticosteroids are given in Table 47.3.

UNWANTED EFFECTS OF GLUCOCORTICOIDS

Pharmacological doses of glucocorticoids given over long periods will produce the typical features of adrenocortical overactivity (Cushing's syndrome). Excessive glucocorticoid actions include:

- Central obesity with "buffalo hump", moon face and abdominal striae.
- Loss of supporting tissue in skin with skin atrophy, bruising, poor wound healing. Local atrophy can be marked at the site of topical steroid application.
- Osteoporosis due to catabolism of protein matrix in the bone.
- Proximal (i.e. shoulder and hip girdle) muscle wasting and weakness.

Table 47.3 Examples of topical steroid administration

Disease	Mode of administration	Chapter
Asthma	Aerosol	11
Vasomotor rhinitis		41
Eczema	Ointment or cream	52
Superficial ocular inflammation	Aqueous solution	53
Ulcerative colitis	Aqueous solution or foam enema	36
Proctitis	Suppository	36
Arthritis	Aqueous solution by intra-articular injection	32

- Hyperglycaemia, which may lead to clinical diabetes mellitus (Chapter 43).
- Peptic ulceration due to gastrointestinal prostaglandin inhibition (Chapters 31 and 35).
- Mood changes, including euphoria and occasionally psychosis.
- Posterior capsular cataracts in the eye, and exacerbation of glaucoma.
- Increased susceptibility to infection with bacteria, viruses or fungi. Activation of latent infection such as tuberculosis can also occur.
- Growth retardation in children with reduced linear bone growth and premature epiphyseal closure.
- After long-term treatment, sudden withdrawal can produce an acute adrenal crisis due to suppression of the hypothalamic–pituitary–adrenal axis (Chapter 46) and adrenal atrophy. Recovery of adrenal responsiveness can take several months. Basal cortisol secretion is restored before maximal responses, leaving patients at risk during stress and intercurrent infection.

Mineralocorticoid effects vary among the different drugs and are detailed below.

CUSHING'S SYNDROME

This syndrome is characterized by the effects of excess glucocorticoid (see unwanted effects of glucocorticoids above). There are four causes:

- Excessive secretion of ACTH by the anterior pituitary (Cushing's disease).
- Excessive secretion of ACTH from an ectopic source (most commonly carcinoma of the bronchus).
- A tumour of the adrenal cortex secreting predominantly cortisol.
- Iatrogenic: administration of glucocorticoid or ACTH in pharmacological doses.

MANAGEMENT OF CUSHING'S SYNDROME

The definitive treatment for excessive pituitary secretion of ACTH (usually from an adenoma) and for unilateral adrenal tumours is surgery, with subsequent radiotherapy in some pituitary cases. Ectopic ACTH secretion is not usually amenable to surgical cure but palliative drug treatment can be helpful. Drug treatment to reduce corticosteroid secretion is desirable for several weeks before surgery to reverse the excessive tissue catabolism and correct the metabolic disturbance.

Control of excessive glucocorticoid secretion is usually achieved by drugs which act on the adrenal cortex to inhibit the synthesis of cortisol.

INHIBITORS OF CORTISOL-SYNTHESIZING ENZYMES AND SELECTIVE ADRENAL CYTOTOXIC DRUGS

AMINOGLUTETHIMIDE

This drug inhibits 20 α-hydroxylation, an early step in steroid hormone synthesis (Fig. 47.2). It also inhibits several other hydroxylase enzymes. Aminoglutethimide is well absorbed orally and is partly metabolized in the liver and partly excreted by the kidney. Skin rashes (which are often transient) and drowsiness are the main unwanted effects. Aminoglutethimide is also useful for the treatment of metastatic carcinoma of breast and advanced carcinoma of prostate which are often dependent on steroid hormone synthesis for growth.

METYRAPONE

The main effect of this drug on corticosteroid biosynthesis is achieved by inhibition of 11β-hydroxylase (Fig. 47.2). It also inhibits cytochrome P450 in the liver which can produce important drug interactions (Chapter 2). Oral absorption is variable and extensive metabolism occurs in the liver. Gastrointestinal upset is the main unwanted effect.

MITOTANE (o, p-DDD)

This drug has a relatively selective cytotoxic effect on adrenocortical cells. Its main use is for metastasizing tumours of the adrenal cortex, either alone or in combination with aminoglutethimide.

MINERALOCORTICOIDS

Aldosterone is the principal mineralocorticoid secreted from the adrenal cortex. Hydrocortisone has much less activity (Table 47.1).

Aldosterone secretion is regulated by several factors, of which the renin–angiotensin system (Chapter 5) and a high plasma potassium are the most important. Angiotensin II acts via specific adrenal receptors which increase intracellular calcium. ACTH has little effect on aldosterone secretion.

Receptors for aldosterone are found in several tissues but its main target is the distal renal tubule. Aldosterone increases the permeability of the apical tubular membrane to sodium and stimulates the Na^+/K^+-ATPase pump which leads to active sodium reabsorption and loss of potassium into tubular urine (Chapter 15). Water is passively reabsorbed with sodium so that extracellular fluid volume and blood pressure are increased.

SYNTHETIC MINERALOCORTICOIDS

Example: fludrocortisone.

Aldosterone is almost completely inactivated at its first passage through the liver and is therefore unsuitable for oral administration. 9α-Fluorohydrocortisone (fludrocortisone) is a synthetic alternative which is well absorbed from the gut and about 10% escapes first-pass metabolism. The half-life is short, but its action is prolonged by slow absorption.

Unwanted effects

- Excessive sodium retention and potassium loss can occur with pharmacological doses. Hypertension can result; however, the expansion of blood volume stimulates atrial stretch receptors leading to secretion of atrial natriuretic peptide. The resulting natriuresis initiates an "escape" mechanism which establishes a new equilibrium between sodium intake and excretion at a higher blood volume. Consequently, oedema does not usually occur.

CLINICAL USES OF MINERALOCORTICOIDS

- Fludrocortisone is given as replacement therapy for patients with defective aldosterone production. This is usually due to primary adrenal pathology with destruction of all three zones of the cortex (Addison's disease).
- Expansion of blood volume by fludrocortisone can be used to raise blood pressure in postural hypotension resulting from autonomic neuropathy. However, it often produces supine hypertension without eliminating the postural fall in blood pressure.

PRIMARY HYPERALDOSTERONISM (CONN'S SYNDROME)

Autonomous over-secretion of aldosterone causes hypertension and a hypokalaemic alkalosis. Most cases are due to an adenoma in the zona glomerulosa of the adrenal cortex and are treated surgically. The remainder are usually due to hyperplasia of both zonae glomerulosa; these are usually less severe clinically and a potassium-sparing diuretic is the treatment of choice (Chapter 15).

48

Female Reproductive System

THE MENSTRUAL CYCLE

The endocrine function of the hypothalamic–pituitary–ovarian axis acts as a series of feedback loops to control the reproductive processes of the menstrual cycle. The ovarian oestrogens and progestogens have many effects (Fig. 48.1 describes those that are important in the actions of the steroidal contraceptives.)

Gonadotrophin-releasing hormones (GnRH)

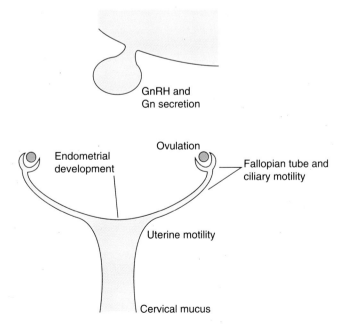

Figure 48.1   Sites of action of synthetic oestrogens and progestogens.

(Chapter 46) cause the release of follicle-stimulating hormone (FSH) and luteinizing hormone (LH) from the anterior pituitary. FSH, LH and oestradiol, which is released by the developing follicle, are responsible for follicle development and maturation during the follicular phase of the menstrual cycle. During the early part of the follicular phase the low levels of oestradiol act on the hypothalamus and anterior pituitary to limit gonadotrophin secretion and FSH and LH release. This allows the slow growth of a small number of follicles but by 5–6 days one of these starts to develop more rapidly to give a single dominant Graafian follicle. LH then stimulates the granulosa cells of this follicle to release oestradiol, which inhibits FSH release, thereby suppressing the other less mature follicles. During this time progesterone also has a weaker inhibitory effect on gonadotrophin secretion. In the latter part of the follicular phase the rising concentrations of oestradiol cause a positive feedback on the hypothalamus and pituitary. This results in a brief surge of LH and FSH release which promotes

ovulation (Fig. 48.2). After expulsion of the ovum the granulosa cells proliferate and the ruptured follicle develops into the corpus luteum which secretes increasing amounts of progesterone and oestradiol (the secretory phase). At the end of this phase and in the absence of pregnancy the corpus luteum starts to degenerate for unknown reasons and secretes less oestradiol and progesterone. This results in shedding of the endometrium and menstruation.

For conception and implantation to occur a precise sequence of events has to occur. Cervical mucus acts as a considerable barrier to passage of sperm and mucus is a reservoir for sperm for many hours after intercourse. Under the dominance of progesterone the mucus becomes less penetrable by sperm. Abnormal fallopian tube, cilia and uterine motility can result in changes in the transport of the sperm and the unfertilized and fertilized oocyte. This may alter the chance of fertilization or the embryo may reach the uterine cavity when the endometrium is not receptive to implantation.

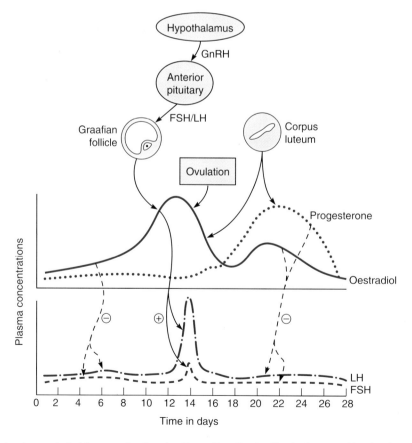

Figure 48.2 Endocrine control of the menstrual cycle. ⊖ ---, Negative feedback; ⊕ —, positive feedback.

Progesterone interferes with both fallopian tube motility and endometrial development. High levels of oestrogen increase tubal motility and accelerate the transport of the embryo into the uterine cavity (Fig. 48.1).

At the menopause, the ovary ceases to produce ova and stops producing oestrogen. Menstruation also stops at this time. Oestrogen levels do not always fall dramatically since various adrenocorticosteroids (such as androstenedione: see Chapter 47) can be converted to oestrogens.

Pregnancy is accompanied by considerable hormonal changes. The feto-placental unit together produce progressively greater quantities of oestrogen (oestriol) and progesterone which reach the maternal circulation. The placenta also produces human chorionic gonadotrophin (HCG) (Chapter 46) which reaches a peak concentration at about 50–60 days of gestation then falls. HCG stimulates progesterone production from the corpus luteum and also maintains the placenta. In pregnancy, oestrogen stimulates uterine growth by effects on cellular enzymes and also produces breast enlargement and ductal growth.

STEROIDAL CONTRACEPTIVES

Oral contraceptives are the most widely used form of contraception and contain either a combination of a synthetic oestrogen and a progestogen (a C-19 synthetic progesterone derivative) or a progestogen alone.

The oestrogen in the majority of contraceptives is ethinyloestradiol although mestranol is used in some formulations; their oestrogenic potency is similar. The progestogens in oral formulations are testosterone derivatives and are either "first generation" compounds such as norethisterone, ethynodiol, levonorgestrel, or newer agents, for example norgestimate, gestodene or desogestrel. The progestational potency of the different progestogens can vary markedly; moreover several have some androgenic, antiandrogenic, oestrogenic or antioestrogenic activity. For example, norethisterone has androgenic activity while the newer compounds, for example norgestimate, gestodene and desogestrel have an antiandrogenic effect. The antiandrogenic action is indirect and is due to an increase in serum sex hormone binding globulin (Chapter 49) which in turn reduces the free testosterone concentration.

MECHANISMS OF CONTRACEPTION

- The combination of oestrogen and progestogen exerts its contraceptive effect mainly through inhibition of ovulation. Progestogen alone inhibits ovulation in only about 40% of users, with variable inhibition in another 40%.
- The oestrogen component, and to a lesser extent the progestogen, suppress LH and FSH secretion and follicular development.
- Progestogen produces asynchronous development of the endometrium with stromal thinning which makes it less receptive to implantation. Fallopian tube motility is increased by oestrogens and decreased by progestogens which may alter transport of the gamete.
- Progestogen alters cervical mucus making it thicker and less copious thereby creating an environment more hostile to sperm penetration.

COMBINED ORAL CONTRACEPTIVE

Monophasic preparations

The "combined oral contraceptive pill" refers to preparations containing 20–35 μg (rarely 50 μg) oestrogen plus 0.5–2.5 mg progestogen (depending upon the progestational potency of the progestogen used). These are given for 21 days followed by 7 days pill-free. Twenty-eight day packs ("every day" preparations) are available which, to improve compliance, include an inert substance such as lactose during the 7 contraceptive-free days. Since the proportions of oestrogen and progestogen are kept constant, these are known as monophasic preparations.

Many combinations of oestrogen and progestogen are available. In some women it may be necessary to change the formulation to reduce minor unwanted effects such as breakthrough bleeding or weight gain during the menstrual cycle. The androgenic or antiandrogenic properties that the progestogen possesses may influence the suitability of an individual preparation to a particular patient.

Biphasic and triphasic preparations

These preparations are designed to mimic more closely the changes in steroid concentrations during the natural menstrual cycle and to reduce the metabolic effects of the progestogen by decreasing the overall intake. Several preparations are available, all of which contain ethinyl-oestradiol in combination with either norethisterone or levonorgestrel. In most preparations the oestrogen doses are kept constant, but the dose often needs to be higher than in the monophasic preparations to inhibit ovulation reliably. Progestogen doses are increased once (biphasic) or twice (triphasic) as the menstrual cycle proceeds. In other preparations both oestrogen and progestogen doses are varied once or twice. Such phasic preparations may become less necessary with the use of newer progestogens such as gestodene in monophasic pills which achieve the same cycle control without metabolic effects.

One-a-month oral preparations

The combination of a very long-acting oestrogen, quinesterol (which is taken up by body fat and is then released slowly) with a faster-acting progestogen, quingestanol acetate, is at an investigational stage. It is given as a single oral dose towards the end of the menstrual cycle and bleeding occurs 3–5 days later when progestogen levels fall. The sustained oestrogen levels then suppress FSH release during the subsequent menstrual cycle.

PROGESTOGEN-ONLY CONTRACEPTIVE

Oral progestogen

The progestogen-only pill is particularly useful for women in whom the administration of oestrogen is considered undesirable, for example, if there is a history of thromboembolic disorders (see below). It is as effective as combined pills containing $30 \mu g$ of oestrogen. A small dose of progestogen is given continuously, without a break, and must be taken within 3 h of the usual time every day. Because the dose of progestogen is low, menstruation does take place but may be irregular. Breakthrough bleeding occurs in up to 40% of women, especially when suppression of ovulation is variable. Some women become amenorrhoeic. Ectopic pregnancy may be increased in women taking the progestogen-only pill, due to impaired tubal transport.

Injectable progestogen

Intramuscular injection of the progestogen medroxy-progesterone acetate can provide contraception for up to 3 months. Although not frequently used in the UK it is widely used in some countries including the USA. Ovulation is prevented more often than with oral progestogen-only contraceptives and there is a high incidence of amenorrhoea when its use is stopped.

Subcutaneous implants of progestogens

Progestogens such as levonorgestrel can be released from implanted silicone-rubber capsules. The implants require surgical insertion and provide contraception for up to 5 years. Unwanted effects are the same as those experienced with the progestogen-only oral contraceptive, but since first-pass metabolism is avoided, lower doses of progestogen are needed.

EMERGENCY POSTCOITAL ("MORNING-AFTER") CONTRACEPTIVE

Only one product is approved for use in the UK and contains $50 \mu g$ ethinyloestradiol and $250 \mu g$ levonorgestrel. Two tablets are taken as soon as possible after unprotected intercourse but not later than 72 h after. A further two tablets are taken 12 h after the first dose. Nausea is a frequent adverse effect occurring in up to 40% of patients; vomiting can occur and an antiemetic (Chapter 34) may be needed. Absorption takes 2 h, so that vomiting after this time will not affect the efficacy of treatment. The mechanism of action may be to accelerate transport of the fertilized ovum so that it reaches the uterine cavity before the endometrium is receptive. The treatment is successful in at least 95% of cases.

PHARMACOKINETICS OF CONTRACEPTIVE STEROIDS

The synthetic oestrogens, like the naturally occurring oestradiol-17β, are well absorbed orally but are less rapidly degraded and undergo a variable amount of enterohepatic recycling. Progesterone itself is inactive orally because of extensive hepatic metabolism.

The pharmacokinetics of individual oestrogens and progestogens vary widely and data on only ethinyloestradiol and norethisterone are summarized.

Ethinyloestradiol is absorbed rapidly from the gut and peak plasma levels are reached in 1 h. It undergoes considerable first-pass metabolism and has an intermediate half-life. Enterohepatic circulation of ethinyloestradiol is responsible for maintaining effective plasma concentrations with low-dose formulations. Norethisterone is rapidly and completely absorbed from the gut and also undergoes extensive first-pass metabolism in the intestinal wall and liver. Peak plasma concentrations occur after 1–3 h and it has an intermediate half-life.

When taken according to the recommended schedule, the failure rate for the combined oral contraceptive is 0.2%. Failure of the progestogen-only pill is age-related and is up to 5% in young women, falling with decreasing fertility to about 0.3% at the age of 40 years. With the combined oral preparations contraceptive protection is lost if there is a delay of more than 12 h in taking the daily dose. In such circumstances the missed pill should be taken and additional contraceptive measures should be used for 7 days. With the progestogen-only contraceptive if there is a delay of only 3 h or more after the normal time of taking the pill then other contraceptive precautions should be taken for 2–3 days.

UNWANTED EFFECTS

Both oestrogen and progestogen have a number of minor and major unwanted effects but the incidence of the major effects, although important, is relatively low:

- Thromboembolism: the incidence of venous thromboembolic disease is increased by taking oestrogens. The risk is independent of age or parity. The mechanism is complex but includes procoagulant activity due to increased production of clotting factors X and II and decreased production of the protective antithrombin (Chapter 10). Fibrinolysis is impaired and reduced prostacyclin generation enhances platelet aggregation (Chapter 10). The risks associated with these changes are greatest in women who smoke, since smoking increases the risk of thrombogenesis.
- Cardiovascular disease: an increased risk of myocardial infarction and cerebrovascular disease occurs with use of the combined oral contraceptive and this is particularly so in women who smoke and are over the age of 35 years. In older patients mortality from cardiovascular disease associated with use of the oral contraceptive is approximately doubled. Older smokers who use the combined oral contraceptive have a six- to ten-fold increase in risk. The risk is related to oestrogen dosage and may be due to adverse changes in the plasma lipoprotein profile when a combined preparation is used (see below). However, this mechanism is speculative, and it has been suggested that enhanced thrombogenesis rather than premature atherogenesis is responsible for the excess cardiovascular effects. If older women use the combined contraceptive pill, then the lowest possible dose of oestrogen should be given with a newer progestogen that does not disturb plasma lipids.
- A small increase in blood pressure is frequently found but a significant rise can occur in about 5% of previously normotensive women and regular monitoring of blood pressure is important. A rise in blood pressure occurs in up to 15% of women with pre-existing hypertension. The mechanism is probably an increase in plasma renin activity (Chapter 5) produced by oestrogen and to a lesser extent progestogen. Blood pressure may remain elevated for some months after the combined contraceptive is stopped.
- Cancer: oral contraceptives reduce the risk of endometrial and ovarian cancers, but the effect on the incidence of cervical cancer is uncertain. Recent evidence suggests that there is little or no effect. Similar doubt exists over a link with breast cancer.
- Nausea, mastalgia, depression, headache and provocation of migraine can occur. They are probably related to the oestrogen content of the pill and can often be minimized by prescribing contraceptives with a low oestrogen content.
- Breakthrough bleeding occurs frequently in some women while in others withdrawal bleeding fails to occur. Gestodene-containing pills or triphasic preparations probably give the best cycle control. Amenorrhoea after stopping the combined contraceptive can last beyond a few months in about 5% of women and a small number can experience amenorrhoea for more than a year. A history of irregular periods

before taking the pill increases the chance of prolonged amenorrhoea.

- Metabolic effects: increased plasma triglycerides and reduced HDL cholesterol (Chapter 51) are produced by the older progestogens which may increase the risk of atherosclerosis. Oestrogens and the newer progestogens increase HDL. Progestogens (apart from the newer agents) can decrease glucose tolerance due to enhanced gluconeogenesis but the effect usually only lasts for a few months. Diabetic patients should be monitored closely when treatment is started.

- Increased skin pigmentation can occur in some women given oestrogens. The androgenic progestogens can sometimes cause or aggravate hirsutism and acne or produce weight gain.

- Effects on the liver are occasionally seen. Cholestatic jaundice can be produced by progestogens, and oestrogens increase the risk of gallstones.

DRUG INTERACTIONS

Drugs which alter the metabolism of oestrogen may cause a reduction in the efficacy of the combined pill which may result in breakthrough bleeding and contraceptive failure. Contraception failure may also occur in patients treated with anticonvulsants (e.g. barbiturates, phenytoin) or rifampicin which induce liver cytochrome P450 (Chapter 2) and some antibiotics for example ampicillin (Chapter 54) which alter the gut flora and thereby decrease the enterohepatic circulation of the oestrogen. A pill containing 50 μg of ethinyloestradiol should be used if these drugs are given long-term and alternative methods of contraception used for the duration of a course of antibiotics and for 7 days after (4 weeks in the case of rifampicin).

NON-CONTRACEPTIVE USES OF CONTRACEPTIVES

The combined contraceptive can be used:

- To reduce excessive blood loss due to menorrhagia.
- To reduce the pain of dysmenorrhoea.
- To treat premenstrual tension.
- To treat endometriosis.

HORMONE REPLACEMENT THERAPY (HRT)

Treatment with oestrogens during the peri- and postmenopausal period is now widespread. HRT is used for two indications:

- Relief of symptoms associated with oestrogen deficiency: these include vasomotor instability (hot flushes and night sweats), and altered sexual and urinary function. Vasomotor instability results from resetting of the hypothalamic temperature set-point so that it perceives that the body is warmer than it is. Vasodilation and sweating result in an attempt to disperse heat. The mechanism is uncertain but may be due to high concentrations of gonadotrophic hormones. Loss of connective tissue in the vagina and trigone of the bladder underlies many of the other problems. Other postmenopausal symptoms such as irritability and depression are less certainly related to oestrogen deficiency.

- Prevention of long-term effects of oestrogen withdrawal: bone loss leading to osteoporosis (Chapter 45) and an increased susceptibility to fracture occurs after the menopause. Cardiovascular and cerebrovascular disease are also increased. The cause of the increased cardiovascular disease is uncertain. Unfavourable changes in lipids may be part of the explanation, due to a reduced HDL$_2$ cholesterol subfraction and increased LDL cholesterol (Chapter 51). However, an independent effect of oestrogen on reducing plasma fibrinogen (a factor in thrombogenesis) may be more important. Oestrogen receptors are also found on the cells of the arterial wall, and stimulation decreases arterial resistance and increases vessel compliance which may also be important.

Oestrogen replacement will reduce the symptoms of postmenopausal deficiency although relief may take up to 3 months. Beneficial effects on bone density have also been clearly demonstrated (Chapter 45) but the effect on cardiovascular disease is less well established. Unopposed oral conjugated equine oestrogens (i.e. without progestogen) in postmenopausal women reduce the risk of cardiovascular disease and stroke by about 50%, but it is not known if the use of combined oestrogen/progestogen preparations has the same effect or if parenteral delivery is effective. The paradoxical effects of hormonal contraception and HRT on cardiovascular disease may be due to the lower oestrogen dose used for HRT. Treatment for symptom relief probably should be given for at least 6 months to perimenopausal women after which withdrawal can be attempted to see if symptoms have spontaneously resolved. The duration of treatment for the prevention of osteoporosis (between 5 and 10 years) is discussed in Chapter 45.

MODE OF ADMINISTRATION

Unopposed oestrogens should only be given for short periods. If treatment is required for more than a few weeks to a woman who has a uterus, then progestogen is also needed to prevent breakthrough bleeding. Continuous oestrogen is supplemented with progestogen for 12 days each calendar month or with continuous progestogen if withdrawal bleeding is to be avoided. One of four routes can be used to administer HRT.

Oral

Natural oestrogen such as oestradiol, or conjugated equine oestrogen are preferred to a synthetic oestrogen such as ethinyloestradiol. Norethisterone or norgestrel are usually given when a progestogen is needed.

A new approach is to give tibolone, a synthetic molecule with combined weak oestrogenic, progestogenic and adrenogenic properties. Tibolone reduces the risk of withdrawal bleeding and progestogenic unwanted effects (see below). Taken continuously, it reduces postmenopausal symptoms and prevents bone loss. Vaginal bleeding can occur in women who still produce some endogenous oestrogen and therefore it is usually reserved for patients who are at least one year postmenopausal.

In a few patients with extensive endometriosis at hysterectomy, unopposed progestogen can be used initially to encourage regression of the residual endometriotic tissue.

Vaginal

Oestrogen cream or pessaries can be used to treat vaginal atrophy and dyspareunia and can relieve perimenopausal urinary symptoms such as frequency and dysuria. Considerable systemic absorption occurs with some formulations and oral progestogen may be needed. They are used daily for 2–3 weeks initially and then applied twice weekly for as long as required.

Subcutaneous implants

Oestradiol can be surgically implanted as pellets which release drug for up to 6 months. The major use for this option is when compliance is poor, perhaps due to nausea with oral oestrogen. Oral progestogen must also be given for 10–12 days each month if the woman has a uterus, and continued for up to 2 years after stopping oestrogen to prevent vaginal bleeding from persistent high oestrogen levels.

Transdermal

Oestradiol patches, which are effective for 3–4 days, have been available for some time. More recently a combined oestradiol/norethisterone patch has been introduced to avoid the need for oral progestogen. Avoidance of first-pass metabolism means that a lower dose of progestogen can be used transdermally, which might reduce unwanted effects.

UNWANTED EFFECTS

- Breakthrough bleeding can be troublesome, but regular withdrawal bleeds during the cycle are common, and may be preceded by symptoms of premenstrual tension.
- Breast pain and abdominal or leg cramps due to the oestrogen or progestogen component.
- Nausea and vomiting, most commonly with ethinyloestradiol.
- Depression, irritability, loss of energy and poor concentration due to progestogen.
- Increased risk of cancer. Endometrial hyperplasia can result from the unopposed use of oestrogen which increases the risk of endometrial carcinoma after 2–3 years of treatment. Progestogen prevents this hyperplastic response. A link with breast cancer is unproven but if it exists the increased risk is small. The effect of HRT in women with previous endometrial or breast cancer is unknown. Although these tumours can be oestrogen-dependent it is not known whether HRT carries a risk after a "curative" procedure.
- Unlike the combined oral contraceptive, HRT does not increase the risk of venous

thromboembolic disease, and is not contra-indicated in patients with a history of such disease. Blood pressure is also rarely increased with most patients actually having a slight fall.

- Because of the low oestrogen dose HRT probably does not provide reliable contraception for the perimenopausal woman.

UTERINE MOTILITY

Plasma concentrations of progesterone and oestradiol increase progressively during pregnancy as placental synthesis increases. Some studies have suggested that progesterone levels fall in the weeks prior to labour. Oestrogens and progesterone appear to contribute in opposing ways to the onset and progress of labour but their roles have not been fully defined. Overall the various actions of oestradiol promote uterine contractility while those of progesterone diminishes contractility:-

- Oestradiol increases the number of uterine oxytocin receptors and oxytocin release from the posterior pituitary; it increases gap junctions; fundal dominance of uterine contractility is increased by enhancing the functioning of the pacemaker at the uterotubular junction; the synthesis of prostaglandins is increased; the sensitivity of the uterus to their effects is also increased.

- In contrast, progesterone decreases gap junctions and diminishes pacemaker activity; it also decreases the sensitivity of the uterus to oxytocin and prostaglandins.

Limited data suggest that oestradiol increases the breakdown of collagen in the cervix thereby promoting softening while progesterone reduces this softening process.

DRUGS THAT STIMULATE UTERINE MOTILITY

Three major types of drugs are used to stimulate uterine activity. Oxytocin and prostaglandins are used to induce labour and late abortion. Ergometrine alone or in combination with oxytocin is used only to prevent postpartum haemorrhage (see below).

OXYTOCIN

Mechanism of action and uses

Oxytocin is a peptide which contains nine amino acids and is secreted from the posterior pituitary gland particularly during the second stage of labour and during breast feeding. Oxytocin is essential for the expulsion of milk from the lumen of the alveolus into the ducts during breast feeding. Without oxytocin the availability of milk to the baby is markedly diminished.

Whether oxytocin is essential for the onset of labour is unclear. The uterus is relatively insensitive to oxytocin until close to term when there is an increase in uterine oxytocin receptors. During the second stage of labour the fetal pituitary also secretes increased amounts of oxytocin and this may contribute to uterine contractility during labour. Oxytocin is used for the induction of labour and to augment contractions when they are deemed inadequate. It is given together with ergometrine (as syntometrine) to prevent postpartum haemorrhage.

Oxytocin, unlike prostaglandin E_2, does not significantly soften the cervix, therefore, it is reserved for inductions near term when the cervix is naturally soft, or when cervical softening has been produced by prior intravaginal administration of a prostaglandin (see below).

Pharmacokinetics

Oral absorption is erratic and oxytocin is administered intravenously by continuous infusion. The dosage is increased at regular intervals until contractions occur at about 2 min intervals. Close monitoring is required throughout labour and the dosage adjusted when necessary.

Unwanted effects

- The main adverse effect is uterine hypertonus, which produces fetal distress due to reduced fetal blood supply; uterine rupture can also occur. Hypertonus can be reversed by stopping drug administration and giving a β_2-adrenoceptor stimulant such as salbutamol (see below).

- Oxytocin differs from vasopressin (antidiuretic hormone) in only two amino acid residues and has only weak antidiuretic activity; however, high doses of oxytocin may cause water retention.

PROSTAGLANDINS

Mechanisms of action and uses

The natural prostaglandins (particularly PGE_2) (Chapter 30) are involved in the physiological onset of labour. They are synthesized by the decidua and fetal tissues. PGE_2 is a potent stimulant of uterine contractions and, unlike oxytocin, it can also soften the cervix.

Inducing very early abortion a few weeks after a missed period can be achieved with PGE analogues but the risk of incomplete abortion is high. Physical methods such as suction are commonly used prior to week 12 of pregnancy.

Prostaglandins (E_2 and $F_{2\alpha}$) or their analogues are given as a single dose intra-amniotically or extra-amniotically to induce abortion in the second trimester. A high success rate is achieved with less adverse effects than intravenous administration, but large doses are used intra-amniotically and even relatively small amounts leaking into the circulation can cause cardiovascular symptoms. $PGF_{2\alpha}$ has about one-tenth the potency of PGE_2. PGE_2 is most widely used in the UK but analogues of $PGF_{2\alpha}$ are used in the USA for inducing late abortion. Gemeprost (a PGE_1 analogue) is given vaginally to soften the cervix prior to surgical abortion. The long-term physical complications of inducing late abortion with prostaglandins (such as cervical incompetence) are less than those using surgical abortion techniques.

Prostaglandin E_2, alone or together with oxytocin, causes delivery in cases of intrauterine fetal death or the induction of labour prior to term. The overall success rate for inducing labour at term is similar for oxytocin and prostaglandins.

Carboprost, a prostaglandin $F_{2\alpha}$ analogue, is used to reduce postpartum haemorrhage in uncontrolled haemorrhage not responding to syntometrine (see below).

Pharmacokinetics

Vaginal suppositories of PGE_2 are administered several hours before a planned induction of labour in order to soften the cervix. This is accompanied by uterine contractions in some women and a significant percentage may go into labour. A continuous intravenous infusion of PGE_2 is given for induction of labour, with the dose rate increased at about 30-min intervals until labour is established. Carboprost is usually given intramuscularly although intra-myometrial fundal injection through the abdominal wall has also been used, and may act faster.

Unwanted effects

- Uterine hypertonus occurs with overdosage and this should be treated by stopping the prostaglandin infusion and administration of a β_2-adrenoceptor agonist; the hypertonus lasts longer than that produced with oxytocin.
- Gastrointestinal disturbances particularly diarrhoea.
- Erythema at the infusion site.

ERGOMETRINE

Mechanism of action and use

Ergometrine is given at the time of delivery of the anterior shoulder of the baby to cause a tonic contraction of the uterus, thereby reducing postpartum haemorrhage. Syntometrine is a mixture of oxytocin and ergometrine which causes a more rapid and sustained contraction with fewer adverse effects.

Pharmacokinetics

Ergometrine is given intravenously or by intramuscular injection.

Unwanted effects

- Hypertension due to α-adrenoceptor stimulation (Chapter 4).
- Nausea, vomiting or headache.

ANTIPROGESTOGENIC AGENTS

Example: mifepristone.

Mechanism of action and effects

Mifepristone is a derivative of the progestogen norethinderone. It is a potent antiprogestogen which also has antiglucocorticoid activity. In the uterus it retards endometrial development, leading to increased stomal activity and inhibition of glandular activity. Endometrial degenerative changes ensue, with menstrual bleeding. These changes reflect withdrawal of progestogenic action. Short-term administration inhibits the release of gonadotrophins from the pituitary.

When mifepristone is given during pregnancy, the withdrawal of progestogenic support for the endometrium results in disruption of placental function and increased myometrial contraction in response to prostaglandins. Synthesis of prostaglandins is also increased and degradation reduced by mifepristone. The uterine cervix is softened and dilated, favouring uterine evacuation.

Pharmacokinetics

Oral absorption of mifepristone is good. It is metabolized slowly by the liver generating an active metabolite. The half-life is long.

Unwanted effects

- Heavy menstrual bleeding.
- Nausea, vomiting, abdominal pain.
- Fatigue, which affects most patients.

Clinical uses

- Abortion: the success of mifepristone given alone is greatest in the first 9 weeks of amenorrhoea. The addition of exogenous prostaglandin increases the successful abortion rate to greater than 90% in early pregnancy.
- Contraception: a theoretical use of mifepristone is either to inhibit ovulation by suppressing the release of luteinizing hormone or to induce menstruation in the late phase of the menstrual cycle. It has also been used as a postcoital contraceptive with success. Mifepristone is not currently licensed in the UK for contraception.
- Treatment of Cushing's syndrome: mifepristone can be given to suppress cortisol secretion induced by excess corticotrophin secretion (Chapter 46).

UTERINE RELAXANTS

Examples: salbutamol, terbutaline, ritodrine.

Prematurity is the largest cause of neonatal morbidity and mortality. β_2-Adrenoceptor agonists such as salbutamol and terbutaline can inhibit uterine contractions. However, the long-term effectiveness of these agents is limited in women undergoing premature labour and the overall impact of the β_2-adrenoceptor stimulants on neonatal morbidity and mortality is small.

Pharmacokinetics

Given by intravenous infusion or intramuscular injection to treat premature labour, and subsequently by mouth until up to the 37th week of pregnancy (see also Chapter 11).

Unwanted effects

- Elevated maternal and fetal heart rate and hypotension at high doses.
- Nausea and vomiting.
- Flushing and sweating.

Androgens and Anabolic Steroids

Naturally occurring androgens are 19-carbon steroids made in the adrenal cortex and gonads, which have characteristic actions on the reproductive tract and other tissues as well as an anabolic effect on metabolism. A number of synthetic androgenic steroids have been developed. When the predominant drug action is anabolic rather than on reproductive tissues the substance is described as an ''anabolic steroid''. Although there are a number of medical uses for such compounds, they have achieved notoriety because of their abuse by athletes to enhance muscle development.

Testosterone is the most powerful and major androgen secreted by the gonads when stimulated by the gonadotrophins (Chapter 46). The adrenal cortex, stimulated by ACTH, releases a greater proportion of dehydroepiandrosterone and androstenedione (Fig. 47.2).

TESTOSTERONE

Actions of testosterone

- Sexual differentiation in the fetus.
- Sexual development of the male at puberty.
- Spermatogenesis in the adult male.
- Metabolic actions: testosterone is a powerful anabolic agent producing a positive nitrogen balance with an increase in the bulk of tissues such as muscle, bone, skin and liver. It also induces several liver enzymes including steroid hydroxylases.
- Haematological actions: testosterone stimulates production of erythropoietin by the kidneys leading to polycythaemia.

Pharmacokinetics

- Oral preparations: testosterone is well absorbed from the gut but is almost completely degraded by first-pass metabolism in the gut wall and liver. The ester testosterone undecanoate is absorbed via lacteals into the lymphatic system, thus avoiding hepatic metabolism.
- Subcutaneous implant: implantation of a pellet of testosterone subcutaneously results in gradual absorption into the systemic circulation over several months. A minor surgical procedure is necessary.
- Testosterone esters for depot injection: the most popular form of replacement therapy for hypogonadal men is a regular intramuscular injection of a testosterone ester which is absorbed gradually from an oily solution. Examples include testosterone enanthate and testosterone propionate.

Circulating androgens are bound largely to a specific transport protein, sex hormone binding globulin (SHBG) which has a greater affinity for androgens than for oestrogen.

Unwanted effects

- In adolescents, initial nitrogen retention and a spurt in linear growth is followed by premature epiphyseal closure.
- Conversion to oestrogens by aromatase results in gynaecomastia in some patients (Fig. 47.2).
- Potentially atherogenic effects on plasma lipids with a rise in LDL cholesterol and a fall in HDL cholesterol (Chapter 51).
- Suppression of gonadotrophin release with diminished testis size and reduced spermatogenesis (Chapter 46).

Clinical use of testosterone

The main clinical use for testosterone is for replacement therapy in hypogonadal males but it is often abused by athletes for its anabolic activity.

DANAZOL

This androgen derivative is described as an "impeded" androgen. It has little androgenic effect on peripheral tissues and is not convertible to an oestrogen. Its main property is feedback inhibition of gonadotrophin and gonadotrophin-releasing hormone secretion. Danazol is well absorbed orally, metabolized in the liver and has a short half-life.

Unwanted effects

- Mainly a consequence of the weak androgenic activity (see testosterone).

Clinical uses of danazol

- To reduce gonadal activity in endometriosis, menorrhagia and premenstrual syndrome (particularly when mastalgia is a problem).
- Like true androgens it has a beneficial effect in angio-oedema and in some cases of idiopathic thrombocytopenic purpura.

ANABOLIC STEROIDS

Examples: nandrolone, stanozolol.

Anabolic steroids are most frequently encountered as drugs of abuse to improve athletic performance. In medical practice there are few indications with little evidence for efficacy. Stanozolol is given orally and nandrolone by intramuscular injections in a depot formulation.

Unwanted effects

- Androgenic effects may be troublesome in women.
- Stanozolol can cause cholestatic jaundice and liver tumours, after long-term use.

Clinical uses

- Nandrolone: the promotion of erythropoiesis in aplastic anaemias, or as palliative therapy in disseminated cancer of the breast.
- Stanozolol: for hereditary angio-oedema and for the vascular manifestations of Behçet's syndrome.

ANTIANDROGENS

CYPROTERONE ACETATE

This 21-carbon steroid is a progestogen, a weak glucocorticoid (Chapter 47), and at high doses it has an inhibitory action on peripheral androgen receptors. Its progestational activity includes feedback inhibition of gonadotrophin secretion.

Pharmacokinetics

It is well absorbed orally, metabolized in the liver and has a long half-life of 2 days.

Unwanted effects

- Inhibition of spermatogenesis and ovulation.
- Reduction in libido and potency in males.

FLUTAMIDE

Flutamide is a relatively "pure" antiandrogen, that is, it is without significant glucocorticoid or progestogenic actions. It is well absorbed orally, metabolized in the liver and has a short half-life. The major metabolite 2-hydroxyflutamide is more active than the parent compound.

Unwanted effects

- Antiandrogenic, for example gynaecomastia.
- Gastrointestinal upset.
- Liver tumours have been reported in animals.

CLINICAL USES OF ANTIANDROGENS

The main use of antiandrogens is in carcinoma of the prostate, often in conjunction with GnRH analogue (Chapter 46). Cyproterone acetate has also been used in male sexual offenders as "chemical castration". In females it can be given for manifestations of hyperandrogenization such as acne, hirsuitism and virilism.

5α-REDUCTASE INHIBITORS

Example: finasteride.

Mechanism of action and effects

5α-Reductase is an enzyme associated with androgen-dependent target cells. It is responsible for the conversion of testosterone to dihydrotestosterone (DHT) which is the hormone responsible for most of the pubertal changes in the male and for prostatic growth. DHT has a greater affinity for and a slower dissociation from the androgen receptor than testosterone. In the adult male finasteride can produce regression of benign prostatic hypertrophy and improve the symptoms of prostatism. Treatment must be continued for several months and only about 50% of patients will show a clinical response.

Pharmacokinetics

A single oral dose of finasteride inhibits 5α-reductase for up to 1 week.

Adverse effects

- Mild sexual dysfunction, for example impotence, decreased libido. This is limited because of the lack of effect on testosterone.

50

Anaemia

A blood concentration of haemoglobin below $135\,\mathrm{g\,l^{-1}}$ in males or $115\,\mathrm{g\,l^{-1}}$ in females constitutes anaemia. The important causes are:

- Blood loss by haemorrhage.
- Increased red cell destruction by haemolysis.
- Inadequate red cell production due to vitamin B$_{12}$ or folate deficiency or to bone marrow replacement (for example by malignancy) or bone marrow depression.

Anaemias are classified by cell size and haemoglobin content:

- Microcytic hypochromic, for example iron deficiency, thalassemia, sideroblastic anaemia.
- Macrocytic, normochromic, for example folate or B$_{12}$ deficiency.
- Normocytic normochromic, for example acute blood loss, haemolysis, bone marrow depression.

IRON

Dietary iron is absorbed from the duodenum and upper jejunum. Most is in the ferric form although ferrous iron is absorbed better; conversion of ferric to ferrous iron is aided by reducing agents such as ascorbic acid, while gastric acid increases its solubility. Absorption is substantially increased in iron deficiency. Iron binds to the protein apoferritin in mucosal cells to form ferritin. Excess iron is transferred to the blood where it is bound to the globulin transferrin and

transported to the bone marrow and iron stores. Most of the iron in the body is found in circulating red cells. When ageing red cells are broken down by the reticuloendothelial system, the released iron is recycled.

IRON DEFICIENCY

The main cause of iron deficiency is abnormal loss of blood, particularly from the gut or exaggerated menstrual loss. Iron malabsorption may result from disease of the upper small intestine, for example coeliac disease, or following partial gastrectomy. Dietary deficiency can be a contributory factor but is rarely the sole cause.

THERAPEUTIC IRON PREPARATIONS

ORAL IRON

Oral supplements are usually preferred and given as ferrous salts, for example sulphate, fumarate or gluconate. Tablets are normally used but some patients find a syrup more acceptable. A dose of 200 mg of elemental iron produces the maximum rate of rise of haemoglobin; about one-third of this dose will be absorbed. Modified-release iron formulations are sometimes given to improve tolerance but much of the iron is released beyond the site where it is best absorbed. Side-effects can often be avoided by reducing the dose of a standard formulation and by taking it with food.

Unwanted effects

- Gastrointestinal intolerance, especially nausea and dyspepsia. The prevalence of these effects depends on both the dose of elemental iron and on psychological factors, rather than the formulation.
- Diarrhoea or constipation. These are not dose-related.
- Patients should be warned that oral iron will turn their stools black.

PARENTERAL IRON

Parenteral iron preparations are used for patients with intractable unwanted effects from oral preparations, those with severe uncorrectable malabsorption or with continuing heavy blood loss, and when compliance with oral treatment is poor. Parenteral iron does not raise the haemoglobin faster than oral iron.

Intramuscular: iron–sorbitol–citric–acid

This complexed iron preparation is rapidly absorbed from an intramuscular site. Transferrin is saturated by high blood concentrations and about one-third of the iron is lost in urine, which may darken on standing. Approximately 30% is incorporated into red cells, the remainder of the retained iron being stored by macrophages in liver, bone marrow, spleen, etc.

Unwanted effects

- Staining of the skin.
- Metallic taste.
- Pain at the injection site.

Intravenous: iron–dextran

It is not bound to transferrin but accumulates in reticulo-endothelial cells. It is usually given as a "total dose" intravenous infusion, when the approximate total body deficit (haemoglobin and body stores) is estimated from the patient's size and haemoglobin concentration then replaced at a single slow infusion. The complex can be used intramuscularly but is very slowly absorbed from the injection site. Iron–dextran has recently been withdrawn in the UK.

Unwanted effects

- Minor side-effects include flushing, headache, bronchospasm, diffuse pains and urticaria.
- Anaphylactoid reactions including cardiovascular collapse. Facilities for resuscitation should always be available.

FOLIC ACID

Folic acid (as conjugated polyglutamates) is ingested mainly in fresh leaf vegetables (in which it is heat labile) and in liver (where it seems less so). It is absorbed principally in the jejunum becoming metabolized to the monoglutamate in the process. This is transported in the blood to the liver, where it is reduced to tetrahydrofolic acid. Tetrahydrofolic acid is involved in synthesis of pyrimidines and purines and hence of DNA (see Chapter 55). The most obvious result of deficiency is a macrocytic anaemia with the presence of megaloblasts in the marrow, a feature which it shares with B_{12} deficiency.

FOLATE DEFICIENCY

Folate deficiency may arise for a number of reasons:

- Dietary: folate stores are adequate for a few weeks only. Lack of folate is uncommon in standard western diets, but may be more common in the diet of elderly patients.
- Pregnancy: increased requirements.
- Malabsorption: coeliac disease, tropical sprue.
- Drugs: anticonvulsants (especially phenytoin (Chapter 24)), methotrexate (Chapter 55), pyrimethamine (Chapter 54).
- Haemolysis: folate is not recycled, unlike iron.

THERAPEUTIC USE OF FOLIC ACID

For most patients with folate deficiency, folic acid tablets are given. Parenteral treatment is rarely needed. For patients receiving drugs which inhibit the enzyme dihydrofolate reductase (e.g. methotrexate; Chapter 55) it is necessary to "by-pass" this enzyme blockade by giving folinic acid (5-formyl tetrahydrofolic acid).

Unwanted effects

- Treatment of combined vitamin B_{12} and folate deficiency with folate alone may correct the anaemia but the neurological damage can continue.

VITAMIN B_{12}

The term vitamin B_{12} is usually used to cover all the cobalamin compounds which have biological activity. Bacteria are the only organisms which can synthesize cobalamin *de novo*. Humans obtain vitamin B_{12} from meat, and particularly liver, but also from dairy products. Absorption is by an unusual mechanism; dietary cobalamin is complexed with a glycoprotein called intrinsic factor which is produced by gastric parietal cells. This complex is absorbed principally from the terminal ileum.

In the blood it is transported by specific binding proteins (transcobalamins) and is rapidly taken up by the tissues, especially the liver, where about 50% of the body content of B_{12} is stored.

Vitamin B_{12} is essential for isomerization of methyl malonyl co-enzyme A to succinyl co-enzyme A and also to convert homocysteine to methionine. Details of how failure of these steps leads to the characteristic haematological and neurological disorders found in B_{12} deficiency are still not well understood.

Vitamin B_{12} deficiency presents with a macrocytic anaemia and a megaloblastic bone marrow. Damage to the neuronal tracts in the spinal cord can also occur, leading to subacute combined degeneration of the cord.

VITAMIN B_{12} DEFICIENCY

- Dietary: strict vegetarians only (vegans).
- Deficiency of intrinsic factor: pernicious anaemia (destruction of gastric parietal cells with achlorhydria), total gastrectomy.
- Intestinal malabsorption: damage to the terminal ileum, for example Crohn's disease, lymphoma.

THERAPEUTIC USE OF VITAMIN B_{12}

Because most patients with vitamin B_{12} deficiency have problems absorbing it from the gut, treatment is usually by intramuscular injection of cobalamin in aqueous solution. Hydroxocobalamin is preferred to cyanocobalamin since it is more highly bound to transcobalamins and less is excreted in the urine. After intitial twice-weekly injections for 2–3 weeks to replenish stores, maintenance treatment with injections every 2–3 months is adequate.

ERYTHROPOIETIN

Erythropoietin is a hormone released from the kidney which controls red cell production. Deficiency of erythropoietin in chronic renal failure contributes to the anaemia that characterizes this disorder. Erythropoietin has been synthesized using recombinant DNA technology (epoetin) and is used to treat anaemia of renal failure after exclusion of other causes such as iron deficiency. Its use is being studied in other situations such as the anaemia associated with certain malignancies or acquired immune deficiency syndrome (AIDS).

Pharmacokinetics

Erythropoietin can be given intravenously, intraperitoneally or, more conveniently, subcutaneously. The red cell response is most rapid after intravenous use, but ultimately greater after subcutaneous injection. Doses are normally given two or three times weekly. Adequate iron stores are essential since erythropoiesis demands large amounts of iron.

Unwanted effects

- Flu-like symptoms early in treatment.
- Hypertension, which can be severe.
- Arteriovenous shunt thrombosis.
- Fits.

Lipids

Lipid metabolism is complex and the following account is a very brief summary, sufficient to establish the mechanism of action of drugs which are used to correct lipid abnormalities.

CHOLESTEROL AND TRIGLYCERIDE

Cholesterol is a sterol which is mainly synthesized in the liver. It is then either transported into the circulation or secreted into the bile after incorporation into bile salt micelles. A small amount of cholesterol is absorbed from the gut, either following dietary ingestion or by enterohepatic circulation of bile salts. Intracellular cholesterol in the liver acts by a negative feedback mechanism to reduce hepatic cholesterol synthesis.

Triglycerides are the major dietary fat. They can also be synthesized in the liver from free fatty acids, and derived from excess carbohydrate in the diet. Triglycerides are stored in adipose tissue from which they can be mobilized as non-esterified free fatty acids to act as an energy substrate during periods of hepatic glycogen depletion.

LIPOPROTEINS

Lipids circulate in plasma bound to specific proteins, known as apolipoproteins which are derived from the liver and intestine. The apolipoprotein–lipid complexes are termed lipoproteins. They are usually classified by the density of the particles into very low density (VLDL), low density (LDL), intermediate density (IDL) and high density (HDL) lipoproteins. The least dense particles, known as chylomicrons, are exclusively concerned with the transport of dietary lipid to the liver. The apolipoprotein constituents and the relative content of lipid on these different particles are summarized in Table 51.1.

IMPORTANT ENZYMES IN LIPID METABOLISM

- Lipoprotein lipase: this is responsible for clearing chylomicrons from the blood (Fig. 51.1). It also hydrolyses most of the triglyceride on VLDL to glycerol and free fatty acids (FFAs), generating IDL and subsequently LDL. Most lipoprotein lipase is found in the blood, although a second form (hepatic lipase) is present in liver. Lipoprotein lipase is activated by apo C in chylomicrons (Table 51.1).

- HMG CoA reductase: synthesis of cholesterol includes a rate-limiting step which is catalysed by the enzyme HMG CoA (β-hydroxy

Table 51.1 The apoprotein and lipid composition of the circulating lipoproteins

Lipoprotein	Major apolipoproteins	Cholesterol (%)	Triglyceride (%)
Chylomicrons	apo A/apo C/apo B_{48}	3	90
VLDL	apo C/apo B_{100}/apo E	20	50
IDL	apo B_{100}/apo E	40	30
LDL	apo B_{100}	50	7
HDL	apo A	40	6

Note: The balance of lipid content of the lipoprotein consists of phospholipids.

β-methylglutaryl-coenzyme A) reductase (Fig. 51.2).

- Lecithin–cholesterol acyl transferase (LCAT): this enzyme is responsible for esterification of circulating cholesterol released from cell membranes. The enzyme is found in association with circulating HDL which accepts esterified cholesterol (Table 51.3). It is activated by apo A in HDL (Table 51.1).

- Cholesteryl ester transfer protein (CETP): this enzyme is responsible for transfer of cholesteryl esters from HDL to VLDL, HDL can then accept triglyceride from VLDL when it is hydrolysed to IDL (Fig. 51.3).

LOW DENSITY LIPOPROTEIN RECEPTORS

Several tissues which take up cholesterol have a genetically controlled cell-surface receptor for LDL. The receptor–LDL particle complex is internalized, the cholesterol released and the receptor returned to the cell surface. As the cell content of cholesterol increases there are two important feedback effects in the cell to limit cholesterol accumulation.

- Reduction of HMG CoA reductase activity.

- Downregulation of LDL receptors. If this occurs in the presence of excess circulating cholesterol, extrahepatic cholesterol uptake

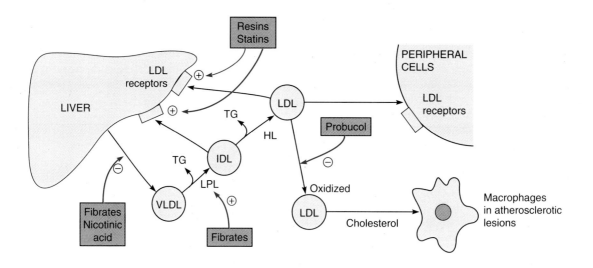

Key

VLDL : Very low density lipoprotein
IDL : Intermidiate density lipoprotein
LDL : Low density lipoprotein
LPL : Lipoprotein lipase
HL : Hepatic lipase

⊖ Inhibition
⊕ Stimulation

Figure 51.1 Metabolism of low density lipoproteins showing the sites of drug action.

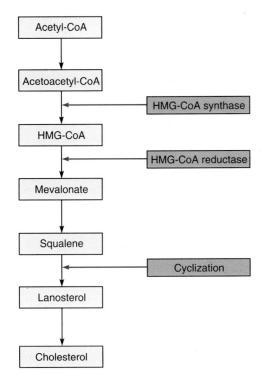

Figure 51.2 Simplified pathway of cholesterol synthesis.

from LDL by non-receptor scavenger mechanisms increases, which enhances atherogenesis (see below). This is due to cholesterol uptake into macrophages which form foam cells in the arterial wall. The chief pathways of LDL metabolism are shown in Fig. 51.1.

HIGH DENSITY LIPOPROTEIN

Most HDL is formed during lipolysis of chylomicrons. Its principal role is to mediate reverse cholesterol transport, carrying cholesterol from peripheral tissues to the liver (Fig. 51.3). This is believed to have a protective role, reducing the risk of atherogenesis. HDL exists in two forms. HDL_3 accepts cholesterol, which is then esterified by LCAT, and is thereby converted to HDL_2 which transfers cholesterol to the liver.

HYPERLIPIDAEMIA

Abnormalities of plasma lipoprotein metabolism produces an excess of circulating choles-

terol and/or triglyceride concentrations. The clinical importance is their relationship to atheroma (mainly cholesterol) and pancreatitis (triglycerides). Excessive amounts of LDL predispose to abnormal lipid deposition in vessel walls initiating plaques of atheroma. LDL cholesterol is believed to become atherogenic after oxidation. By contrast, the HDL concentration shows an inverse relationship to atheroma, presumably due to its involvement in reverse cholesterol transport. High plasma triglycerides are associated with low levels of HDL cholesterol and are usually associated with increased production of VLDL, the main carrier of triglycerides in plasma. Variations in the pattern of lipoproteins can result from:

- Dietary factors which contribute to most hyperlipidaemias.
- Primary (inherited) disorders of enzymes or receptors involved in lipid metabolism. Most inherited hyperlipidaemias are polygenic. However, an important inherited defect is familial hypercholesterolaemia, a single recessive gene disorder which affects 1 in 500 of the population who have reduced synthesis of LDL receptors.
- Secondary disorders when hyperlipidaemia results from diseases which affect lipid metabolism, for example liver disease, nephrotic syndrome, hypothyroidism.

The WHO has adopted a classification for the various patterns of hyperlipidaemia which is shown in Table 51.2.

DRUGS FOR HYPERLIPIDAEMIA

BILE ACID BINDING (ANION-EXCHANGE) RESINS

Example: cholestyramine.

Mechanism of action

These insoluble, non-absorbable compounds bind bile salts in the gut and prevent enterohepatic recirculation of cholesterol-derived bile acids. There is a compensatory increase in bile acid synthesis in the liver leading to further elimination of cholesterol. LDL receptors in the liver are up-regulated due to intracellular cholesterol depletion and as a result LDL

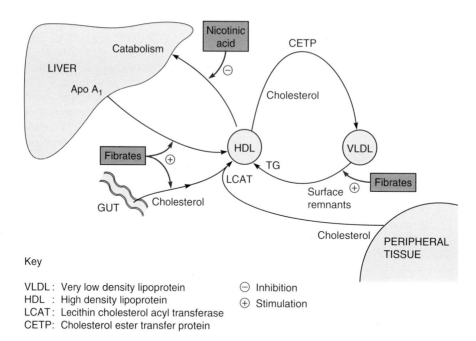

Key

VLDL : Very low density lipoprotein
HDL : High density lipoprotein
LCAT : Lecithin cholesterol acyl transferase
CETP : Cholesterol ester transfer protein

⊖ Inhibition
⊕ Stimulation

Figure 51.3 Metabolism of high density lipoprotein showing the sites of drug action.

cholesterol in blood is cleared more rapidly, with a fall in circulating levels. Stimulation of VLDL synthesis produces a small rise in plasma triglycerides.

Unwanted effects

- Unpalatability: sachets containing several grams of powder have to be taken, usually mixed with food. The taste and texture limit patient acceptability.
- Interference with the absorption of certain drugs, for example digoxin (Chapter 8), warfarin (Chapter 10).
- Diarrhoea.

FIBRIC ACID DERIVATIVES ("FIBRATES")

Examples: bezafibrate, gemfibrozil.

Mode of action

The main effect of these drugs is to decrease the synthesis of VLDL. The release of free fatty acids from adipose tissue (required for hepatic triglyceride synthesis) is reduced, so that less is available to incorporate into VLDL. Activation of the enzyme lipoprotein–lipase also increases the clearance of triglycerides from plasma (Fig. 51.1). When LDL cholesterol is high, its reduced catabolic rate is restored to normal which decreases circulating

Table 51.2 The Fredrickson classification of dyslipidaemia

Type	Triglyceride	Total cholesterol	LDL cholesterol	Raised lipoprotein
I	+++	+	N	Chylomicrons
IIa	N	++	++	LDL
IIb	++	++	++	LDL/VLDL
III	++	+	N	IDL and chylomicron remnants
IV	++	N/+	N	VLDL
V	+++	+	N	VLDL/chylomicrons

N, Normal; +, slightly raised; ++, moderately raised; +++, extremely raised.

LDL concentrations. The increased LDL cholesterol uptake by the liver reduces the activity of HMG CoA reductase and therefore reduces cholesterol synthesis. This is often accompanied by an increase in HDL, possibly due to increased conversion of VLDL remnants to HDL and to reduced clearance of HDL by the liver.

Pharmacokinetics

Fibrates are well absorbed from the gut and highly protein bound in the plasma. Excretion is primarily by the kidney although some metabolism occurs in the liver. The half-lives of the fibrates are short.

Unwanted effects

- Gastrointestinal upset.
- Increased lithogenicity of bile theoretically increases the risk of gallstones but this has not been a problem with the drugs mentioned here.
- Myalgia or myositis is uncommon.
- Drug interactions include potentiation of warfarin (Chapter 10).

HMG CoA REDUCTASE INHIBITORS ("STATINS")

Examples: simvastatin, pravastatin.

Mechanism of action

These drugs competitively inhibit the enzyme which catalyses the rate-limiting step in synthesis of cholesterol by the liver (Fig. 51.2). The fall in cholesterol available for bile acid synthesis produces a compensatory up-regulation in the number of LDL receptors on the cell surface, with increased clearance of circulating LDL cholesterol. LDL particles also contain triglyceride, so circulating triglyceride will fall. A modest increase in HDL cholesterol is often seen.

Pharmacokinetics

The statins are well absorbed from the gut. Pravastatin is active, but simvastatin is a prodrug (Chapter 2) which is activated by first-pass metabolism in the liver. Further metabolism inactivates the drug and little active compound reaches the circulation. Pravastatin is hydrophilic and crosses the blood–brain barrier less readily than the lipophilic simvastatin. Its half-life is short and elimination is mainly renal, partly by metabolism.

Unwanted effects

- Gastrointestinal upset.
- CNS effects, for example dizziness, blurred vision, headache (may be less common with pravastatin).
- Transient disturbance of liver function tests.
- Myalgia or myositis particularly when used in combination with fibrates or nicotinic acid.

NICOTINIC ACID AND DERIVATIVES

Examples: nicotinic acid, acipimox.

Mechanism of action

Nicotinic acid is a B vitamin which when used in pharmacological doses has effects on lipids. Decreased VLDL synthesis in the liver appears to be the major effect, and results from reduced free fatty acid mobilization (see fibric acid derivatives). Circulating triglycerides are substantially reduced and LDL cholesterol modestly reduced. HDL cholesterol is increased possibly as a result of hepatic lipase inhibition.

Pharmacokinetics

Nicotinic acid is well absorbed from the gut. Hepatic metabolism occurs at low doses but is saturable, and large doses are excreted unchanged in the urine. It has a very short half-life. Acipimox is a synthetic derivative of nicotinic acid which is longer acting, but rather less effective for lowering LDL cholesterol.

Unwanted effects

- Nicotinic acid is often poorly tolerated but unwanted effects can be minimized by gradual dosage increases. Acipimox is better tolerated.
- Cutaneous vasodilation (mediated by prostaglandins) is particularly troublesome. A small dose of aspirin 30 min before nicotinic acid, or taking the drug with food will reduce this.

- Gastrointestinal upset.
- Glucose intolerance with high doses of nicotinic acid (not seen with acipimox).

FISH OILS

Long-chain polyunsaturated omega-3 fatty acids, for example eicosapentaenoic acid (EPA) and docosahexaenoic acid (DHA), are found in high quantities in oily fish such as mackerel, sardines, etc. They reduce the synthesis of the apolipoprotein portion of VLDL, and therefore reduce plasma triglycerides. They also increase conversion of VLDL to LDL, and increase circulating LDL cholesterol. Other effects of fish oils may be important for reducing coronary artery disease, for example reduced plasma fibrinogen and impaired platelet aggregation (Chapter 10). Large quantities are necessary, which frequently cause gastrointestinal upset.

PROBUCOL

Mechanism of action

Probucol has an antiatherogenic effect which may be independent of its actions on total lipid concentrations. It stimulates transfer of cholesterol esters from HDL to VLDL by enhancing the action of cholesteryl ester transfer protein (CETP), thereby reducing "protective" HDL concentrations. LDL synthesis is reduced but a more important action may be its powerful antioxidant effect. Oxidation of LDL is believed to promote its accumulation in atheromatous lesions and subsequent phagocytosis by macrophages.

Pharmacokinetics

Oral absorption is poor and the drug is excreted unchanged in the bile. Probucol accumulates in fat from where it is released gradually over several months.

Unwanted effects

- Prolongation of the QT interval on the ECG may predispose to arrhythmias.
- Diarrhoea.

MANAGEMENT OF HYPERLIPIDAEMIA

Raised LDL cholesterol and low HDL cholesterol are independent risk factors for coronary heart disease and peripheral vascular disease. Epidemiological studies suggest that the total cholesterol : HDL ratio is one of the most sensitive indicators of risk, an ideal ratio being less than 3.5. Raised triglycerides may also be atherogenic, particularly in the presence of abnormal cholesterol concentrations. A more immediate risk of hypertriglyceridaemia is acute pancreatitis.

Dietary modification, with reduction in saturated fat intake, is important if the cholesterol profile is unfavourable, while reduction of triglycerides can often be achieved by weight loss and alcohol restriction.

Underlying causes of secondary hyperlipidaemia such as diabetes, hypothyroidism or nephrotic syndrome should be treated as necessary.

The place of drug treatment in primary prevention of coronary artery disease is controversial. There is evidence for a reduction in the incidence of coronary heart disease when drugs such as nicotinic acid, gemfibrozil or resins are given to middle-aged males with high total cholesterol concentrations. However, trials have been too small and too short to show an effect on mortality. As a consequence many clinicians reserve drugs for patients with familial hypercholesterolaemia, severe hypertriglyceridaemia or for raised plasma cholesterol in the presence of several other risk factors for coronary artery

Table 51.3 Percentage changes in plasma lipid concentrations produced by drug therapy

	Total cholesterol	HDL cholesterol	Triglycerides
Fibrates	−15 to 20%	+15 to 30%	−35%
Resins	−20%	+5 to 10%	0 to +5%
Nicotinic acid	−25%	+30%	−40%
Statins	−35%	+10%	−15%

disease (such as hypertension, smoking, diabetes or a history of premature coronary artery disease in a first-degree relative).

There is increasing interest in the use of drugs for secondary prevention of coronary heart disease. Statins, resins and nicotinic acid have all been shown to produce regression of atheroma in coronary arteries. It is not yet known how this will affect outcome in patients with angina. After myocardial infarction, reducing cholesterol appears to improve survival if ventricular function is good enough to avoid early mortality.

If plasma LDL cholesterol is elevated with normal triglycerides, then resins or statins are appropriate. For mixed hyperlipidaemia, a fibrate is usually given with the addition of a resin or statin if the cholesterol is not reduced sufficiently. Hypertriglyceridaemia can be treated with a fibrate. Alternatives include nicotinic acid and marine oils (Table 51.3).

It is important to remember that any intervention to reduce lipids for the prevention of coronary artery disease should form part of a programme to manage all co-existing risk factors.

Skin Disorders

52

Skin Disorders

TOPICAL APPLICATIONS

Topical treatments for skin disorders usually have two components: a base and the active ingredient, for example corticosteroid, antifungal agents, tar. Four types of base are used:

- Ointments are greases such as white or yellow soft paraffin.
- Creams are emulsions of water in a grease or grease in water which are less greasy than ointments. They are absorbed more quickly into the skin and are often used as a vehicle for active ingredients. The choice between an ointment or cream depends on patient preference unless the skin is very dry when an ointment is better.
- Pastes are suspensions of powder in an ointment. Pastes will stay where they are put on the skin. Their main use is to apply noxious chemicals which should be confined to one area of the skin.
- Lotions are any kind of liquid. They are used on wet surfaces and hairy areas. The main advantage is that they do not make a mess.

ECZEMA/DERMATITIS

Dermatitis is a syndrome that has several possible causes:

- Contact dermatitis to an external agent results from direct irritation or sensitization involving a delayed hypersensitivity response (Chapter 40). The latter can be a response to topical application of drugs. Once the skin has been sensitized, the potential for reaction persists indefinitely.
- Atopic eczema is often associated with asthma and hayfever and has a familial tendency. Affected skin is red, scaly and extremely dry. There may be vesicles and weeping and crusting over the skin surface. Scratching produces excoriation and thickening of the skin.

TREATMENT OF CONTACT DERMATITIS

- Providing a barrier to an irritant, for example wearing gloves, or removing an allergen may be sufficient.
- Dilute topical corticosteroid ointment (Chapter 47).
- Potassium permanganate soaks can help to dry up exudative lesions.

TREATMENT OF ECZEMA

- Emollients act as hydrophobic agents which seal the surface of the skin and reduce water loss. Paraffin derivatives are most effective but are greasy and not well accepted by patients. Alternatives, such as aqueous cream, are more cosmetically acceptable.

- Topical corticosteroid ointment (Chapter 47). In general, the least potent corticosteroids should be used whenever possible to minimize unwanted effects. The anti-inflammatory effect of these drugs makes them the mainstay of treatment.

- Sedative antihistamines (Chapter 41) taken orally at night ensure that the patient can sleep although they have little direct effect on itching.

- Systemic antibiotics are given for secondary infection.

- Tar bandages on the limbs are messy but aid healing and prevent scratching.

PSORIASIS

The psoriatic skin lesion is produced by a very rapid proliferation of epidermal cells. Cell turn-over is increased from about 28 days to 3–4 days which prevents adequate maturation. Instead of producing a normal keratinous surface layer the skin thickens, forming a silvery scale with dilated upper dermal blood vessels. Leucocytes infiltrate into the dermis. The basic defect is genetically determined.

TOPICAL THERAPY

- Dithranol is an anthroquinone which decreases cell division and is very effective in healing psoriatic plaques. In hospital it is applied in a stiff paste so that the dithranol does not contact and burn normal skin, and is left in contact with the plaque for 24 h. At home dithranol is used as a cream which is applied to the plaque for half-an-hour and then washed off. The breakdown products of dithranol stain the skin brown, leaving discoloration of healed areas. They also stain bedding and clothes a mauve colour that will not wash out. Since dithranol irritates normal skin it should not be used in flexures.

- Coal tar preparations: crude coal tar is a mixture of a large number of hydrocarbons which have a cytostatic action. It enhances the effect of ultraviolet B radiation on psoriatic lesions. The main disadvantages are its mess and smell. More refined tar preparations have greater patient acceptability but are less effective.

- Keratolytics: these break down keratin and soften skin which improves penetration of other treatments. Salicylic acid ointment is most frequently used.

- Phototherapy: ultraviolet light produces improvement in most patients but should not be used on individuals who are very fair and who burn in the sun. Ultraviolet B ("sunburn" wavelength 290–320 nm) is very useful if patients have extensive small plaques of psoriasis. Long wavelength ultraviolet A (320–400 nm) requires more specialized equipment and prior administration of an oral photosensitizing drug such as psoralen (photochemotherapy). Psoralen probably acts by locating between base pairs in the DNA helix and inhibiting cell replication. Photochemotherapy with ultraviolet A (PUVA) is usually reserved for severe, resistant psoriasis. Psoralen can produce nausea, and the long-term risks of PUVA include accelerated skin ageing and an increased incidence of skin cancer.

- Topical corticosteroid preparations: should not be used because their withdrawal can produce a rebound phenomenon and even generalized pustules.

SYSTEMIC TREATMENTS

These are reserved for the most severe forms of disease.

- Methotrexate (Chapter 55): this is the most common treatment for resistant and widespread disease. Its main actions are cytostatic and immunosuppressant. Oral or intramuscular dosing is usually used once a week; bone marrow and hepatotoxicity are the main complications. (The latter mainly occurs in conjunction with alcohol.) Blood counts are checked every 2–3 months and liver biopsies every 1–2 years to monitor treatment. Other cytotoxic drugs which are used include azathioprine (Chapter 42) and hydroxyurea.

- Retinoids: these are synthetic vitamin A derivatives such as etretinate and its active metabolite acitretin. Given orally, they are anti-inflammatory and cytostatic. The half-life of etretinate is very long, up to several weeks due to sequestration in fat, while that of acitretin is about 2 days. However, in about 50% of patients reverse metabolism of acitretin occurs to etretinate. Unwanted effects are almost universal and include dry lips and nasal mucosa, dryness of skin with localized peeling over the digits and transient thinning of hair. These effects are dose-dependent and reversible. Longer-term problems include ossification of ligaments, increased plasma triglycerides and to a lesser extent plasma cholesterol. There is a high risk of teratogenesis and women must use adequate contraception and stop treatment for 2 years before conception. Response is delayed by up to 2 months.

- Cyclosporin A (Chapter 42): its effectiveness in psoriasis occurs at lower doses than those required for prevention of allograft rejection.

ACNE

This is a condition most commonly arising in adolescence which often regresses in the late teens or early twenties. Acne affects areas of skin with large numbers of sebaceous glands: the face, back and chest. There is increased production of sebum which distends the pilosebaceous duct producing a small papule (comedone) called a whitehead. Hyperkeratosis at the mouth of the hair follicle blocks the duct. If the duct then opens, melanin at the tip gives the appearance of a blackhead. The bacterium, *Propionibacterium acnes*, degrades triglycerides in sebum to free fatty acids and glycerol. Free fatty acids are irritant and produce inflamed lesions of pustules, nodules or multilocular cysts if the lesions coalesce. The inflammatory lesions can scar with permanent disfigurement.

There is a genetic background to acne which determines the rate of sebum production. Androgens which are produced at puberty induce hypertrophy of sebaceous glands and the excess secretion rate in predisposed individuals triggers the acne. The duct also becomes abnormally corneified, perhaps in response to hormonal stimulation and altered fatty acid content of the sebum which obstructs the duct.

TREATMENT OF ACNE

There are several effective treatments for acne. The choice will depend on the nature of the lesions and their severity:

- Benzoyl peroxide has antibacterial and keratolytic actions which reduce the numbers of comedones. It produces scaling and skin irritation which limit its use to short treatment periods.
- Topical antibiotics for example clindamycin, erythromycin, tetracycline (Chapter 54): they are less effective than oral antibiotics but with fewer unwanted effects. Efficacy is similar to benzoyl peroxide with less skin irritation; tetracycline is least likely to cause bacterial resistance. They are used for mild to moderate acne and are particularly useful in pregnant women since there is no systemic absorption.
- Oral antibiotics are used for inflammatory acne (papules/pustules), producing some improvement after 2–3 months, but requiring 4–6 months for maximal benefit. Treatment should be given for extended periods since relapse is common if it is stopped. Among the more useful antibiotics are tetracyclines, for example oxytetracycline and doxycycline, erythromycin or cotrimoxazole (Chapter 54).
- Azelaic acid is an aliphatic dicarboxylic acid which has an antibacterial action against propionibacteria, and is effective against bacteria that have become resistant to erythromycin and tetracycline. It also inhibits the division of keratinocytes which may reduce follicular plugging and prevent the development of comedones. It is applied topically; the most fequent unwanted effects are local burning, scaling or itching. Azelaic acid is most effective for mild to moderate acne, especially of the face.
- The antiandrogen cyproterone acetate (Chapter 49) is useful in women with moderate or severe acne and is usually given in combination with ethinyloestradiol (Chapter 48). It reduces sebum flow by 40%.
- Isotretinoin is a vitamin A derivative which has a keratolytic action that unblocks the pilosebaceous follicles and allows flow of sebum to extrude the plug. It also reduces sebum production by up to 90% and has an antibacterial action. Topically it produces erythema and scaling, which can be minimized by starting with a low concentration. It is used orally in severe acne and gives an almost 100% chance of complete remission. Unwanted effects include dry lips, nose and eyes, muscle aches and increased plasma triglycerides. Teratogenesis is a major problem and conception should be avoided during and for 1 month after stopping treatment.

The Eye

53

The Eye

AUTONOMIC NERVOUS SYSTEM CONTROL OF THE EYE

The autonomic nervous system innervates the ciliary muscle which controls visual accommodation, and the iris, which determines the size of the pupil. Indirectly this will also influence the drainage of aqueous humour from the anterior chamber of the eye (Fig. 53.1).

- Accommodation: the ciliary muscle is a circular or constrictor muscle which is attached to the lens by suspensory ligaments. The ciliary muscle receives parasympathetic innervation.

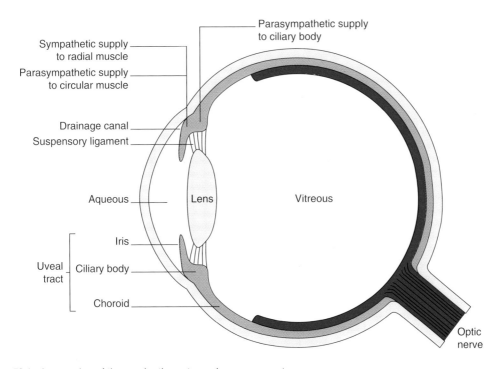

Figure 53.1 Innervation of the eye by the autonomic nervous system.

When the muscle is relaxed, tension on the suspensory ligaments stretches and flattens the lens inside its capsule, which adjusts visual acuity for distant vision. Stimulation of the parasympathetic innervation contracts the ciliary muscle which relaxes the suspensory ligaments. The lens assumes a more globular shape which accommodates the eye for near vision. Contraction of the ciliary muscle also aids drainage of aqueous humour through the canals of Schlemm. If drainage of this fluid is impaired, the intraocular pressure rises leading to glaucoma and progressive loss of vision. Paralysis of the ciliary muscle is known as *cycloplegia*.

- Pupil size: this is determined by the relative tone in the two muscles of the iris. The circular (constrictor) muscle is the more powerful and receives parasympathetic nervous innervation. The radial (dilator) muscle is sympathetically innervated. Constriction of the pupil is known as *miosis*, dilation is called *mydriasis*. The light reflex and accommodation for near vision both invoke a response in the parasympathetic nervous system producing pupillary constriction. Dilation of the pupil narrows the angle between the iris and the cornea, which restricts drainage of aqueous humour through the canals of Schlemm. This predisposes to primary acute-angle closure glaucoma.

GLAUCOMA

This is a group of disorders, characterized by raised intraocular pressure, which lead to ischaemia of the optic nerve head and damage to retinal nerve fibres. Progressive visual defects occur, initially as scotomas (blind spots) in the peripheral visual field. These scotomas enlarge, coalesce and eventually lead to reduced visual acuity. Glaucoma can be due to a developmental defect or degenerative process (primary glaucoma) or secondary to another disease process.

Two types of glaucoma are recognized. Open angle glaucoma is due to changes in the endothelium of the canals of Schlemm which drain the anterior chamber of the eye. Closed angle glaucoma which is usually acute in onset is due to the peripheral iris blocking access to the canal of Schlemm in a subject with a shallow anterior chamber, especially long-sighted individuals. Chronic closed angle glaucoma is much less common.

TOPICAL APPLICATION OF DRUGS TO THE EYE

Drugs applied in solution to the anterior surface of the eye can penetrate to the anterior chamber and the ciliary muscle, principally via the cornea. The high water content of the cornea makes lipid solubility less important for adequate penetration compared with transdermal drug delivery, but formulation of the carrier is important to avoid irritation of the conjunctivae. There is little diffusion to more posterior structures of the eye.

Systemic absorption of drug can occur either via conjuctival vessels, or from the nasal mucosa after drainage via the tear ducts.

MYDRIATIC AND CYCLOPLEGIC DRUGS

PARASYMPATHETIC ANTAGONISTS

Examples: atropine, homatropine, cyclopentolate, tropicamide (Chapter 4).

These are both mydriatic and cycloplegic. Tropicamide is weak and short-acting (about 3 h) which makes it useful for fundal examination. Cyclopentolate and homatropine both last for up to 24 h and are more powerful; the former has a more rapid onset of action. Atropine is long-acting, the effect persisting for up to 7 days. The longer-acting compounds are used to prevent adhesions (posterior synechiae) in patients with iridocyclitis.

The degree of cycloplegia will depend on the dose of drug; small doses produce pupil dilation with insufficient diffusion to profoundly affect accommodation. Patients should not drive after receiving a cycloplegic and care must be taken in patients predisposed to acute angle-closure glaucoma.

SYMPATHETIC AGONISTS

Examples: phenylephrine, adrenaline, dipivefrine (Chapter 4).

These compounds are mydriatic, by acting as α_1-adrenoceptor agonists, but are not cycloplegic. Adrenaline is rarely used now. The prodrug dipivefrine is converted to adrenaline in the eye and has the advantage of substantially greater penetration through the cornea. The α-agonist action of the drug is useful in glaucoma by improving aqueous outflow.

Sympathomimetic drugs are often used in combination with β-adrenoceptor antagonists, an apparently antagonistic combination which does, however, appear to be complementary in effectiveness.

MIOTIC DRUGS

MUSCARINIC AGONISTS

Example: pilocarpine (Chapter 4).

This is usually given for closed-angle glaucoma to contract the ciliary muscle and open up the drainage channels in the anterior chamber of the eye. The miotic effect is an inevitable consequence. Ciliary muscle spasm produces blurred vision and an ache over the eye (especially in younger patients). The miotic effect lasts about 4 h, but prolonged miosis can be achieved by the use of Ocuserts, a small plastic reservoir that releases drug in the lower fornic of the eye for up to a week.

ANTICHOLINESTERASES

Example: physostigmine (Chapter 29).

Physostigmine is more potent than pilocarpine and is often used in combination with it. Diffusion around the eye can produce twitching of the eyelids due to the effects of ACh at the neuromuscular junction. Actions in the eye resemble those of pilocarpine.

β-ADRENOCEPTOR ANTAGONISTS

Example: timolol, betaxolol.

These drugs are useful in glaucoma and probably act by reducing the formation of aqueous-humour or by increasing uvoscleral drainage of fluid. They have no effect on accommodation or pupil size which makes them the treatment of first choice for glaucoma. However, systemic absorption can produce the typical unwanted effects associated with these compounds (Chapter 6) and the same contraindications apply as for oral use. Timolol is a non-selective blocker, betaxolol is "cardioselective".

OTHER TOPICAL APPLICATIONS

Several other drugs are used topically in the eye:

- *Antibacterial agents*: (Chapter 54). These are given for local infection such as blepharitis, conjuctivitis or trachoma. Aqueous solutions are rapidly diluted or flushed away by lachrimation; ointments are often given for longer action, for example at night. Examples of broad spectrum agents are gentamicin, chloramphenicol, neomycin and tetracycline (the last for trachoma).

- *Antiviral agents*: (Chapter 54). These are mainly used for herpes simplex infection, which causes dendritic corneal ulcers. Examples include idoxuridine and acyclovir.

- *Corticosteroids*: for example dexamethasone or prednisolone (Chapter 47). These are given for local inflammatory conditions such as uveitis and scleritis. Care must be taken to exclude local viral infections and glaucoma since these can be exacerbated by corticosteroids.

- *Antiallergic agents*: topical antihistamines (Chapter 41). These are used for allergic conjunctivitis. Sodium cromoglycate (Chapter 11) can also be given.

- *Local anaesthetics*: (Chapter 19). Lignocaine eye drops provide surface anaesthesia; cocaine also produces mydriasis and local vasoconstriction.

Chemotherapy

Chemotherapy of Infections

Antimicrobial agents are natural or synthetic chemical substances which suppress the growth of or destroy microorganisms including bacteria, fungi and viruses. The widely used term antibiotic strictly should be used for antimicrobial agents derived from microorganisms.

ANTIBACTERIAL AGENTS

Antibacterial agents form the largest group of antimicrobials. They can be classified in several ways. First, they can be considered bacteristatic or bactericidal:

- Bacteristatic antimicrobials inhibit bacterial growth but do not destroy the cell. The natural immune mechanisms of the body are used to eliminate the organism. Such drugs will be less effective in immunocompromised individuals or when organisms are dormant (e.g. in carrier states) and may, by preventing cell division, make bactericidal antimicrobials less effective. Some of these agents may be bactericidal if used in high doses.

- Bactericidal antimicrobials kill bacteria.

Second, they can be classified by chemical structure, and they are discussed in this format below. Third, they can be grouped according to mechanisms of action:

- Agents which inhibit the synthesis of the bacterial cell wall or activate enzymes which disrupt it.
- Agents that act directly on the cell membrane and affect permeability, leading to leakage of intracellular contents.
- Agents that alter the functioning of ribosomes thereby causing a reversible inhibition of protein synthesis. The process of bacterial protein synthesis is shown in Fig. 54.1.
- Agents that block metabolic pathways which are essential for survival of the microorganisms.

Fourth, antimicrobials may be classified according to whether their spectrum of activity against bacteria is limited ("narrow spectrum") or extensive ("broad spectrum").

RESISTANCE TO ANTIMICROBIAL AGENTS

When an antimicrobial is ineffective against a microorganism the latter is said to be resistant. There are several ways by which resistance to antimicrobial agents arises; it may be inherent in the organism or be acquired genetically. The three major mechanisms of acquired resistance are:

- *Spontaneous mutation.* In this process a single-step genetic mutation in a bacterial population leads to selective growth of the resistant strain in the presence of an antimicrobial.
- *Transduction.* Bacteria are susceptible to infection by viruses known as bacteriophages. During phage replication the host cell's DNA (containing resistance genes) may be replicated along with viral DNA and taken

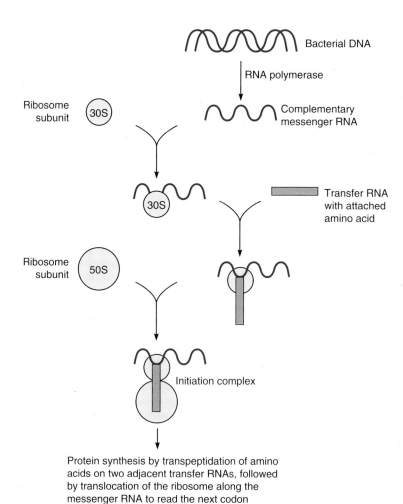

Protein synthesis by transpeptidation of amino acids on two adjacent transfer RNAs, followed by translocation of the ribosome along the messenger RNA to read the next codon

Figure 54.1 Bacterial protein synthesis.

into the virus. The phage carrying the resistance genes may then infect other bacterial cells thus spreading resistance.

- *Conjugation.* Direct cell to cell contact is the best way of exchanging genetic material and usually involves transfer of extrachromosomal fragments of DNA called plasmids, which can contain resistance genes.

β-LACTAM ANTIMICROBIALS

All of these compounds have a β-lactam ring in common which is responsible for their activity but is susceptible to enzymic attack by β-lactamases (penicillinases) that are produced by certain bacteria (Fig. 54.2). Two groups of β-lactam antimicrobials are used: the penicillins and the cephalosporins.

PENICILLINS

Examples: benzylpenicillin, phenoxymethylpenicillin, ampicillin, flucloxacillin, amoxycillin, azlocillin, mecillinam.

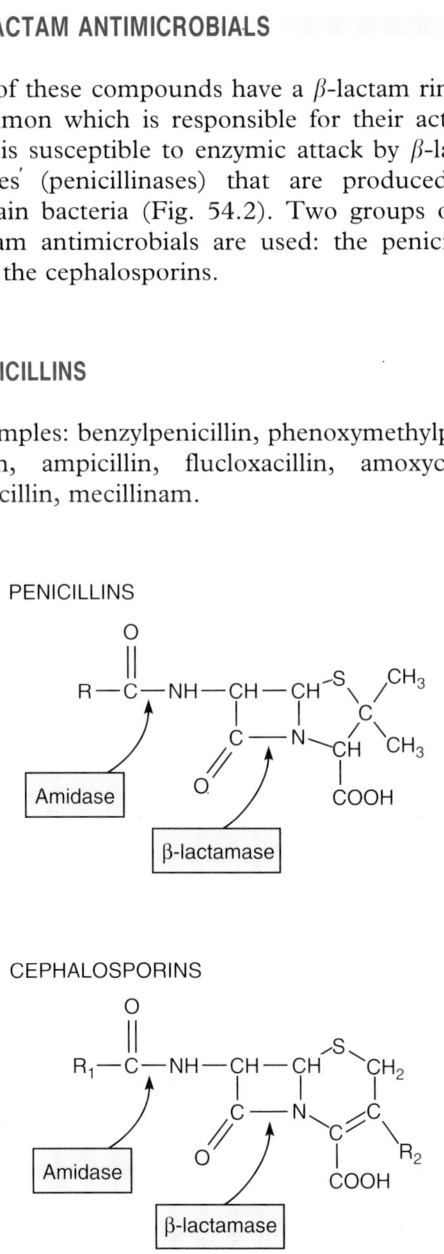

Figure 54.2 Core structures of penicillins and cephalosporins.

Mechanism of action

Penicillins consist of a thiazolidine ring connected to a β-lactam ring to which is attached a side-chain. The latter determines many of the antibacterial and pharmacological characteristics of a particular type of penicillin. β-Lactam antimicrobials inhibit synthesis of the peptidoglycan layer of the cell wall which surrounds certain bacteria and is essential for their survival. Peptidoglycan synthesis occurs in three stages and the last stage of cross-linking is inhibited by penicillin. The β-lactam ring is a structural analogue of one of the constituents of the peptidoglycan layer; it binds to enzymes such as transpeptidase involved in the cross-linking process. The antimicrobial effect is confined to growing cells which become unable to maintain their transmembrane osmotic gradient; this leads to cell swelling which is followed by rupture and cell death. Their bactericidal action is confined to dividing cells.

Spectrum of activity

Penicillins differ considerably in their spectrum of activity (Table 54.1). Thus, benzylpenicillin is active against aerobic Gram-positive bacteria, Gram-negative cocci and many anaerobic microorganisms. Gram-negative bacilli are not sensitive. Benzylpenicillin is susceptible to the action of β-lactamase. The addition of an acyl side-chain to the β-lactam nucleus produces derivatives such as flucloxacillin which prevent the access of β-lactamase. Although the spectrum of activity of flucloxacillin is similar to that of benzylpenicillin, it is far less effective against most bacteria. Flucloxacillin is therefore usually reserved for treating β-lactamase producing staphylococci which are particularly common in hospitals.

Ampicillin and amoxycillin are aminopenicillins which have an extended spectrum of activity to include many Gram-negative bacteria. They are destroyed by β-lactamase and are somewhat less effective than benzylpenicillin against Gram-positive cocci. Other extended spectrum penicillins include ureidopenicillins (eg. azlocillin) which are active against *Pseudomonas aeruginosa* and amidinopenicillins (e.g. mecillinam) which are active mainly against Gram-negative bacteria. Carboxy-penicillins (e.g. ticarcillin) are not widely used now, but have some activity against pseudomonas species.

Table 54.1 Examples of penicillins and their properties

	Oral absorption	β-Haemolytic streptococci	*Staphylococcus aureus*	Coliforms	*Pseudomonas aeruginosa*
			Activity against		
Natural					
Benzylpenicillin	Poor	++	+/o*	o	o
Phenoxymethylpenicillin	Incomplete	+	+/o	o	o
β-Lactamase-resistant					
Flucloxacillin	Good	++	++/o	o	o
Aminopenicilins					
Ampicillin	Incomplete	++	+/o*	++	o
Amoxycillin	Good	++	+/o*	++	o
Carboxypenicillins					
Ticarcillin	Poor	++	+/o*	++	+
Ureidopenicillins					
Azlocillin	Poor	++	+/o*	+	++

Guide to spectrum of activity: ++, very active; +, active; o, inactive.
*Most strains have a β-lactamase which destroys these penicillins.

Clavulanic acid is structurally related to the β-lactam antibiotics but has little intrinsic antibacterial activity. It is, however, a potent inhibitor of β-lactamase. When given in combination with other penicillins such as amoxycillin and ticarcillin they can be used to treat infections caused by β-lactamase-producing organisms which are otherwise insensitive to penicillins.

Resistance

Resistance to penicillins is most often due to the production of β-lactamase which hydrolyses the β-lactam ring. Gram-positive bacteria release extracellular β-lactamases. In Gram-negative bacteria the β-lactamases are located between the inner and outer cell membranes in the periplasmic space. The information for β-lactamase production is encoded in a plasmid and this may be transferred by transduction or conjugation to other bacteria.

Pharmacokinetics

• Benzylpenicillin and phenoxymethylpenicillin: only about one third of an orally administered dose of benzylpenicillin (penicillin G) is absorbed, the rest is destroyed in the stomach. Benzylpenicillin is therefore admin-

istered intramuscularly or intravenously. The phenoxymethyl derivative (penicillin V) is more stable in an acid environment and is better absorbed from the gut. Maximum concentrations in blood occur rapidly in 30–60 min.

Penicillins are widely distributed throughout the body, although transport across the meninges is poor, unless they are acutely inflamed (e.g. in meningitis) when penetration by the antibiotic is improved. The half-life of these penicillins is very short at 30 min and they are very rapidly eliminated by the kidneys mainly by active tubular secretion. Effective plasma concentrations of penicillin are usually maintained by frequent administrations. An alternative method is combining penicillin with a local anaesthetic such as procaine for intramuscular injection. Penicillin is then released slowly from the intramuscular depot, maintaining plasma concentrations for up to 24 h. A second method for prolonging effective plasma concentrations is to co-administer probenecid which blocks the tubular secretion of penicillin by competitive inhibition (Chapter 2).

• Flucloxacillin, ampicillin and amoxycillin: flucloxacillin is rapidly and well absorbed from the gut with peak plasma concentrations attained 1 h after the dose. Flucloxacillin has a short half-life. Ampicillin is incompletely absorbed from the gut but the absorption of amoxycillin is almost complete. Both drugs have short half-lives. These penicillins all can be administered parenterally if required, and are eliminated by the kidney.

- The amidinopenicillins (e.g. mecillinam) and carboxypenicillins (e.g. ticarcillin) are available for parenteral use and also as prodrug formulations which are absorbed orally. The ureidopenicillins (e.g. azlocillin) are given parenterally. Biliary excretion eliminates about a quarter of ureidopenicillins which show dose-dependent kinetics due to reduced renal and biliary clearances at high dose. All have short half-lives.

Unwanted effects

Penicillins are normally very safe antimicrobials with a high therapeutic index.

- Hypersensitivity reactions. Manifestations of allergy to penicillins include rashes, fever, vasculitis, serum sickness, exfoliative dermatitis, Stevens–Johnson syndrome and severe anaphylactic shock. Cross-allergy among various penicillins and to a lesser extent cephalosporins is found. Penicillins and their breakdown products bind to proteins and act as haptens, stimulating the production of antibodies which mediate the allergic response (Chapter 56).
- Aminopenicillins (e.g. ampicillin) frequently produce a non-allergic maculopapular rash in patients with glandular fever.

- Reversible neutropenia and eosinophilia can occur with prolonged high doses.
- Grand-mal seizures can occur with excessively high cerebrospinal fluid concentrations of penicillin (a risk in patients with renal failure).
- Diarrhoea due to disturbance of normal colonic flora, especially with broad-spectrum penicillins.

CEPHALOSPORINS

Examples: cefadroxil, cephradine, cefuroxime, cefotaxime, cefixime.

Mechanism of action

Cephalosporins, like penicillins, have a β-lactam ring to which is fused a dihydrothiazine ring which makes them more resistant to hydrolysis by β-lactamases. They inhibit bacterial cell wall synthesis in a manner similar to that of the penicillins.

Spectrum of activity

Cephalosporins are often classified by "generations". The members of each generation share similar antibacterial activity and pharmacokinetics. Succeeding generations tend to have increased activity against Gram-negative bacilli usually at the expense of Gram-positive activity (Table 54.2).

The first-generation oral cephalosporins (e.g. cefadroxil) have good activity against staphylococci and most streptococci except enterococci.

Table 54.2 Examples of cephalosporins and their spectrum of activity

	Staphylococcus aureus	Haemophilus influenzae	Coliforms	Pseudomonas aeruginosa	Bacteroides fragilis
First generation					
Oral: cefadroxil/cephradine	+	o	+	o	o
Parenteral: cephradine	+	o	+	o	o
Second generation					
Oral: cefuroxime	++	++	++	o	o
Parenteral: cefuroxime	++	++	++	o	o
Third generation					
Oral: cefixime	o	+++	++	o	o
Parenteral: cefotaxime	++	+++	+++	o	+

Key: +++, very active; ++, active; +, variable activity; o, inactive.

They do not cross the blood–brain barrier. Second-generation oral cephalosporins such as cefuroxime are also active against some Gram-negative organisms such as Haemophilus species. Third-generation oral cephalosporins have improved β-lactamase stability and are able to penetrate the cerebrospinal fluid in useful quantities. Cefixime, which belongs to this group, improves on the Gram-negative activity of the other two generations and adds proteus and klebsiella species to its spectrum. It has no activity against staphylococci however.

The same principles apply to the generations of parenteral cephalosporins. First-generation compounds such as cephradine have a similar spectrum to oral equivalents. Cefuroxime is a second-generation agent which is active against *Staphylococcus aureus*, most Gram-negative bacilli, *Haemophilus influenzae* and *Neisseriae gonorrhoea*. By contrast, the third-generation cefotaxime is also active against *Pseudomonas aeruginosa* but has only modest activity against *Staphylococcus aureus*. Some newer third-generation agents also inhibit *Staphylococcus aureus* and have activity against anaerobes such as *Bacteroides fragilis*.

Resistance

Cephalosporins can be destroyed by enzymatic hydrolysis of the β-lactamase ring but susceptibility is less with the later "generations".

Pharmacokinetics

The pharmacokinetics of the cephalosporins vary greatly. First-generation oral cephalosporins are usually well absorbed. Several, for example cefuroxime and cefotaxime, are acid labile and only available for parenteral use. Cefuroxime has been formulated as a prodrug (cefuroxime axetil) for oral use, which has good absorption and is hydrolysed at first-pass through the liver to cefuroxime. Cephalosporins are primarily excreted by the kidney, and have short half-lives. Cefixime is mainly eliminated by biliary excretion.

Unwanted effects

- Cephalosporins can produce hypersensitivity reactions similar to those observed with the penicillins. Between 6 and 18% of patients who are allergic to penicillin show cross-allergy to cephalosporins. A history of a serious reaction to penicillin precludes the administration of cephalosporins.
- Diarrhoea due to disturbance of normal bowel flora. This is more common with the poorly absorbed oral drugs such as cefuroxime axetil and cefixime.
- Nausea and vomiting.

MONOBACTAMS

Example: aztreonam.

Aztreonam is another β-lactam antimicrobial related to the penicillins but with a single ring structure. It has little cross-allergenicity with the penicillins and has been successfully administered to patients with proven penicillin allergy. Its spectrum of activity is limited to Gram-negative bacteria with none against Gram-positive bacteria or anaerobes. Aztreonam is given parenterally and is β-lactamase resistant.

CARBAPENEMS

Example: imipenem.

Imipenem is a β-lactam agent which has broad spectrum antimicrobial activity and is potent against Gram-positive cocci, Gram-negative bacilli including *Pseudomonas aeruginosa*, *Neisseria suppurans* and bacteroides species and many anaerobes. It can penetrate the blood–brain barrier and is resistant to β-lactamases. Imipenem is rapidly metabolized by dihydropeptidases in the kidney and so is given in combination with cilastatin, a compound which inhibits its renal destruction.

AMINOGLYCOSIDES

Examples: gentamicin, netilmicin, streptomycin.

Mechanism of action

Aminoglycosides inhibit protein synthesis in bacteria by binding irreversibly to the 30S ribosomal subunit. This inhibits translation from messenger RNA to protein and also increases the frequency of misreading of the genetic code. Aminoglycosides are bactericidal.

Spectrum of activity

Aminoglycosides are active against many Gram-negative bacteria (including pseudomonas species) but are less effective against Gram-positive organisms and inactive against anaerobes. They are particularly useful for serious Gram-negative infections, when they have a complementary spectrum to and synergistic action with the penicillins. Streptomycin is mainly used to treat *Mycobacterium tuberculosis*.

Resistance

Resistance is transferred by plasmids and is principally due to the production of degradative enzymes which acetylate, phosphorylate or adenylate aminoglycosides in the bacterial periplasmic space. Bacterial uptake of the modified drug is poor. Changes in the ribosomal proteins can also inhibit drug binding. Netilmicin is effective against many gentamicin-resistant bacteria.

Pharmacokinetics

Aminoglycosides are poorly absorbed from the gut and are therefore given parenterally. They have short half-lives and are rapidly excreted by the kidney. They do not cross the blood–brain barrier but administration in late pregnancy may result in accumulation of the drug in foetal plasma or amniotic fluid. Blood concentrations should always be measured to guide dosing. Peak concentrations and trough concentrations are both important to ensure bactericidal efficacy and to minimize the risk of toxic effects.

Unwanted effects

Most unwanted effects of aminoglycosides are dose-related and reversible, probably related to high trough concentrations of the drug.

- Ototoxicity can lead both to vestibular and auditory dysfunction. Repeated courses lead to accumulation of aminoglycoside in the inner ear resulting in irreversible deafness.
- Renal damage occurs due to retention of aminoglycosides in the proximal tubular cells of the kidney. It is usually reversible and is manifest initially by a defect in the concentrating ability of the kidney with mild proteinuria followed by a reduction in the glomerular filtration rate.
- Acute neuromuscular blockade, usually if the aminoglycoside is used in association with anaesthesia (Chapter 18) or administration of other neuromuscular blocking agents (Chapter 28). It is caused by inhibition of prejunctional acetylcholine release in association with reduced postsynaptic sensitivity, and it is reversed by intravenous calcium salts.

TETRACYCLINES

Examples: tetracycline, oxytetracycline, doxycycline, minocycline.

Mechanism of action

Tetracyclines enter bacteria mainly by an active uptake mechanism not found in human cells. They are bacteristatic and inhibit bacterial protein synthesis by binding reversibly to the 30S subunit of ribosomes.

Spectrum of activity

Tetracyclines have a broad spectrum of activity and are active against many Gram-positive and Gram-negative bacteria, rickettsiae, mycoplasma, amoebae, *Chlamydia psittici*, and *Trachomatis coxiella* and cholera. Minocycline is active against *Neisseria meningitidis*, unlike other tetracyclines.

Resistance

Resistance to the tetracyclines develops slowly but for most Gram-positive and several Gram-negative organisms is now widespread. Microorganisms which have developed resistance to one tetracycline frequently display resistance to the others. In most cases it is mediated by plasmids and is due to decreased uptake of the drug into bacteria. In other cases the effect of tetracyclines on bacterial ribosomes is decreased.

Pharmacokinetics

Tetracyclines are incompletely absorbed from the gut, particularly if taken with food. Absorption is also impaired by milk, aluminium, calcium or magnesium salts (antacids, Chapter 35), iron and increased intestinal pH; tetracyclines bind to divalent and trivalent cations forming inactive chelates. A parenteral formulation of tetracycline is available.

The tetracyclines diffuse reasonably well into sputum, urine and peritoneal and pleural fluid and cross the placenta. They have poor penetration into the cerebrospinal fluid. All of the tetracyclines have intermediate or long half-lives; doxycycline and minocycline have the longest.

Tetracyclines are concentrated in the liver and excreted via the bile into the small intestine from which they are partially reabsorbed. Drug concentrations in the bile may be three to five times higher than in the plasma.

Tetracyclines are eliminated unchanged in the urine, with the exception of doxycycline which is largely metabolized in the liver.

Unwanted effects

- Nausea, vomiting and epigastric discomfort commonly occur after oral administration.

- Intravenous tetracycline can cause thrombophlebitis.

- Tetracyclines in children depress bone growth, produce permanent discoloration of the teeth and enamel hypoplasia. They should be avoided during the latter half of pregnancy and in children in the first 8 years of life.

- Antianabolic effects from inhibition of protein synthesis in human cells (*not* seen with doxycycline or minocycline). In patients with impaired renal function this can lead to uraemia.

SULPHONAMIDES

Examples: sulfadiazine, sulphamethoxazole.

Mechanism of action

Unlike man, bacteria cannot utilize external folic acid, a nutrient which is essential for growth, and have to synthesize it from para-aminobenzoic acid (PABA). Sulphonamides are structurally similar to PABA and inhibit the enzyme dihydrofolate synthetase in the synthetic pathway for folic acid (Fig. 54.3). High concentrations of PABA antagonize the effectiveness of sulphonamides.

Spectrum of activity

Sulphonamides have a bacteristatic action against a wide range of Gram-positive and Gram-negative organisms and are also active against toxoplasma, nocardia species and chlamydia. Resistance is common and sulphonamides alone are usually reserved for treatment of nocardiosis or toxoplasmosis.

Resistance

Resistance is common and is due to the production of dihydrofolate synthetase which has reduced affinity for binding of sulphonamides, and is transmitted in Gram-negative bacteria by plasmids. Resistant strains of *Staphylococcus aureus* can synthesize more PABA than normal.

Pharmacokinetics

Sulphonamides are well absorbed orally although parenteral preparations of some (e.g. sulfadiazine) are available. They are widely distributed in the body and cross the blood–brain barrier and placenta.

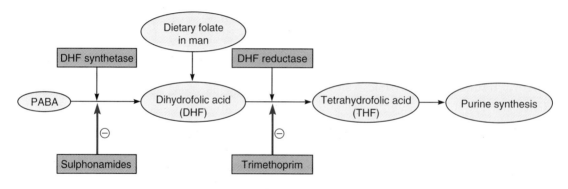

Figure 54.3 Bacterial synthesis of folic acid. ⊖, Inhibition.

Sulphonamides are metabolized in the liver, initially by acetylation which shows genetic polymorphism (Chapter 2). The acetylated product has no antibacterial action but retains toxic potential. Substantial amounts of parent drug and *N*-acetyl metabolite are excreted by the kidney. Most sulphonamides have intermediate half-lives.

Unwanted effects

- Nausea and vomiting.
- Hypersensitivity reactions include rashes, vasculitis, and Stevens–Johnson syndrome.
- Sulphonamides can precipitate haemolysis in patients with glucose-6-phosphate-dehydrogenase deficiency (Chapter 56).
- Crystalluria is unusual with newer sulphonamides, which are more soluble than earlier compounds, but is a potential problem with overdose or with acid urine.
- Sulphonamides should not be used in the last trimester of pregnancy or in neonates because they compete for bilirubin binding sites on albumin. This can raise the concentration of unconjugated bilirubin which increases the risk of kernicterus.

TRIMETHOPRIM AND CO-TRIMOXAZOLE

Mechanism of action

Trimethoprim inhibits dihydrofolate reductase which converts dihydrofolate to tetrahydrofolate (Fig. 54.3). The bacterial enzyme is inhibited at much lower concentrations than the mammalian equivalent. The combination of trimethoprim with the sulphonamide sulphamethoxazole (co-trimoxazole) acts synergistically to prevent folate synthesis by bacteria. However, resistance to the sulphamethoxazole component, and the incidence of unwanted effects limit the value of this combination.

Spectrum of activity

Trimethoprim has a wide spectrum of activity against Gram-positive and Gram-negative bacteria. The combination with sulphamethoxazole is also effective against the protozoan *Pneumocystis carinii* and this is now its major indication.

Resistance

Resistance to trimethoprim is due to the same process as that for sulphonamides.

Pharmacokinetics

Trimethoprim is well absorbed from the gut. Most is excreted unchanged by the kidney and it has an intermediate half-life. Both trimethoprim and co-trimoxazole are available for intravenous use.

Unwanted effects

- Nausea, vomiting and diarrhoea, which are usually mild.
- Skin rashes.
- Folate deficiency leading to megaloblastic changes in the marrow is rare except in patients with depleted folate stores.
- Marrow depression with agranulocytosis.

MISCELLANEOUS ANTIBACTERIAL AGENTS

CHLORAMPHENICOL

Mechanism of action

Chloramphenicol inhibits protein synthesis in bacteria by binding reversibly to the 50S subunit of bacterial ribosomes. It inhibits peptide bond formation by impairing the reading of messenger RNA. The effect is bactericidal to some organisms, bacteristatic to others.

Spectrum of activity

Chloramphenicol is a broad-spectrum antimicrobial active against many Gram-positive cocci (both aerobic and anaerobic) and Gram-negative organisms. The sensitivities of all bacteria are variable but *Escherichia coli*, *Streptococcus pneumonia*, *Haemophilus influenzae* and *Neisseria meningitidis* are killed. *Bordetella pertussis*, salmonellae, shigellae, *Vibrio cholerae*, bacteroides species and some streptococci and staphylococci are inhibited.

Because of its toxicity, chloramphenicol is reserved for life-threatening infections, particularly with *Haemophilus influenzae* or typhoid fever.

Resistance

Resistance is due to the production of an enzyme which inactivates the drug by acetylation. This enzyme is plasmid-mediated. It is produced by many Gram-negative bacteria but can also be induced in Gram-positive bacteria.

Pharmacokinetics

Chloramphenicol is well absorbed orally but an ester prodrug is used to disguise its bitter taste when given as a syrup. Intramuscular injection leads to inadequate plasma concentrations and so the intravenous route is preferred for parenteral administration. Chloramphenicol is widely distributed into many tissues including the cerebrospinal fluid and the biliary tree. It crosses the placenta and is present in breast milk.

Chloramphenicol is almost completely metabolized in the liver and has a short half-life.

Unwanted effects

- The most important unwanted effect is bone marrow toxicity. Reversible anaemia, thrombocytopenia or neutropenia can occur particularly in patients receiving high or prolonged dosing. Aplastic anaemia is rare and usually fatal.
- Premature infants and babies of less than 2 weeks old have immature hepatic enzymes, particularly glucuronyl transferase, plus reduced renal elimination and chloramphenicol can accumulate causing the "grey baby syndrome". Initial symptoms include vomiting and cyanosis followed by hypothermia, vasomotor collapse and an ashen grey discoloration of the skin.

QUINOLONES

Example: ciprofloxacin.

Mechanism of action

Quinolones inhibit replication of bacterial DNA. They block the activity of DNA gyrase, the enzyme which forms DNA supercoils and is essential for DNA replication and repair. The effect is bactericidal.

Spectrum of activity

Ciprofloxacin has a broad spectrum of activity and is active against many organisms resistant to penicillins, cephalosporins and aminoglycosides. Its spectrum includes most Gram-negative bacteria including *Haemophilus influenzae* and *Pseudomonas aeruginosa*. It has only moderate activity against streptococci but is active against β-lactamase producing staphylococci. Ciprofloxacin has poor activity against anaerobic cocci and bacilli.

Resistance

Resistance to ciprofloxacin is uncommon and may be due to a mutation which results in a DNA gyrase that is less susceptible to the drug's action. Plasmid-mediated resistance has not been found.

Pharmacokinetics

Oral absorption of ciprofloxacin is variable but adequate. It is widely distributed in body tissues and fluids; but cerebrospinal fluid penetration is poor unless there is meningeal inflammation. The majority of the drug is eliminated unchanged by the kidney, partly by tubular secretion, but about 20% is excreted in the bile and a similar amount is metabolized in the liver. An intravenous formulation is available. Ciprofloxacin has a short half-life.

Unwanted effects

The incidence of unwanted side-effects is low:

- Gastrointestinal upset.
- CNS effects: dizziness, headache, tremors.
- Drug interaction: the plasma concentrations of theophylline are increased, which can produce toxicity.

MACROLIDES

Example: erythromycin, azithromycin.

Mechanism of action

Erythromycin interferes with bacterial protein synthesis by binding reversibly to the 50S subunit of the bacterial ribosome. The action is primarily bacteristatic.

Spectrum of activity

Erythromycin has a narrow spectrum of activity and is effective against Gram-positive organisms and *Haemophilus influenzae*. It is the drug of choice for legionella and mycoplasma infections.

Although erythromycin is primarily bacteristatic, it is bactericidal for some Gram-positive species such as group A streptococci and pneumococci at high concentrations. Azithromycin has a similar spectrum of activity.

Resistance

Bacteria become resistant by a mutation which modifies the target sites on the ribosome.

Pharmacokinetics

Erythromycin is adequately absorbed from the gut. It is destroyed at acid pH and is therefore given as an enteric coated tablet or as an ester prodrug (erythromycin ethyl succinate) which is acid stable. It can also be administered intravenously. Azithromycin is acid stable and well absorbed from the gut.

Erythromycin is metabolized in the liver and it has a short half-life. Azithromycin is released slowly from the tissues and has a long half-life.

Unwanted effects

- Epigastric discomfort, nausea, vomiting and diarrhoea are common with the oral preparation of erythromycin. Azithromycin is better tolerated which is its main advantage.
- Cholestatic jaundice can occur with erythromycin, usually if treatment is continued for more than 2 weeks.

METRONIDAZOLE

Mechanism of action

Metronidazole acts via an intermediate metabolite which inhibits bacterial DNA synthesis and breaks down existing DNA. It is bactericidal. The intermediate metabolite is not produced in human cells.

Spectrum of activity

Metronidazole is mainly active against anaerobic bacteria and protozoa, including bacteroides and clostridium species, *Trichomonas vaginalis*, *Giardia lamblia* and *Entamoeba histolytica*.

Resistance

Acquired resistance is unusual.

Pharmacokinetics

Metronidazole is well absorbed orally and can also be given intravenously or as vaginal or rectal suppositories. Rectal absorption is high, and this route is often preferable to intravenous administration if the drug cannot be taken by mouth. It penetrates well into body fluids including vaginal, pleural and cerebrospinal fluids and can cross the placenta. Metronidazole is mostly metabolized by the liver and has an intermediate half-life.

Unwanted effects

- Mild gastrointestinal symptoms often occur and patients not uncommonly complain of a metallic taste.
- Intolerance to alcohol may occur which is similar to the disulfiram reaction (Chapter 58).

POLYMYXINS

Example: polymyxin B.

Mechanism of action

Polymyxin binds to bacterial membrane phospholipids and alters permeability to potassium and sodium ions. The cell's osmotic barrier is lost, and susceptible organisms are killed by lysis.

Spectrum of activity

Polymyxin is active against Gram-negative organisms including pseudomonas species, but is inactive against Gram-positive bacteria and most fungi.

Resistance

Acquired resistance is rare.

Pharmacokinetics

Polymyxin is very poorly absorbed from the gut and is given parenterally or topically to the skin. Penetration into joint spaces or CSF is poor. It is excreted unchanged in the kidney with an intermediate half-life.

Unwanted effects

Substantial toxicity limits the use of polymyxin:

- Nephrotoxicity produces a dose-related but reversible renal impairment.

- Neurotoxicity produces dizziness, circumoral parasthesiae, convulsions. Rarely, neuromuscular blockade can produce respiratory paralysis.

GLYCOPEPTIDES

Examples: vancomycin, teicoplanin.

Mechanism of action

Vancomycin and teicoplanin act by inhibiting bacterial cell wall synthesis, but may have other effects on RNA synthesis. They are bactericidal.

Spectrum of activity

Vancomycin and teicoplanin are active only against Gram-positive bacteria, particularly staphylococci. They are reserved for serious staphylococcal infection or for bacterial endocarditis not responding to other treatments. Vancomycin is also effective against *Clostridium difficile* which colonizes the colon when normal flora are disturbed in antibiotic-associated colitis but metronidazole is now preferred for this indication.

Resistance

Acquired resistance is rare.

Pharmacokinetics

Both drugs are very poorly absorbed orally and are therefore usually given by intravenous infusion or in the case of teicoplanin by intramuscular injection. Oral administration of vancomycin is only useful for treating antibiotic-associated colitis. They are excreted by the kidneys; vancomycin has an intermediate half-life, teicoplanin a long half-life.

Unwanted effects

- Ototoxicity occurs with very high plasma levels but nephrotoxicity is uncommon. These effects may be enhanced if vancomycin or teicoplanin are used in combination with an aminoglycoside.
- Thrombophlebitis at the site of infusion.
- Skin rashes. Rapid intravenous injection of vancomycin produces generalized erythema, the "red man" syndrome.

- Blood disorders, including leucopenia, thrombocytopenia with teicoplanin.
- Gastrointestinal upset.

FUSIDIC ACID

Mechanism of action

Fusidic acid is a steroid which inhibits bacterial protein synthesis by preventing binding of transfer RNA to the ribosome.

Spectrum of activity

Activity is mainly against Gram-positive organisms, particularly *Staphylococcus aureus*. It is bactericidal.

Resistance

This is not infrequent when fusidic acid is used alone. It occurs either by mutation or by plasmid conjugation.

Pharmacokinetics

Oral absorption is complete, but an intravenous formulation is available. Penetration into synovial fluid and soft tissues is good. It is extensively metabolized in the liver and has an intermediate half-life.

Unwanted effects

- Cholestatic jaundice.
- Gastrointestinal intolerance.
- Thrombophlebitis with intravenous infusions.

NITROFURANTOIN

Mechanism of action

The probable mode of action is a consequence of reduction of nitrofurantoin to unstable metabolites inside the bacteria leading to DNA disruption. It is bactericidal, especially to organisms in acid urine.

Spectrum of activity

Nitrofurantoin is active against most Gram-positive cocci and *Escherichia coli* which infect the urinary tract; pseudomonas species are naturally resistant, as are many *Proteus* species.

Resistance

Chromosomal resistance occurs but is not common.

Pharmacokinetics

Nitrofurantoin is well absorbed from the gut. The half-life is short in the plasma where therapeutic concentrations are not achieved. It is excreted unchanged in the urine by both glomerular filtration and tubular secretion, but also appears in the bile. Urinary concentrations are high enough to treat lower urinary tract infections but the low tissue concentrations are often inadequate for acute pyelonephritis.

Unwanted effects

- Gastrointestinal upset is common including anorexia, nausea and vomiting.
- Pulmonary toxicity with long-term use includes acute allergic pneumonitis or chronic interstitial fibrosis.

ANTITUBERCULOUS DRUGS

RIFAMPICIN

Mechanism of action and spectrum of activity

Rifampicin acts by inhibition of DNA-dependent RNA polymerase and has a bactericidal action. It has a broad spectrum of activity which in addition to mycobacteria species includes brucella, legionella species and staphylococci. In tuberculosis it is considered an essential drug in the UK.

Resistance

This develops rapidly which limits its wider use as an antibacterial agent apart from the treatment of tuberculosis. It is a one-step process of mutation.

Pharmacokinetics

Oral absorption is good, and an intravenous formulation is also available. For tuberculosis, it is often given as a combination tablet with isoniazid to enhance compliance. Rifampicin is metabolized in the liver and has a short half-life.

Unwanted effects

- Nausea and anorexia.
- Hepatotoxicity, usually only producing a transient rise in plasma of transaminases.
- Induction of drug-metabolizing enzymes in the liver (Chapter 2). Important interactions include those with oral contraceptives (Chapter 48), phenytoin (Chapter 24), warfarin (Chapter 10) and sulphonylureas (Chapter 43).
- Various "toxicity syndromes" occur commonly with intermittent use, due to sensitization. They include renal failure, a shock-like syndrome and acute haemolytic anaemia.

ISONIAZID

Mechanism of action and spectrum of activity

Isoniazid inhibits production of long-chain mycolic acids which are unique to the cell wall of mycobacteria species. It is bactericidal against dividing organisms.

Resistance

Resistance is due to random mutation. It is uncommon in developed countries, but can be troublesome in developing countries.

Pharmacokinetics

Oral absorption is good, but reduced by food. Isoniazid is metabolized by acetylation in the liver, which is subject to genetic polymorphism (Chapter 2). Rapid acetylators show extensive first-pass metabolism and slow acetylators achieve twice the blood concentrations to those in rapid acetylators. The half-life is short but varies according to acetylator status.

Unwanted effects

- Nausea and vomiting.
- Peripheral neuropathy with high doses. This can be prevented by prophylactic use of oral pyridoxine supplements in high risk patients, for example those with diabetes, alcoholism, chronic renal failure or malnutrition. Neuropathy is more common in slow acetylators.

- Hepatotoxicity.
- Systemic lupus erythematosus like syndrome. Positive antinuclear antibodies are found in 20% of patients during long-term treatment, but fewer develop symptoms.

PYRAZINAMIDE

Mechanism of action and spectrum of activity

The action may be due to metabolism of pyrazinamide by an enzyme pyrazinamidase found inside *Mycobacterium tuberculosis*. The product pyrazinoic acid works at an acid intracellular pH to destroy the cell. It is bactericidal to semi-dormant cells.

Resistance

This develops rapidly if pyrazinamide is used as a sole treatment for tuberculosis.

Pharmacokinetics

Oral absorption is good and metabolism occurs in the liver. Pyrazinamide has a long half-life.

Unwanted effects

- Hepatotoxicity. A rise in plasma bilirubin usually requires cessation of treatment.
- Nausea and vomiting.
- Gout due to inhibition of uric acid excretion by the kidney.

ETHAMBUTOL

Mechanism of action and spectrum of activity

This is uncertain, but involves impaired synthesis of the cell wall of mycobacteria. Ethambutol is primarily bacteristatic.

Resistance

Resistance develops slowly but is common during prolonged treatment of tuberculosis if ethambutol is used alone.

Pharmacokinetics

Oral absorption is good. Only a small amount is metabolized and most is eliminated unchanged by the kidney. The half-life is long.

Unwanted effects

- Headache, dizziness.
- Optic neuritis produces initial red/green colour blindness, then reduced visual acuity. It is dose-related, but usually reversible.

STREPTOMYCIN

This is discussed above (see aminoglycosides). It is not used in the UK as first-line treatment for tuberculosis due to toxicity and the need for parenteral administration.

THIACETAZONE

Mechanism of action and spectrum of activity

Thiacetazone is a bacteristatic compound which is believed to form copper complexes within mycobacteria and interfere with copper enzyme carriers.

Resistance

This develops in about 30% of mycobacteria if thiacetazone is used alone.

Pharmacokinetics

Oral absorption is slow and most thiacetazone is metabolized in the liver. The half-life is usually long but shows wide interindividual variation.

Unwanted effects

- Gastrointestinal upset including nausea, vomiting, anorexia, abdominal pain and diarrhoea are common.
- Blurred vision, giddiness.
- Hypersensitivity reactions with severe cutaneous reactions and hepatitis.

DRUG TREATMENT OF TUBERCULOSIS

Mycobacterium tuberculosis readily develops resistance to single drug therapy. Three or four drugs are used for the first 2 months until bacterial sensitivities are known when treatment is continued with two drugs for a further 6–9 months to achieve a cure. A standard regimen in the UK includes rifampicin and isoniazid for

6 months with ethambutol and pyrazinamide for 2 months only. Ethambutol is not used for children, while streptomycin is substituted in some countries. In countries which cannot afford rifampicin, thiacetazone is often used in combination with isoniazid and initially streptomycin.

PRINCIPLES OF ANTIBACTERIAL THERAPY

Treatment of individual infections will not be discussed here. The following guidelines outline the principles that should be considered in the choice of a safe and effective therapy:

- Most antibacterial therapy is started "blind" without prior identification of the organism and its antimicrobial drug sensitivities. Such treatment should be guided by the clinical diagnosis and a knowledge of the most common pathogenic organisms in that situation. Local information about patterns of antimicrobial resistance should be considered.

- A drug with a narrow spectrum of activity should be used in preference to a broad-spectrum drug whenever possible. Unnecessary use of broad-spectrum drugs encourages the development of resistant organisms. This can present problems for the individual with selection of resistant pathogens or overgrowth of resistant commensal organisms. For. the community, the selection of resistant pathogens can create a substantial hazard, and render standard antimicrobial therapy less reliable. However, broad-spectrum cover is sometimes more appropriate, for example "blind" therapy of seriously ill patients.

- Combination therapy with more than one antimicrobial agent should not be used routinely. It may, however, be valuable to provide broad-spectrum cover in serious illness, for example the combination of cefotaxime and metronidazole to cover aerobic and anaerobic organisms in suspected Gram-negative septicaemia. When resistance is likely to develop readily to the first choice drug during protracted treatment, use of combination therapy can minimize that risk, for example in infective endocarditis or tuberculosis.

- In some situations bactericidal drugs are preferred to bacteriostatic agents, for example infective endocarditis or when the patient is immunocompromised. In most other situations the choice is probably not important.

- The site of infection may determine the choice of drug, for example some antimicrobials penetrate poorly into the biliary tree, urine, bone or cerebrospinal fluid.

- Oral therapy is preferred to parenteral treatment unless the drug is only available in parenteral formulation, for example some cephalosporins, or if gastrointestinal absorption may be unpredictable or unreliable, for example after abdominal surgery or in serious systemic infections.

- The duration of therapy should be as short as is compatible with adequate treatment of the infection. The decision is often arbitrary, for example 7–10 days in many infections. Some infections can be effectively treated over much shorter periods, for example 3-day courses are usually adequate for lower urinary tract infections. For other infections, long periods of treatment may be necessary to eliminate semi-dormant organisms or those in "privileged sites" to which antimicrobial penetration is poor, for example infective endocarditis, tuberculosis, osteomyelitis.

- Chemoprophylaxis with antimicrobials is used to prevent infection in many situations. Common examples include prevention of meningococcal meningitis in close contacts of an infected patient, prevention of infectious endocarditis in patients with diseased or artificial heart valves undergoing surgery and preoperative prophylaxis before gut, biliary, thoracic or orthopaedic surgery.

ANTIFUNGAL AGENTS

Compared with antibacterial drugs only a few agents have been developed which have activity against fungi, and most are toxic. Most fungal infections occur because of an underlying defect in host resistance such as immunosuppression which increases the need for effective agents.

POLYENES

Examples: nystatin, amphotericin B.

Mechanism of action

Polyenes bind to sterols in the cell wall of fungi and promote leakage of intracellular ions and disruption of membrane active transport mechanisms. They can be fungistatic or fungicidal.

Spectrum of activity

Nystatin is particularly effective against candidal infections and amphotericin B is active against all common systemic fungi (candida, aspergillus, mucor and cryptococcus).

Resistance

Acquired resistance is rare.

Pharmacokinetics

Nystatin is too toxic for systemic use and is not absorbed from the gastrointestinal tract. It is therefore used topically, for example cream, vaginal pessaries for superficial infections, or by mouth for oral and bowel infections.

Amphotericin B is poorly absorbed from the gut and is administered intravenously, or topically for oral and bowel infections. It can also be given intrathecally for fungal meningitis. Amphotericin B is eliminated slowly via the biliary tract and kidney and has a very long half-life of 1–2 days. Recently a new delivery vehicle amphotericin B liposomes has been developed. This delivers drug in a lipid environment which helps to concentrate it at the site of infection and reduces the toxicity of large doses.

Unwanted effects

- Nystatin is virtually free of both toxic and allergic side-effects when used topically.

Intravenous infusion of amphotericin B is commonly associated with:

- Fever and rigors during the first week of therapy.
- Anorexia, nausea and vomiting.
- Nephrotoxicity, which is the major limiting factor in treatment. It is dose-related, reduces glomerular filtration rate and produces hypokalaemia due to tubular leakage of potassium. Amphotericin B liposomes substantially reduce the risk of nephrotoxicity and are particularly useful to treat patients with pre-existing renal impairment.

N-SUBSTITUTED IMIDAZOLES

Example: ketoconazole.

Mechanism of action

These agents damage the cell membranes of fungi by inhibiting enzymes involved in membrane sterol synthesis, which inhibits fungal growth.

Spectrum of activity

The imidazoles are active against a wide variety of filamentous fungi and yeasts, including candida species.

Resistance

The development of resistance is rare.

Pharmacokinetics

Absorption of imidazoles from the gastrointestinal tract is incomplete but adequate blood concentrations of ketoconazole can be achieved. Topical formulations are available for superficial infections, for example skin and vagina. The imidazoles are metabolized in the liver and have intermediate half-lives.

Unwanted effects

- Nausea.
- Itching.
- Hepatitis. Asymptomatic elevation of liver enzymes is common, but more severe reactions are unusual.
- High doses of ketoconazole suppress androgen production in males and can cause oligospermia or gynaecomastia.

TRIAZOLES

Examples: fluconazole, itraconazole.

These compounds have a similar mechanism of action and spectrum of activity to the imidazoles (see above).

Pharmacokinetics

Oral absorption is good. Intravenous (fluconazole) and topical (itraconazole) formulations are also available. The triazoles are metabolized in the liver and have long half-lives.

Unwanted effects

- Abdominal pain and nausea.

5-FLUCYTOSINE

Mechanism of action

5-Flucytosine is converted to 5-fluorouracil selectively in fungal cells. This acts as an antimetabolite which competes with uracil for incorporation into fungal RNA. If some 20–40% of uracil is replaced by 5-fluorouracil this inhibits protein synthesis. Inhibition of DNA synthesis also occurs.

Spectrum of activity

5-Flucytosine is only active against yeasts such as candida and cryptococcus species. It is used for systemic infections.

Resistance

Resistance occurs readily and is due to a mutation which produces a deficiency of an enzyme which metabolizes 5-flucytosine or an excess synthesis of uracil which competes with the antimetabolite.

Pharmacokinetics

Flucytosine is well absorbed from the gut, and is also available for intravenous use. It is mainly eliminated unchanged in the urine and has a short half-life.

Unwanted effects

- Gastrointestinal intolerance is usually limited to diarrhoea.
- High concentrations produce reversible bone marrow depression.

GRISEOFULVIN

Mechanism of action

Griseofulvin inhibits dermatophyte mitosis by affecting the polymerization of microtubule protein.

Spectrum of activity

Griseofulvin is active against dermatophytes such as microsporum, epidermophyton and trichophyton species.

Resistance

Resistance has not been shown.

Pharmacokinetics

Griseofulvin is well absorbed from the gut and selectively concentrated in skin; only low concentrations are found in serum. Elimination is by metabolism in the liver and the half-life is long.

Unwanted effects

- Headache, nausea and diarrhoea.

ANTIVIRAL AGENTS

Viruses are intracellular parasites and share many of the host's metabolic processes. It is therefore difficult to damage the virus without damaging the host itself. In addition, the drugs are only effective while the virus is replicating, so the earlier they are given the more likely they are to work. An outline of the replication of RNA and DNA viruses is shown in Fig. 54.4. Since the mechanisms involved are distinct, antiviral drugs are often specific for one or other class of virus.

ZIDOVUDINE (AZT OR AZIDOTHYMIDINE)

Mechanism of action

Zidovudine inhibits RNA viral replication by an action on the viral enzyme reverse transcriptase which generates viral DNA for insertion into the host DNA sequence.

Spectrum of activity

It is mainly used for the palliation of acquired immunodeficiency syndrome (AIDS, human immunodeficiency virus (HIV) infection). Early suggestions that it may retard the progression of asymptomatic HIV disease have not been supported by recent studies.

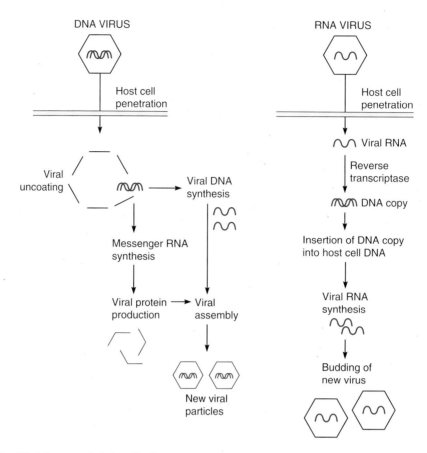

Figure 54.4 Simplified diagram of viral replication.

Pharmacokinetics

Zidovudine is almost completely absorbed from the gut, and about a third undergoes first-pass metabolism in the liver. Elimination is by hepatic metabolism and the half-life is short.

Unwanted effects

- Neutropenia and anaemia are the most frequent unwanted effects, usually occurring in patients with advanced AIDS.
- Headache, nausea, insomnia.
- Myalgia or myositis, especially with high doses.

AMANTADINE

Amantadine is discussed in Chapter 25. It acts by inhibiting viral DNA replication at the stage of uncoating after entry into the cell. The clinically useful activity of amantadine is limited to the treatment of influenza A. It will reduce the incidence of influenza A when used prophylactically and will shorten the symptoms and duration of the established illness, if given early enough.

ACYCLOVIR

Mechanism of action

Selective phosphorylation of acyclovir by viral thymidine kinase produces compounds which are potent inhibitors of viral DNA polymerase, and prevent viral DNA synthesis.

Spectrum of activity

Acyclovir is most active against herpes viruses (both simplex and zoster). It is only active against cytomegalovirus at high doses. Treatment of herpes infections is only successful if it is given at the start of the illness.

Pharmacokinetics

Acyclovir can be given topically, orally or intravenously but absorption from the gut is poor. The drug is widely distributed, but concentrations in the cerebrospinal fluid are low compared to plasma. Most elimination is via the kidney, and the half-life is short.

Unwanted effects

Most adverse effects occur with intravenous use:

- Severe local phlebitis at an infusion site.
- Encephalopathy occurs in 1% of patients.
- Nephrotoxicity due to crystallization of drug in the kidney. This can be limited by a high fluid intake.

GANCICLOVIR

Mechanism of action

Ganciclovir is related to acyclovir. It is activated in infected cells by intracellular kinases to a triphosphate derivate which inhibits viral DNA polymerase.

Spectrum of activity

Ganciclovir is active against all herpes viruses including cytomegalovirus. Because of its toxicity it is mainly used to treat serious infection with cytomegalovirus in immunosuppressed patients.

Pharmacokinetics

Ganciclovir is given intravenously. It is eliminated unchanged in the urine, and has a short half-life.

Unwanted effects

- The commonest side-effect is bone marrow suppression with neutropenia occurring in up to 40% of patients, and thrombocytopenia less frequently. The neutropenia may be prevented in some patients by the use of granulocyte-macrophage colony stimulating factor (Chapter 55).

IDOXURIDINE

Idoxuridine is used topically to treat superficial eye and skin infections caused by herpes simplex. For use on the skin penetration is enhanced by dissolving it in dimethylsulphoxide (DMSO). Its phosphorylated metabolite is incorporated into viral DNA and impairs transcription.

HUMAN INTERFERON α

Interferons are glycoproteins produced as part of the natural host defences to virus infections. There are three types: α, β and γ. Interferons α and β are produced by most cells in response to viral infection but production of interferon γ is limited to T lymphocytes. Administration of interferon α produced by *Escherichia coli* can prevent, but not cure, certain viral infections. They have several actions including binding to receptors on both RNA and DNA viruses and enhancing synthesis of intracellular enzymes which affect RNA translation.

Interferons have additional effects on human malignant cells (Chapter 55), reducing their rate of multiplication, possibly by reimposing normal control mechanisms. Macrophage and natural killer-cell activity is enhanced (Chapter 40).

Pharmacokinetics

Interferon α is not absorbed orally and must be given intramuscularly or subcutaneously. It is inactivated in renal tubular cells and also in target tissue cells. The half-life is short.

Unwanted effects

- An influenza-like illness with fever, chills, headache and myalgia.
- Bone marrow suppression is common.
- Neurological effects include confusion and seizures.

Clinical uses of interferon α

- Chronic hepatitis.
- Condylomata acuminata.
- AIDS-related Kaposi's sarcoma.
- Hairy cell leukaemia.
- Recurrent or metastatic renal cell carcinoma.

ANTIPROTOZOAL AGENTS

MALARIA

Four species of the protozoan plasmodium produce malaria in man: *P. vivax*, *P. ovale*, *P. malariae* and *P. falciparum*. After entry of sporozoites into blood from the *Anopheles* mosquito, the parasite is sequestered in the liver and divides to form tissue schizonts (Fig. 54.5). When the pre-erythrocytic sexual cycle is complete, merozoites escape into the blood and invade erythrocytes. They then multiply asexually in the erythrocytes which rupture and release merozoites to invade new cells. Symptoms usually occur after several such cycles; the duration of the incubation period varies between different parasites. *P. vivax* and *P. ovale* continue to multiply in the liver: drugs which treat the erythrocytic phase will not produce a radical cure (elimination of all parasites) in these patients and relapsing infection can occur. *P. falciparum* and *P. malariae* only multiply in erythrocytes, but disease can "recrudesce" if parasites are not completely eliminated from the blood.

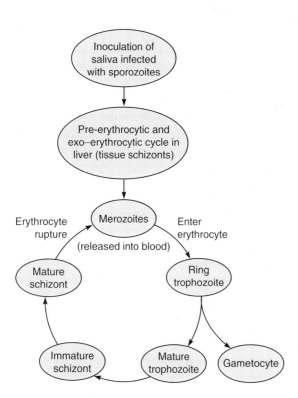

Figure 54.5 The life-cycle of malaria parasites in man.

Clinical symptoms include chills as merozoites enter blood from ruptured erythrocytes. Nausea, vomiting and headache are common. A fever follows and the attack concludes with sweating. *P. falciparum* produces the most severe symptoms due to agglutination of red cells which produce capillary thrombosis, especially in the brain leading to cerebral malaria.

ANTIMALARIAL DRUGS

CHLOROQUINE AND HYDROXYCHLOROQUINE

Mechanism of action

Erythrocytes infected by malaria parasites concentrate large amounts of chloroquine or hydroxychloroquine, since it is actively transported across the membrane of the parasites. Three mechanisms of action have been proposed:

- Both compounds are bases which may raise lysosomal pH. This will reduce the ability of the parasite to digest haemoglobin, thus inhibiting its growth.

- The drugs also interact with ferriprotoporphyrin IX which is formed during digestion of haemoglobin, an action which prevents further degradation by the parasite.

- A third possibility is inclusion of chloroquine among the nucleic acids in DNA, inhibiting gene expression.

Both chloroquine and hydroxychloroquine also possess slow-onset anti-inflammatory activity which is useful in the treatment of rheumatoid arthritis (Chapter 32).

Pharmacokinetics

Chloroquine and hydroxychloroquine are 4-aminoquinolines which are completely absorbed from the gut, or can be given intravenously. They have a very high volume of distribution due to selective concentration in melanin-containing tissues, for example the retina of the eye, in the liver, spleen and kidney. About half is converted in the liver to active metabolites, the rest is excreted unchanged by the kidney. The half-life is very long during chronic dosing; an initial half-life of up to 6 days is followed by a second slow phase of tissue elimination with a half-life greater than 1 month.

Unwanted effects

- Nausea, vomiting, diarrhoea, abdominal pain, which may be due to anticholinesterase activity (Chapters 4 and 29).
- Cardiovascular depression after intravenous use with hypotension and heart block; these are quinidine-like effects (Chapter 9).
- Retinopathy with cumulative doses producing retinal pigmentation and visual field defects.
- Skin rashes and itching.

MEFLOQUINE

Mechanism of action

This is similar to chloroquine, although binding to DNA does not occur.

Pharmacokinetics

Mefloquine is an amino alcohol which is well absorbed from the gut and has a high affinity for lung, liver and lymphoid tissue. Extensive metabolism occurs in the liver but the elimination half-life is very long, in excess of 20 days.

Unwanted effects

- CNS effects: dizziness, vertigo, headache.
- Gastrointestinal effects, similar to chloroquine.

PRIMAQUINE

Mechanism of action

Unlike structurally related drugs, primaquine only affects the exoerythrocytic parasite. It enters the parasite in the liver, and may inhibit mitochondrial respiration. The active metabolites also bind to parasitic DNA (cf. chloroquine).

Pharmacokinetics

Primaquine is an 8-aminoquinolone which is completely absorbed from the gut and rapidly metabolized in the liver, producing active compounds. The half-life is intermediate.

Unwanted effects

- Intravascular haemolysis in patients with glucose-6-phosphate dehydrogenase (G6PD) deficiency (see Chapter 56).
- Gastrointestinal effects similar to chloroquine.
- Chest pain.
- Discoloration of urine.

Primaquine is available in the UK only for individual "named" patients.

QUININE

Mechanism of action

Similar to chloroquine, but does not bind to DNA.

Pharmacokinetics

Quinine is well absorbed from the gut, but can also be given by intravenous infusion. Metabolism in the liver is extensive and the half-life is intermediate in healthy subjects, becoming long in severe malaria.

Unwanted effects

- "Cinchonism": tinnitus, headache, nausea, visual disturbances with vertigo and hearing loss if severe.
- Stimulation of insulin secretion producing hypoglycaemia.
- Quinidine-like effects on the heart (Chapter 9) with bradycardias, heart block or ventricular tachycardia. Most often this occurs with intravenous loading doses.

PYRIMETHAMINE

Mechanism of action

Selective dihydrofolate reductase inhibition in the parasite reduces folic acid synthesis (Fig. 54.3). It is usually given as a combination formulation with a sulphonamide derivative, either sulfadoxine or dapsone.

Pharmacokinetics

Pyrimethamine is well absorbed from the gut and undergoes extensive hepatic metabolism. The half-life is very long at about 3–4 days.

Unwanted effects

Pyrimethamine is usually well tolerated.

- Photosensitive rashes.
- Megaloblastic anaemia with chronic therapy.

PROGUANIL

Mechanism of action

Proguanil inhibits plasmodial dihydrofolate reductase (Fig. 54.3), mainly through its active metabolite. This inhibits folate production in both pre-erythrocyte and erythrocyte parasites. It is only used for prophylaxis.

Pharmacokinetics

Absorption of proguanil from the gut is good, and extensive metabolism occurs in the liver to cycloguanil, a potent active derivative. The half-life of proguanil is long, that of cycloguanil is short.

Unwanted effects

- Mouth ulcers.
- Epigastric discomfort.

DRUG TREATMENT OF MALARIA

The recommended drug depends on the type of parasite and the pattern of resistance where the infection was acquired. If the infecting organism is unknown, it is assumed to be *P. falciparum* which carries the greatest risk. Latest recommendations should be obtained from regional tropical disease advisory centres.

Examples of current recommended treatments include:

- *P. falciparum*: chloroquine resistance is common. Oral quinine or mefloquine are given initially (intravenous quinine is used for serious infections). This is followed by pyrimethamine with sulfadoxine (Fansidar) or by tetracycline if the plasmodia are Fansidar-resistant.
- Benign malaria: chloroquine is given initially. For *P. vivax* and *P. ovale*, primaquine is then given to destroy hepatic parasites.

PROPHYLAXIS AGAINST MALARIA

The recommendations for prophylaxis depends on patterns of resistance in the area to be visited. Where resistance is low, chloroquine or proguanil are often recommended. For many areas a combination of both drugs is desirable. Mefloquine is recommended in some areas for short-term travellers. Specific prophylaxis must also take into account the unwanted effects of the drugs and other factors such as pregnancy, renal or hepatic impairment. Prophylaxis must be continued for 1 month after leaving a malarious area to protect against infection acquired immediately prior to departure.

OTHER PROTOZOAL INFECTIONS

Details of these infections are not given here: an outline is given in Table 54.3. Important drugs available in the UK for these conditions are discussed below.

Table 54.3 Protozoal infections

Organism	Disorder	Drug examples
Entamoeba histolytica	Acute amoebic dysentery	Metronidazole
	Chronic intestinal amoebiasis	Diloxanide
	Amoebic liver abscess	Metronidazole
Trichomonas vaginalis	Vaginitis	Metronidazole
Giardia lamblia	Giardiasis	Metronidazole
Leishmania	Visceral leishmaniasis	Sodium stibogluconate
Pneumocystis carinii	Pneumocystis pneumonia	Pentamidine

PENTAMIDINE

Indications: *Pneumocystis carinii*, leishmania species.

Mechanism of action

Pentamidine undergoes active uptake into the cell where it probably inhibits DNA synthesis and ribosomal synthesis of protein and phospholipid. It is cytotoxic to *Pneumocystis carinii* in the non-replicating state.

Pharmacokinetics

Pentamidine is given intravenously or inhaled as an aerosol. The latter route is particularly useful for *Pneumocystis* pneumonia (which affects immuno-compromised patients, especially those with AIDS), since lung concentrations are low after intravenous administration. Pentamidine is metabolized in the liver and has an intermediate half-life.

Unwanted effects

- Inhaled pentamidine produces bronchial irritation with cough and bronchospasm.
- Intravenous pentamidine is nephrotoxic, can produce irreversible hypoglycaemia and life-threatening arrhythmias such as ventricular tachycardia.

SODIUM STIBOGLUCONATE

Indication: visceral leishmaniasis.

Mechanism of action

Sodium stibogluconate is an organic pentavalent antimony derivative which may act by binding to thiol groups in the parasite.

Pharmacokinetics

It must be given parenterally, either by intramuscular injection or slow intravenous infusion. It has a short half-life and is eliminated by the kidney.

Unwanted effects

- Anorexia and vomiting.
- Cough and substernal pain during intravenous infusion.

DILOXANIDE FUROATE

Indication: *Entamoeba histolytica*.

Mechanism of action

Unknown.

Pharmacokinetics

Hydrolysis in the gut liberates diloxanide and furoic acid; 90% of the diloxanide is then absorbed and rapidly conjugated in the liver. Diloxanide has a short half-life. The unabsorbed fraction of diloxanide may contribute to the drug's effectiveness in amoebic dysentery.

Unwanted effects

Usually well tolerated.

- Gastrointestinal effects: flatulence, anorexia, nausea, diarrhoea.

ANTIHELMINTHIC AGENTS

Details of helminth infections are not given here, but an outline of the more commonly encountered conditions is given in Table 54.4. Drugs specifically for helminth infections are discussed below.

THIABENDAZOLE

Indications: threadworm, mixed worm infestations (not filariasis).

Mechanism of action

Thiabendazole inhibits the mitochondrial fumarate reductase system, which is specific to helminths. It is active against the adults, larvae and eggs.

Table 54.4 Helminthic infections

Helminth	Common name	Drug examples
Enterobius vermicularis	Threadworm	Mebendazole Piperazine Pyrantel
Ascaris lumbricoides	Roundworm	Mebendazole Pyrantel Piperazine
Toxocara canis	Dog roundworm	Thiabendazole Diethylcarbamazine
Taenia species	Tapeworm	Niclosamide
Ancylostoma species Necator species	Hookworm	Bephenium Pyrantel Mebendazole
Microfilariae (e.g. loa loa, *Wuchereria bancrofti, Brugia malayi*)		Diethylcarbamazine
Strongyloides stercoralis		Thiabendazole

Pharmacokinetics

Oral absorption is almost complete and metabolism in the liver is extensive. The half-life is short.

Unwanted effects

- Gastrointestinal effects are common: anorexia, nausea, vomiting.
- Dizziness.

DIETHYLCARBAMAZINE

Indication: filariasis.

Mechanism of action

Diethylcarbamazine may paralyse the neuromuscular system of the filariae and also expose antigens on the surface coat, leading to their destruction in the reticuloendothelial system.

Pharmacokinetics

Oral absorption is good, and about half the drug is metabolized in the liver, the rest excreted unchanged in the kidney. The half-life is intermediate.

Unwanted effects

- Most problems are due to release of antigens from dying filariae. The subsequent reaction includes fever, headache, nausea, muscle and joint pains, itching and postural hypotension. The onset is about 2 h after dosing and is almost diagnostic of the disease. The reaction is occasionally severe and life-threatening.

MEBENDAZOLE

Indications: threadworm, roundworm, hookworm.

Mechanism of action

Mebendazole produces selective, irreversible blockade of glucose uptake by sensitive worms, depleting their main source of energy.

Pharmacokinetics

Oral absorption is poor; drug which is absorbed is rapidly metabolized in the liver. Most of the drug acts from within the gut.

Unwanted effects

• Diarrhoea and colic.

PIPERAZINE

Indications: threadworm and roundworm.

Mechanism of action

Piperazine competitively inhibits the effect of acetylcholine at the smooth muscle of the worm, producing a reversible flaccid paralysis.

Pharmacokinetics

Absorption is rapid from the gut, but little is known about its handling after absorption.

Unwanted effects

• Gastrointestinal upset.

PYRANTEL

Indications: roundworm, threadworm, hookworm.

Mechanism of action

Pyrantel acts as a depolarizing neuromuscular blocking agent in the worm (see Chapter 28). Poor absorption limits the effect on the host.

Pharmacokinetics

Absorption from the gut is very low.

Unwanted effects

• Gastrointestinal effects: nausea, vomiting, diarrhoea, abdominal cramps.

NICLOSAMIDE

Indication: tapeworm.

Mechanism of action

Niclosamide inhibits generation of ATP by preventing phosphorylation of ADP in the mitochondrion. Purgatives are usually given after niclosamide to remove viable ova from the gut.

Pharmacokinetics

Some oral absorption (up to 20%) occurs with subsequent liver metabolism.

Unwanted effects

• Gastrointestinal upset.
• Lightheadedness.
• Pruritis.

BEPHENIUM

Indication: hookworm.

Mechanism of action

Bephenium reduces the concentration of histamine in the worm by interference with its metabolism.

Pharmacokinetics

Oral absorption is negligible. The taste is extremely bitter.

Unwanted effects

• Gastrointestinal upset: vomiting, nausea, diarrhoea, abdominal pain.
• CNS effects: vertigo, headache.

55

Chemotherapy of Malignancy

Approximately 20–25% of people in the western world die from cancer. Surgery and radiotherapy are valuable in treating localized cancers, but are less effective in prolonging the patient's life once the tumour has spread to produce metastases. The successful treatment of cancer frequently involves a multidisciplinary approach which also includes necessary psychological and social support. The introduction of cytotoxic chemotherapy to kill rapidly proliferating neoplastic cells has had a major impact on the successful treatment of malignant disease, especially diffuse tumours.

A wide range of different chemicals with a variety of mechanisms and sites of action within the cell has been introduced into clinical practice in the past three decades. Although the agents may differ in their specific cellular targets they nearly all rely on the rapid rate of growth and division of cancer cells to provide a measure of selectivity between normal and malignant tissue. Thus they share a number of properties and characteristics, both beneficial and adverse, which will be discussed first as general considerations. Information on the major groups of chemicals will then be given with information on mechanisms of action and specific unwanted effects.

The rate of introduction of new anticancer drugs has decreased in recent years largely because effective agents are already in widespread use. A placebo-controlled clinical trial of a single new cytotoxic drug is now unethical and the efficacy of any new agent has to be assessed by its addition to the best available current therapy. Therefore, a major benefit would be necessary for a new agent to have a clinically or statistically significant effect. There are a number of *in vivo* animal tests for detecting antineoplastic activity, but these frequently over-predict the likely effectiveness in clinical use because the animal tumours used as models have a much higher growth fraction (see later). Therefore most recent advances in cancer chemotherapy have arisen from the more effective use of existing agents, by optimizing drug combinations and regimens and by minimizing toxicity, rather than the introduction of novel compounds.

Considerable attention is currently being given to the products of proto-oncogene activation, since these are often related to cell growth factors and may provide a useful target for future drug development. Proto-oncogenes are normal gene sequences which control cell proliferation and differentiation; they are capable of being activated to oncogenes, the expression of which leads to tumour development. Identification of the protein sequence and tertiary structure of the growth factor may allow new drug molecules to be designed to interact with the specific structure of the growth factor (analogous to recent developments in the field of receptor pharmacology). However, whether this will increase the selectivity of drugs for neoplastic cells is unknown as this may still be based on rates of growth and division. Another possible future approach for therapy is to increase the effectiveness of tumour suppressor genes.

GENERAL CONSIDERATIONS

CLINICAL USE OF ANTINEOPLASTIC AGENTS

Different forms of cancer differ in their sensitivity to chemotherapy. The most responsive include lymphomas, leukaemias, choriocarcinoma and testicular carcinoma, while solid tumours such as colorectal, adrenocortical and squamous cell bronchial carcinomas generally show a poor response. An intermediate response is shown by other cancers, for example bladder, head and neck, and oat cell bronchogenic tumours and sex-related cancers, for example breast, ovary, endometrium and prostate. The sensitivity within a patient may change due to the development of resistance (see later).

MECHANISMS OF ACTION

The majority of antineoplastic agents act on the process of DNA synthesis within the cancer cell, as summarized in Fig. 55.1. Therefore, target selectivity is determined by the rate of cell division. Resting cells, that is those in the G_o phase (Fig. 55.2), are resistant to many anticancer drugs, such as the antimetabolites; these are termed cell-cycle specific agents because the cells have to be in the appropriate phase of the cell cycle at the time of treatment

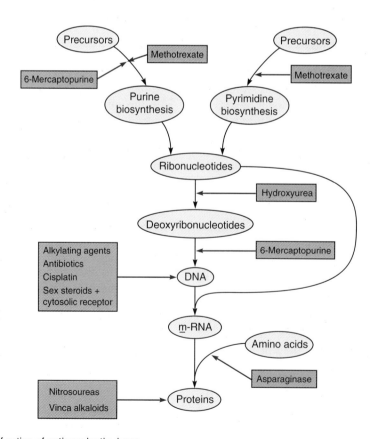

Figure 55.1 Sites of action of antineoplastic drugs.

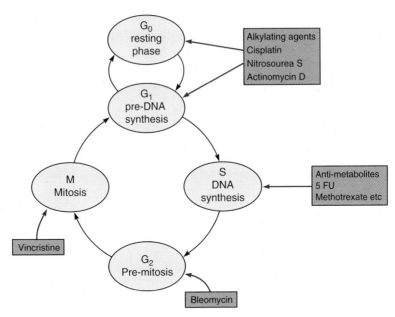

Figure 55.2 Anticancer drugs and the cell cycle.

for the drug to work (Fig. 55.2). However, other drugs, such as the alkylating agents, nitrosoureas and cisplatin have a "hit and run" action on the DNA and their effect becomes apparent later when the cells attempt to undergo division.

The sensitivity of a cancer to treatment depends therefore on the growth fraction — that is the fraction of cells undergoing mitosis at any time. For example in Burkitt's lymphoma almost 100% of neoplastic cells are undergoing division and the tumour is very sensitive and shows a dramatic response to a single dose of cyclophosphamide. In contrast the growth fraction represents less than 5% of cells in a carcinoma of the colon resulting in its resistance to chemotherapy. However, metastases from colonic carcinoma deposited in the liver and elsewhere initially have a high growth fraction and are sensitive to chemotherapy, which is frequently given following surgical removal of the primary tumour.

Studies using *in vitro* cancer cell lines have shown that:

- Anticancer drugs produce a proportional cell kill, for example 99% of the cells present, so that multiple treatments may be necessary with each treatment producing an exponential decrease in the number of viable cells remaining.

- Essentially complete eradication of tumour cells is necessary to prevent regrowth.

- Increased efficacy is obtained if treatment with cell-cycle specific drugs is timed to coincide with appropriate phases of cell division within the cell population.

Although these concepts also apply to *in vivo* therapy the situation is complicated because there are risk:benefit considerations to be taken into account and these change with successive treatments. In addition the immune system probably contributes to the final removal of residual malignant cells, and most cytotoxic drugs compromise immunoresponsiveness. Finally, the periodicity of doses is less critical *in vivo* because cancer cell cycles are not synchronized within the target population between treatments.

RESISTANCE

Resistance to chemotherapeutic agents may develop in a number of ways:

- Use of alternative metabolic pathways and salvage mechanisms to circumvent the blocked biochemical process; such mechanisms are usually drug-specific.

- Increased inactivation of the compound within the cancer cell.

- Increased removal of the chemical from the cancer cell; this may involve increased transcription of the gene for P-glycoprotein which acts as a carrier for the elimination from the cell of a number of cytotoxic compounds. The carrier can be blocked by calcium channel antagonists, such as nifedipine or verapamil, cyclosporine and tamoxifen and these drugs may be added to cytotoxic drug regimens to minimize resistance.

ADVERSE EFFECTS

Anticancer drugs are among the most toxic compounds given to humans with a therapeutic index of approximately 1, that is the toxic dose usually *is* the therapeutic dose. Because drug selectivity is for tissues with a high growth fraction it is not surprising that a number of normal non-malignant tissues are also affected:

- Gastrointestinal tract — mucosal cells have a rapid turnover. Toxicity may produce anorexia, mucosal ulceration or diarrhoea. Nausea and vomiting are common especially with alkylating agents and cisplatin and this may limit the patient's ability to tolerate an optimal dosage regimen.

- Bone marrow — myelosuppression is a serious consequence of treatment and can lead to severe leucopenia, thrombocytopenia and sometimes anaemia. These haematological consequences may limit the drug dosage prescribed for the patient. There is a high risk of both infection and haemorrhage following chemotherapy.

- Hair follicle cells — partial or complete alopecia may occur but this is usually temporary.

- Reproductive toxicity — both sexes are affected and sterility can result; women frequently show dysmenorrhoea or amenorrhoea. Because of the mechanism of action of cytotoxic drugs it must be considered that most would exhibit teratogenic activity — pregnant women should not be exposed to cytotoxic drugs as patients, doctors or nurses.

Dosage regimens are usually established so that the normal tissues, especially bone marrow and gut, can recover between doses (Fig. 55.3).

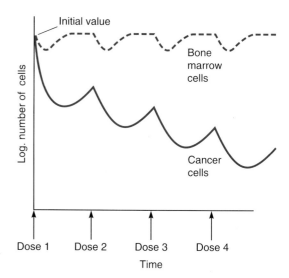

Figure 55.3 Hypothetical dosing schedule to allow recovery of normal tissues. The malignant cells show a greater proportional kill because a greater fraction are in division at any time. Theoretically the response of the malignant cells to dose 2 would be greater than for dose 1 if cell cycles became synchronized and dose 2 was given during the correct phase of the growth cycle. A typical dose interval would be 3–4 weeks. A minimum of 10^9 tumour cells are usually present when tumours are first detectable.

DRUG COMBINATIONS

It is common practice to treat many cancers with a mixture of different antineoplastic drugs simultaneously, and there are numerous permutations used clinically, for example MOPP (mustine, oncovin (vincristine), procarbazine, prednisolone) for Hodgkin's lymphoma. Criteria for selecting combinations are:

- Each drug should be an active anticancer drug in its own right (e.g. a second drug would not be given simply to increase the formation of an active metabolite of the first).

- Each drug should have a different mechanism of action and target site within the cancer cell — this will increase efficacy while reducing the likelihood of resistance.

- Each drug should have a different site for any organ-specific toxicity (obviously all agents will affect tissues with a high growth factor).

- (Another criterion apparent to cynics is that one of the drugs should preferably start with a vowel so that the acronym for the combination is more memorable! (e.g. "oncovin" which is a trade name for "vincristine" in MOPP).)

SPECIFIC CHEMOTHERAPEUTIC AGENTS

ALKYLATING AGENTS

Examples: cyclophosphamide, melphalan, busulphan, chlorambucil.

These drugs were developed from the sulphur mustard gases

$$S \begin{array}{c} \diagup CH_2CH_2Cl \\ \diagdown CH_2CH_2Cl \end{array}$$

used in the First World War trenches and which caused bone marrow suppression in addition to the respiratory toxicity for which they were developed. Replacement of the sulphur atom by nitrogen allowed the introduction of more complex side-chains which has given rise to a range of more stable non-volatile therapeutic agents.

Mechanism of action and uses

The important functional groups are the chloroethane side-chains

$$R{-}N \begin{array}{c} \diagup CH_2CH_2Cl \\ \diagdown CH_2CH_2Cl \end{array}$$

which are highly reactive and undergo rearrangement to produce a chemical species which can bind covalently to sites within DNA such as N7 of guanine

$$R{-}N \begin{array}{c} \diagup CH_2CH_2Cl \\ \diagdown CH_2CH_2Cl \end{array} \quad \overset{\displaystyle \rightharpoonup}{Cl^{\ominus}} \quad R{-}\overset{\oplus}{N} \begin{array}{c} CH_2{-}CH_2 \\ | \\ CH_2CH_2Cl \end{array}$$

$$\longrightarrow R{-}N \begin{array}{c} CH_2CH_2 \text{ Guanine} \\ | \\ \diagdown CH_2CH_2Cl \end{array}$$

The alkylated guanine in DNA may either be repaired or interfere with DNA replication by (i) being misread; (ii) undergoing further metabolism via ring opening; or (iii) cross linking to another guanine via the remaining CH_2CH_2Cl group.

Cyclophosphamide and chlorambucil are commonly used for chronic lymphocytic leukaemia and chlorambucil is also given for lymphomas. Melphalan is useful for myeloma and busulphan for chronic myeloid leukaemia.

Cyclophosphamide is also used for immunosuppression in non-malignant disorders (Chapter 42).

Pharmacokinetics

These depend on the nature of the R-group in the general formula given above. The original and simplest drug is mustine in which $R = -CH_3$; it is very unstable and solutions have to be injected soon after preparation since decomposition occurs in minutes; care is necessary when handling the toxic dosing solutions.

A major advance was achieved with the introduction of cyclophosphamide which is a chemically stable solid which can be given orally: it is a prodrug which undergoes metabolic activation in the R-group:

$$R = \begin{array}{c} O \quad O{-}CH_2 \\ \parallel \\ -P \quad \quad CH_2 \\ \diagdown \\ N{-}CH_2 \\ | \\ H \end{array}$$

Two toxic metabolites are produced from cyclophosphamide, acrolein ($CH_2{=}CH{-}CHO$) and phosphoramide mustard which contains the $-N(CH_2CH_2Cl)_2$ group: the drug has an intermediate half-life due to its metabolism but toxic metabolites are excreted in the urine. Melphalan and chlorambucil have an aromatic substituent as the R-group: they have short or very short half-lives and may be excreted in the urine unchanged.

Unwanted effects

- Generalized cytotoxicity is common.
- Cyclophosphamide also causes bladder toxicity with haemorrhagic cystitis which may be prevented by prior treatment with MESNA (Chapter 56); bladder cancer may develop years after cyclophosphamide therapy.
- Fertility is reduced due to impaired gametogenesis.
- A particular problem with the long-term use of alkylating agents, especially if combined with radiotherapy, is the development of acute myeloid leukaemia.

NITROSOUREAS

Examples: BCNU (carmustine), CCNU (lomustine).

Mechanism of action and uses

Nitrosoureas inhibit the synthesis of DNA, RNA and protein; they contain a reactive group:

$$X—N—C—NH—R$$

(with NO and O groups on the N—C)

which is exposed by non-enyzmatic degradation and covalently binds to nucleic acids and protein to produce a carbamylated product:

$$Protein—NH—C—NH—R$$

(with O group on the C)

Both BCNU and CCNU also contain an active chloroethane ($–CH_2CH_2Cl$) side-chain in the above general formula at X (CCNU) or X and R (BCNU), and therefore also react by the alkylating mechanism given above. They are mainly used for Hodgkin's lymphoma.

Pharmacokinetics

The drugs are well absorbed from the gut and have short half-lives, and are eliminated by the kidney. BCNU is given as a short term (1–2 h) infusion to provide a more extended exposure profile.

Unwanted effects

These drugs, like the alkylating agents, have a typical general toxicity profile.

ANTIMETABOLITES

FOLIC ACID ANTAGONISTS

Example: methotrexate.

An astute clinical observation, that the administration of folic acid to children with leukaemia exacerbated their condition, led to the development of a folate antagonist methotrexate, which represents an important landmark in cancer chemotherapy.

Mechanism of action and uses

Folic acid in its reduced form (tetrahydrofolic acid; THF) is an important biochemical intermediate. It is essential for synthetic reactions which involve the addition of a single carbon atom, such as the introduction of the methyl group into thymidylate and the synthesis of the purine ring system. During such reactions THF is oxidized to dihydrofolic acid (DHF) which has to be reduced by dihydrofolate reductase back to THF before it can accept a further 1-carbon group. Methotrexate has a very high affinity for and inhibits the active site of mammalian dihydrofolate reductase, thereby blocking purine and thymidylate synthesis and inhibiting the synthesis of DNA, RNA and protein.

Mechanisms of resistance of cancer cells include altered or increased cellular levels of dihydrofolate reductase, increased salvage of thymidine and impaired uptake of methotrexate. Leucovorin (formyl THF or folinic acid) is frequently administered shortly after high-dose methotrexate to rescue normal tissues and enhance selectivity for tumour cells.

Methotrexate is given for acute lymphoblastic leukaemia, non-Hodgkin's lymphomas and various other malignancies. It is also used in non-malignant conditions such as psoriasis (Chapter 52).

Pharmacokinetics

Methotrexate is well absorbed from the gut but can also be given intravenously or intrathecally. It has an intermediate elimination half-life and is eliminated by renal excretion. A small amount may be retained for longer periods both strongly bound to the dihydrofolate reductase and as polyglutamate conjugates.

Unwanted effects

- The general forms of tissue toxicity are produced (especially of the bone marrow).
- Hepatotoxicity following chronic therapy (as in psoriasis).
- Toxicity is increased in the presence of reduced renal excretion, and methotrexate should be avoided if there is significant renal impairment.

BASE ANALOGUES

Examples: 5-fluorouracil (5-FU), cytarabine (cytosine arabinoside), 6-mercaptopurine.

A number of useful chemotherapeutic agents have been produced by simple modifications to the structures of normal purine and pyrimidine bases.

5-fluorouracil(5-FU)

azacytidine

6-mercaptopurine

cytosine arabinoside (cytarabine)

Mechanisms of action and uses

Nucleic acid biosynthesis is inhibited by a variety of actions.

- Synthesis of purine or pyrimidine e.g. thymidylate synthetase involves the addition of a methyl group on carbon-5 of deoxyuridine-monophosphate, and this is blocked by the introduction of a fluorine substituent (5-FU).
- Inhibition of DNA polymerase leading to impairment of DNA synthesis. This action will be cell-cycle specific for the S-phase (cytosine arabinoside).
- Incorporation into DNA and misreading (5-FU).
- Many of these drugs require bioactivation by conversion to the corresponding nucleotides before they can exert their intracellular effects.

5-FU is given for colon and breast cancers, cytosine arabinoside for acute myeloblastic leukaemia and mercaptopurine for various acute leukaemias.

Pharmacokinetics

Base analogues tend to be absorbed and metabolized (where possible) by the pathways involved with the corresponding normal base. Oral absorption is often erratic, and most are given intravenously. The urine is a minor route of elimination (up to 1% of the parent drug) and half-lives are short to intermediate.

Unwanted effects

- Typical cytotoxic effects are common.
- Allopurinol (Chapter 33) interferes with the metabolism of 6-mercaptopurine, and the dose should be reduced if these drugs are used concurrently.

MITOTIC INHIBITORS

Examples: vincristine, vinblastine, etoposide.

The vinca alkaloids are complex natural chemicals isolated from the periwinkle plant. They are structurally very similar but have different spectra of clinical use and side-effects. Etoposide has a similar mechanism of action.

Mechanism of action and uses

They bind to tubulin to produce metaphase arrest and therefore are cycle specific. They are used for various lymphomas and the vinca alkaloids for acute leukaemia. All are effective in some solid tumours.

Pharmacokinetics

Absorption of oral doses is unpredictable and these drugs are usually given intravenously. Etoposide can be given orally. Elimination is largely by metabolism with little renal excretion. They have long half-lives.

Unwanted effects

- General cytotoxicity occurs, although vincristine produces little marrow toxicity.
- Neurological effects, such as peripheral neuropathy and neuromuscular problems, occur especially with vincristine and with patients who have hepatic dysfunction.

ANTIBIOTICS

Examples: doxorubicin, bleomycin, actinomycin D.

Some antibiotics which do not show a high selectivity for bacteria have proved to be useful for cancer chemotherapy rather than infections.

Mechanisms of action and uses

These compounds intercalate between base pairs in the DNA double-helix stabilizing its structure and inhibiting DNA replication. Increased scission of DNA also occurs with bleomycin and doxorubicin, possibly by enhanced free radical attack. Toxicity is increased by simultaneous radiotherapy. Doxorubicin is widely used for acute leukaemias, lymphomas and solid tumours. Bleomycin is also given for lymphomas and some solid tumours, and actinomycin is reserved for paediatric cancers.

Pharmacokinetics

They are poorly absorbed from the gut and therefore given intravenously. They have very long half-lives of 1–2 days (except that of bleomycin which is short) and are eliminated by either metabolism (doxorubicin) or renal excretion (actinomycin and bleomycin).

Unwanted effects

- Generally cytotoxicity can occur.
- Doxorubicin produces dose-related irreversible myocardial damage due to free radical attack.
- Bleomycin can rarely cause a fatal pulmonary fibrosis, but produces little bone marrow suppression.

HORMONES AND HORMONE ANTAGONISTS

Cancers that arise from cell lines with steroid receptors which promote their growth and cell division are frequently susceptible to inhibitory steroids:

- Glucocorticoids (Chapter 47) — suppress lymphocyte mitosis and are used in leukaemia and lymphoma; also helpful in reducing oedema around a tumour.

- Oestrogens (Chapter 48) — suppress prostate cancer cells both locally and metastases, and provide symptomatic improvement; gynaecomastia is a common side-effect.
- Progestogens (Chapter 48) — suppress endometrial cancer cells and lung secondaries.
- Oestrogen antagonists (e.g. tamoxifen) — suppress breast cancer cells. Tamoxifen is active orally and binds competitively to oestrogen receptors. It has an active metabolite with a long half-life which may take several weeks to achieve steady-state concentrations. Unwanted effects include hot flushes and amenorrhoea in premenopausal women and vaginal bleeding in postmenopausal women.
- Androgen antagonists (e.g. flutamide, Chapter 49) — suppress prostate cancer cells. Unwanted effects include gynaecomastia, decreased spermatogenesis and decreased libido.
- Gonadotrophin-releasing hormone antagonists (Chapter 46) — suppress prostate cancer cells.
- Aromatase inhibitors (e.g. formestane) — aromatase is the enzyme which converts androgens to oestrogens (Fig. 47.2). Inhibition of aromatase reduces oestrogen production in postmenopausal women who produce oestrogen mainly from andostenedione and testosterone in many tissues such as adipose tissue, skin, muscle and liver. Aromatase is also present in the cells of two-thirds of breast carcinomas and many breast cancers are oestrogen-dependent. In postmenopausal women, treatment with formestane by deep intramuscular injection every 2 weeks may be useful if antioestrogen treatment, e.g. with tamoxifen, is unsuccessful. It is a potential alternative to the non-specific aromatase inhibitor aminoglutethimide (Chapter 47). Unwanted effects include itching, pain, irritation and painful lumps at the injection site, symptoms of oestrogen withdrawal, e.g. hot flushes and lethargy, dyspepsia, nausea, alopecia.

MISCELLANEOUS AGENTS

In addition to the main groups given above there have been both conspicuous successes and failures in the search for anticancer compounds.

CIS-PLATIN

A platinum derivative $(Cl_2Pt_{II}(NH_3)_2)$ which is reactive and binds to DNA and proteins. It has made a significant impact on the treatment of testicular teratoma and ovarian tumours. It is inactive orally and has a long half-life due to extensive protein binding and slow elimination by the kidney. Renal toxicity is a major problem that can be minimized by maintaining a good diuresis. Severe nausea and vomiting are often troublesome.

HYDROXYUREA

A simple compound

$$\begin{matrix} O \\ \parallel \\ (H_2N-C-NHOH) \end{matrix}$$

which blocks the conversion of ribonucleotides to deoxyribonucleotides. It is used for chronic myeloid leukaemia. The compound is rapidly absorbed from the gut and has a short half-life. The general unwanted effects of cytotoxic drugs are common.

PROCARBAZINE

A cytotoxic hydrazine derivative

$$R_1-NH-NH-R_2$$

which inhibits the synthesis of DNA, RNA and proteins; well absorbed orally and eliminated via metabolism which is essential also for its bioactivation

$$\begin{matrix} O \\ \uparrow \\ R_1-N=N-R_2 \end{matrix}$$

It is used as a standard treatment for lymphomas and produces the usual unwanted effects of cytotoxic drugs.

MITOTANE

A selective cytotoxic chemical for the adrenal cortex (see Chapter 47).

ASPARAGINASE

Asparagine is an essential amino acid for cancer cells which require circulating asparagine for growth. This observation led to the use of L-asparaginase from *Escherichia coli* to remove the circulating asparagine. Although this promised true selectivity between normal and malignant cells the agent is only effective in acute lymphoblastic leukaemia. It has to be given by infusion and causes severe toxicity to liver and pancreas in addition to anaphylactic reactions.

INTERFERON α

Interferon α has proved to be a disappointing agent despite the vast resources committed to its isolation in sufficient amounts for early clinical trials. The main clinical benefit may be its use in combination with conventional immunosuppresive cancer chemotherapeutic drugs described above. It is discussed in Chapter 54.

INTERLEUKIN 2 (ALDESLEUKIN)

Interleukin 2 is a lymphokine produced by T lymphocytes which activates cytotoxic killer cells (Chapter 40). Aldesleukin, made by recombinant DNA technology, has been given by intravenous infusion for the treatment of patients with metastatic renal carcinoma. Its efficacy has yet to be established but toxic effects include hypotension and oedema due to capillary leakage, flu-like symptoms, nausea, vomiting, diarrhoea, anaemia and thrombocytopenia.

LAETRILE

A natural product present in apricot kernels which has received considerable media attention as an "alternative medicine" but has been shown in clinical trials to be without therapeutic benefit but of great potential toxicity. It is hydrolysed by the intestinal bacteria to release cyanide and was used in ancient Egypt to execute condemned prisoners (where its efficacy was established!).

GRANULOCYTE AND GRANULOCYTE-MACROPHAGE COLONY STIMULATING FACTORS (G-CSF AND GM-CSF)

Examples: filgrastim, molgramostim.

Mechanism of action and uses

Colony stimulating factors for granulocytes (G-CSF; filgrastim) and granulocyte-macrophages (GM-CSF; molgramostim) which increase haemopoiesis have been synthesized by recombinant DNA technology. They promote the development of marrow stem cells into distinct cell lineages and enhance cell differentiation and release of mature cells from bone marrow stores. They also enhance the chemotactic and phagocytic action of released cells. The actions are largely, but not exclusively, confined to the cell types indicated by their names.

Administration produces a sustained rise in white cell count. Their main potential use is to reduce the extent and duration of neutropenia after intensive chemotherapy for cancer and thereby reduce the risk of infection. The clinical value and cost-effectiveness of these agents are currently uncertain.

Currently they have a place in mobilizing bone marrow cells prior to harvesting for bone marrow transplantation.

Pharmacokinetics

The CSFs are given by intravenous infusion or subcutaneous injection, starting 24 h after chemotherapy to minimize damage to dividing stem cells. The effects of a single dose persist for up to 3 days.

Unwanted effects

- Musculoskeletal pain is common.

- Reversible elevation of liver enzymes or plasma urate.

Drug Toxicity and Abuse

56

Drug Toxicity

Most therapeutic drugs are developed for their ability to interfere with human homeostatic mechanisms in order to produce a beneficial response; only antimicrobial agents and parasiticides hold the possibility of a therapeutic response without some effect on the human body. Many therapeutic agents, for example atropine (belladonna), tubocurarine (curare), ergot alkaloids (St Anthony's Fire), digoxin (digitalis) and dicoumarol (haemorrhagic disease in cattle) were first recognized in relation to poisoning — either accidental or intentional. It is hardly surprising therefore that all drugs are capable of producing adverse effects.

The relationship between a drug and a poison was recognized five centuries ago when Paracelsus stated: "all things are toxic and it is only the dose which makes a thing a poison". Many of the medicines prescribed today were first used as plant extracts, for example cardiac glycosides and opium extracts. It was the identification and isolation of the active chemical entity in such plant extracts that allowed the dose to be controlled sufficiently to optimize the risk:benefit analysis. Recent interest in "natural, herbal remedies" represents a step back to the middle of the last century as far as safety and efficacy are concerned.

The toxic effects of drugs are more numerous than their beneficial properties. Therefore this chapter aims to provide a framework into which different adverse effects can be classified rather than being an apparently endless catalogue. Prescribers should be alert to both anticipated and unexpected reactions to the medicines prescribed. Patients should also be informed of the risk:benefit balance inherent in their treatment. Prescription information leaflets included in the dispensed medicine represent a useful way of providing such advice (Chapter 59).

It should be appreciated that there are almost no absolute value judgements possible in drug toxicity; except causing fatalities! The acceptability of toxicity is inversely related to the severity of the disease being treated; for example, rare idiosyncratic reactions with an incidence of 1 in 10 000 have led to the withdrawal of NSAIDs whereas cancer chemotherapeutic agents may result in toxicity in nearly all patients. In addition "one man's cure is another man's poison" because the beneficial effects in one situation (e.g. opiate-induced constipation or respiratory depression) may be an adverse effect in other circumstances (e.g. when used for pain relief). Thus, even classification of the nature of effect into beneficial or adverse may depend on the disease being treated.

A useful indication of the safety margin available to the physician (and patient) is given by the therapeutic index (TI):

$$\text{Therapeutic index} = \frac{\text{Dose resulting in toxicity}}{\text{Dose giving therapeutic response}}$$

Drugs such as diazepam have a TI of about 50 and it is almost impossible for even the most inept doctor to poison patients with diazepam. In contrast, digoxin has a TI of only about 2 and in such cases toxicity may be precipitated by relatively small changes in dosage regimen, bioavailability of the tablet or the patient's clearance of the drug.

THE SAFETY ASSESSMENT AND REGULATION OF MEDICINES

Therapeutic drugs are assessed for *safety, quality* and *efficacy* before they are approved for clinical use. In the UK these assessments are made by the Committee on Safety of Medicine (CSM), a body of independent experts which advises the Department of Health and the Medicines Control Agency. European harmonization will provide a similar pan-European assessment system. In the USA these aspects are the responsibility of the Food and Drugs Administration (FDA).

Each year a vast number of synthetic novel compounds (new chemical entities) and pure compounds isolated from plant sources are screened for useful and/or novel pharmacological activities. Potentially valuable compounds are then subjected to a sequence of *in vitro* and *in vivo* animal studies and clinical trials to investigate safety and therapeutic benefit.

PRECLINICAL STUDIES

These define three areas:

- Pharmacological effects — the receptor binding characteristics; *in vitro* effects using isolated cells/organs; *in vivo* effects in animals and/or animal models of human diseases; prediction of potential therapeutic use.

- Pharmacokinetics — identification of metabolites (since these may be the active form); evidence of bioavailability (to assist with the design of both clinical trials and *in vivo* animal toxicity studies); establishment of principal route and rate of elimination.

- Toxicological effects — a battery of *in vitro* and *in vivo* studies is undertaken with the aim of weeding out toxic compounds as early as possible and before there is extensive *in vivo* exposure of animals or subsequently humans.

The extent of animal toxicity testing considered necessary depends on the proposed duration of human exposure and population to be treated. Thus all drugs are subjected to an initial *in vitro* screen for mutagenic potential and if satisfactory this is followed by acute and subacute studies up to 14 days of administration to two animal species.

Recent EC guidelines have proposed the following duration of *in vivo* animal studies:

Intended human exposure (days)	Duration of animal study (days)
1	14
2–10	28
10–30	90
>30	180

Teratogenicity and reproductive toxicity studies are required if the drug is to be given to women of child-bearing age. Carcinogenicity testing is necessary for drugs which may be used for long periods, for example over 1 year. The use of animals for the establishment of chemical safety is an emotive issue and there is extensive current research to replace *in vivo* studies with *in vitro* tests based on known mechanisms of toxicity. Despite these advances, toxicology as a predictive science is still in its infancy. *In vivo* studies remain essential to investigate interference with integrative functions, and complex homeostatic mechanisms. At the present it is impossible to replicate the complexity of mammalian physiology and biochemistry by *in vitro* systems and carefully controlled safety studies in animals are essential in preventing extensive human toxicity. Although toxicology has failed in the past to prevent some tragedies, such as the phocomelia (developmental limb abnormalities) produced by thalidomide, these have led to improvements of methods, for example the use of rabbits as the second species for teratology studies.

Toxicity tests include:

- *Mutagenicity* — a variety of *in vitro* tests using bacteria and mammalian cell lines are employed to define any potential effect on DNA which may be linked to carcinogenicity or teratogenicity.

- *Acute toxicity* — single dose by the route proposed for human use; this may reveal a target for toxicity, and is essential in defining the initial dose for human studies.

- *Subacute toxicity* — repeated doses for 14 or 28 days; this will usually reveal the target for toxic effects, and comparison with single dose data may indicate any potential for accumulation.
- *Chronic toxicity* — repeated doses for up to 6 months; this reveals the target for toxicity (except cancer); the aim is to define a dose regimen associated with both adverse effects and a no-observed effect level ("safe dose").
- *Carcinogenicity* — repeated doses throughout the lifetime of the animal.
- *Reproductive toxicity* — repeated doses from prior to mating and throughout gestation to assess any effect on fertility, implantation, foetal development and neonatal growth.

Although such studies are not infallible they have provided an effective predictive screen. It is interesting to note that in recent years the few cases where drugs have been withdrawn after initial approval have mostly been because of rare, idiosyncratic reactions which may have an immunological mechanism (see later) and which are not detected adequately in preclinical studies.

CLINICAL STUDIES

There are four phases of clinical research which are aimed at providing evidence of both safety and efficacy. These are discussed in Chapter 3.

TYPES OF DRUG TOXICITY

Toxicity is frequently divided into two main types:

- Type A — dose-related and largely predictable.
- Type B — not dose-related, idiosyncratic and unpredictable.

Our understanding of the processes involved in toxicity has increased greatly in recent years, and a subdivision based on the mechanisms of toxicity provides a useful framework for students to integrate future knowledge:

- Pharmacological — type A.
- Biochemical — type A and some type B.
- Immunological — type B.
- Unknown — mostly type B?

PHARMACOLOGICAL TOXICITY

The toxic reaction is an extension of the known pharmacological properties of the drug at its site(s) of action.

There are numerous examples in this book where the adverse effects listed at the end of a section are a direct consequence of excessive therapeutic effects (drug A in Fig. 56.1). Examples of this type of effect include:

Warfarin	— Haemorrhage
Insulin	— Hypoglycaemia
β-Adrenoceptor antagonists	— Heart block when used as an anti-arrhythmic
Loop diuretics	— Hypokalaemia
General anaesthetics	— Medullary depression
AChE inhibitors	— Muscle weakness (note — in this case the dose-response is bell shaped).

The change from subtherapeutic → therapeutic → toxic has given rise to the concept of a "therapeutic window" within which most patients should show a beneficial response. This

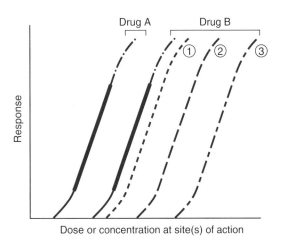

Figure 56.1 Dose–response relationships in relation to toxicity. Drug A, low doses (——) give a subtherapeutic response; median doses (——) give the desired therapeutic response; high doses (–·–·–·) give a toxic response. Drug B, therapeutic effect (——); toxic effect 1 (······) normally accompanies a therapeutic response; toxic effect 2 (-----) frequently seen when there is also toxicity due to an excessive therapeutic response; toxic effect 3 (— - — -) only normally seen in massive overdose or in subjects particularly susceptible.

concept is particularly valuable in the interpretation of measurements of drug concentrations in plasma to monitor both compliance and response (Table 56.1).

In many cases the toxicity may be caused by a secondary or alternative effect which is not the primary aim of the treatment given (drug B in Fig. 56.1). This toxicity would usually be present to a limited extent in patients receiving therapeutic doses (e.g. toxic effect 2 in Fig. 56.1), for example:

Opiate analgesics	—	Respiratory depression
β-Adrenoceptor antagonists	—	Reduction in heart rate when used for hypertension
Antiepilepsy drugs	—	Sedation.

The effect of separation of therapeutic and toxic dose–response curves is a measure of the therapeutic index. If these are very close (e.g. toxic effect 1 in Fig. 56.1) then there is little safety margin and most patients will exhibit some degree of toxicity, for example:

| Cytotoxic anticancer drugs | — | Myelosuppression. |

A wide therapeutic index (toxic effect 3 in Fig. 56.1) results in a form of toxicity which would not be seen with normal therapeutic doses, for example:

| β-Adrenoceptor antagonists | — | Bronchoconstriction. |

However, some patients may be uniquely sensitive to the toxic effect due to either genetic constitution or their physical condition, for example:

| β-Adrenoceptor antagonists | — | Bronchoconstriction in asthmatics (in whom the toxicity response curve resembles toxic effect 1 rather than 3 in Fig. 56.1). |

Pharmacological toxicity is the most common cause of adverse effects. Such toxicity can be minimized by an assessment of the risk : benefit balance for the individual patient. This should take into account factors which may influence both pharmacokinetics and sensitivity including age, physiological status (e.g. renal function), concurrent medication, disease processes, environmental aspects (e.g. smoking), etc.

BIOCHEMICAL TOXICITY

The toxicity or tissue damage is caused by an interaction of the drug, or an active metabolite, with cell components, especially macromolecules. A generalized scheme is given in Fig. 56.2.

Table 56.1 Therapeutic windows based on plasma concentrations

Drug	Therapeutic concentration range		Toxic response
	Minimum	Maximum	
Aspirin (analgesia)	$20\,\mu g\,ml^{-1}$	$300\,\mu g\,ml^{-1}$	Tinnitus, metabolic acidosis
Carbamazepine	$4\,\mu g\,ml^{-1}$	$10\,\mu g\,ml^{-1}$	Drowsiness, visual disturbances
Digitoxin	$15\,ng\,ml^{-1}$	$30\,ng\,ml^{-1}$	Bradycardia, nausea
Digoxin	$0.8\,ng\,ml^{-1}$	$3\,ng\,ml^{-1}$	Bradycardia, nausea
Gentamicin	$2\,\mu g\,ml^{-1}$	$12\,\mu g\,ml^{-1}$	Ototoxicity, renal toxicity
Kanamycin	$10\,\mu g\,ml^{-1}$	$40\,\mu g\,ml^{-1}$	Ototoxicity, renal toxicity
Phenytoin	$10\,\mu g\,ml^{-1}$	$20\,\mu g\,ml^{-1}$	Nystagmus, lethargy
Theophylline	$10\,\mu g\,ml^{-1}$	$20\,\mu g\,ml^{-1}$	Tremor, nervousness

Notes:
The maximum concentration may be based on toxicity related to the primary therapeutic response (e.g. carbamazepine) or an unrelated effect (e.g. gentamicin).
The values given represent average values only; patients will vary in their inherent sensitivity and response to particular concentrations.
The concept of a therapeutic window also applies to cases where the response can be measured directly (e.g. blood clotting control with warfarin and hypoglycaemia with oral hypoglycaemics).

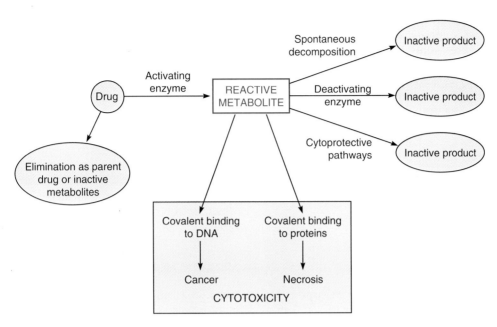

Figure 56.2 Metabolism and cytotoxicity. The extent of cytotoxicity depends on (i) the balance between the activation process and alternative pathways of elimination of the parent drug, and (ii) the balance between inactivation of the reactive metabolite and the production of biochemically adverse effects. Therapeutic interventions are aimed at either increasing elimination of the parent drug or enhancing cytoprotective pathways.

In most cases this form of toxicity is excluded in approved drugs during both preclinical studies in animals and early clinical trials, for example by monitoring changes in serum enzyme levels.

In some cases an understanding of the mechanism of toxicity has allowed the development of appropriate treatments. A key observation was the discovery that the thiol (–SH) group of the tripeptide glutathione provides a cytoprotective mechanism by preventing the cell damage caused by highly reactive chemical species. The nature of the cytotoxic effect depends to some extent on the stability of the reactive species, since extremely unstable metabolites may bind covalently to and inactivate the enzyme which forms them, while more stable species may diffuse to a distant site, for example DNA.

PARACETAMOL

Paracetamol-induced hepatotoxicity represents the results of an imbalance between inactivation (by conjugation) and activation (by oxidation). Low doses are safe because they are eliminated by conjugation with little oxidation. However, in overdose the conjugation reactions are saturated and there is increased cytochrome P450 mediated oxidation to an unstable quinone-imine metabolite. Initially much of this is inactivated by a cytoprotective pathway involving glutathione, but as this is used up, so there is increased covalent binding and cell death. This mechanism explains the site of toxicity (centrilobular necrosis in the liver because of the large amounts of cytochrome P450 present), the increased toxicity seen in patients treated with inducers of cytochrome P450 and the value of treatment with *N*-acetylcysteine (which has an –SH group) to enhance the cytoprotective processes prior to irreversible covalent binding (Chapter 57).

CYCLOPHOSPHAMIDE

This is converted to highly toxic metabolites which are eliminated in the urine, and cause haemorrhagic cystitis (Chapter 55). This may be prevented by prior treatment with MESNA (mercaptoethane sulphonic acid) which possesses both an –SH group for cytoprotection and a polar sulphonic acid group to give high renal excretion of the parent compound. Because of its polarity, MESNA is slowly and incompletely absorbed from the gut but rapidly eliminated. It is therefore given intravenously prior to cyclophosphamide and to cover the period of maximum excretion of toxic metabolites. It is not yet known if MESNA will also protect the urinary bladder from the delayed consequence of cyclophosphamide, that is bladder cancer about 10–20 years after initial treatment.

ISONIAZID

This very rarely causes hepatitis (Chapter 54), which is believed to be due to increased formation in susceptible patients of a reactive metabolite — N-acetylhydrazine. The biochemical basis for the idiosyncratic sensitivity of some patients is not known, and is not related directly to acetylator status.

CHLOROFORM

Chloroform is no longer used clinically due to hepatotoxicity mediated by the generation of reactive free radicals.

SPIRONOLACTONE

Spironolactone (Chapter 15) is oxidized by cytochrome P450 including that in the testes, where the metabolite formed binds to and destroys the enzyme; this decreases testosterone formation which results in gynaecomastia and decreased libido.

AROMATIC AMINES AND NITRITES

These may cause both haemolysis and methaemoglobinaemia, which are linked to the generation of toxic metabolites (probably in the liver with release into the circulation). In the presence of oxygen, the active metabolite oxidizes haemoglobin to methaemoglobin and is oxidized itself (Fig. 56.3). Because of the large amounts of

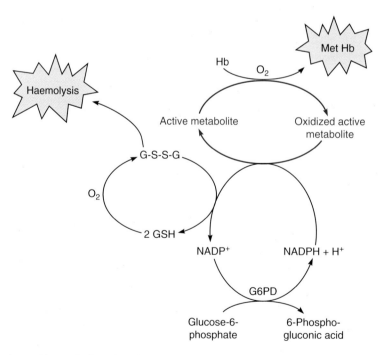

Figure 56.3 Mechanisms of haemolysis and methaemoglobinaemia. Hb, Haemoglobin; G6PD, glucose-6-phosphate dehydrogenase; GS-SG, glutathione dimer (oxidized form); GSH, glutathione (reduced form). High concentrations of reduced glutathione are necessary for maintaining cell membrane integrity; a build-up of oxidized glutathione is associated with haemolysis. The active metabolite may also react with glutathione directly to lower GSH concentrations.

haemoglobin in the blood this would be inconsequential except that the oxidized active metabolite can be reduced by NADPH in the erythrocyte back to the active metabolite. Thus one molecule of the metabolite is able to oxidize many molecules of haemoglobin via NADPH and its formation from glucose-6-phosphate via G6PD (Fig. 56.3). In addition the resulting depletion of NADPH leads to haemolysis. The amounts of G6PD are determined genetically and the incidence of G6PD deficiency is high in Blacks and very high in Mediterranean races, such as the Kurds. Such patients have limited NADPH reserves and are very susceptible to drug-induced haemolysis (but show less methaemoglobinaemia); it is ironic therefore that the amino groups linked with this form of toxicity are present in antimalarials (e.g. primaquine) and the main antileprosy drug (dapsone) in addition to some sulphonamides and antibiotics. Newborn infants also have very low levels of G6PD and may show haemolysis after treatment with vitamin K analogues.

IMMUNOLOGICAL TOXICITY

This is frequently referred to as "drug allergy" and is the form of toxicity with which patients may be most familiar, for example penicillin allergy, etc. Immunological mechanisms are implicated in a number of common adverse effects such as rashes and fever, but may also be involved in organ-directed toxicity. Although the term "allergy" may not be strictly correct for all forms of immunologically mediated toxicity it is probably better than "hypersensitivity" which has also been used to describe an elevated sensitivity to any mechanism or effect.

The ability of low molecular weight compounds (<1100 Da) to elicit an allergic response is dependent on the formation of a stable product with a macromolecule, a process that has been recognized for many years. The process is summarized in Fig. 56.4.

Immunologically mediated toxicity shows a wide range of characteristics:

- Unrelated to pharmacological effects but has been implicated in some forms of "biochemical" toxicity following the formation of a reactive, covalently binding metabolite.
- Unrelated to dose; once the antibody has been developed even very small amounts of antigen can trigger a reaction.

- There is usually a lag of at least 3 days between initial exposure and the development of symptoms; however, the first dose of a subsequent treatment may give an immediate reaction.
- Cross-reactivity is possible between compounds that share the same antigen-determinant or antibody-recognition moiety such as the penicilloyl group of penicillins.
- The incidence varies between different drugs, for example from about 1 in 10 000 for phenylbutazone induced granulocytosis to 1 in 20 for ampicillin-related skin rashes.
- The response is idiosyncratic but genetically controlled. Individual responsiveness cannot be predicted, but individuals who have a history of atopic disease are more likely to develop a drug allergy.

The effects produced may be subdivided into the classical four types of allergic reaction (see also Chapter 40):

- *TYPE I — immediate or anaphylactic reactions —* mediated via IgE antibodies attached to the surface of basophils and mast cells: the release of numerous mediators, for example histamine, 5HT and leukotrienes, produces effects which include urticaria, bronchial constriction, hypotension, oedema and shock. A skin-prick challenge test usually produces an acute inflammatory response; for example, penicillins and peptide drugs such as streptokinase.
- *TYPE II — cytotoxic reactions —* the antigen is formed by the drug binding to a cell membrane; subsequent interaction of this antigen with circulating IgG, IgM or IgA antibodies activates complement and initiates cell lysis. Loss of the carrier cell can result in: thrombocytopenia (e.g. digitoxin, cephalosporins, quinine), neutropenia (e.g. phenylbutazone, metronidazole), and haemolytic anaemia (e.g. penicillins, rifampicin and possibly methyldopa).
- *TYPE III — immune-complex reactions —* the antigen–antibody interaction occurs in serum and is deposited on endothelial cells, basement membranes, etc. to initiate a more localized inflammatory reaction, for example arteritis, nephritis, serum sickness (urticaria, angio-oedema, fever), LE (lupus erythematosus)-like syndrome with hydralazine and procainamide (especially in slow acetylators) and penicillin and possibly NSAID-related nephropathy.

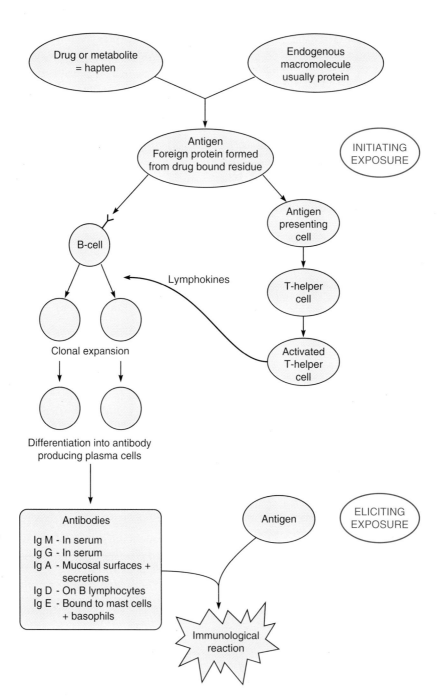

Figure 56.4 Mechanisms of drug allergy. The initial exposure produces an antigen which results in the production of antibodies via B-cell clonal expansion and differentiation, which is stimulated by activated T-helper cells. The eliciting exposure occurs later (usually at least 3 days later during which time therapy may or may not be continuing); antigen–antibody interaction exposes a complement binding site which triggers the reaction. The nature of the immunological reaction depends on the nature of the antibody and/or localization of the antigen (see Chapter 40). Immunosuppressant drugs such as cyclophosphamide, methotrexate and azathioprine act primarily to block the clonal expansion stage; cyclosporine is highly selective and prevents helper T-cell activation without myelosuppression.

- *TYPE IV* — *cell-mediated reactions* — reaction to the eliciting exposure is delayed. They occur mostly in skin due to reaction of the drug with skin proteins and an infiltration by sensitized T lymphocytes which recognize the antigen, and release lymphokines to produce local inflammation, oedema and irritation, for example contact dermatitis.

In addition to true immunologically mediated toxicity, as described above, there are examples of so-called "allergic" reactions such as aspirin hypersensitivity, which show many of the characteristics given above (e.g. rashes, induction of asthma in susceptible patients, cross-reactivity with other aromatic acids such as benzoates) but for which a true immunological basis has not been demonstrated.

It has been estimated that "drug allergy" accounts for about 10% of adverse drug reactions and that severe reactions are very rare. For example only about 5 patients in 10 000 develop an anaphylactic reaction to penicillins. About one half of these are sufficiently serious to warrant hospital treatment which is aimed at blocking the effects on the airways and heart and preventing further mediator release (see Chapter 41). Given the large numbers of patients receiving drugs such as penicillins, "drug allergy" is an important source of iatrogenic morbidity.

57

Drug Poisoning

Self-poisoning can be either accidental or deliberate. Approximately a quarter of a million episodes are believed to occur each year, although less than 40% of these reach hospital. Deaths from self-poisoning still average about 2000 each year in England and Wales. Accidental poisoning is common in the under fives at which age it often involves household products as well as medicines. A second peak of self-poisoning occurs in the teens and early twenties when it is more frequent in girls. The incidence then progressively falls with increasing age.

Most deliberate self-poisoning represents "parasuicide" or attention-seeking behaviour. However, it is important to recognize that the severity of poisoning bears little relationship to suicidal intent. True suicide attempts comprise a minority of events, occurring most frequently in patients over 45 years. About 30% of the deaths are in the over-65-year-olds. Self-poisoning at this age occurs most often in response to depression or specific life events such as bereavement. The drugs most frequently used are benzodiazepines, analgesics and antidepressants. Alcohol is often taken together with these drugs. It is important to attempt to identify the cause of the poisoning since it may influence treatment. However, it should be remembered that the history of how much was taken, and when, is frequently unreliable.

IMMEDIATE MEASURES

- Obtain a clear history if possible. Preserve any evidence, for example bottles, written notes.
- Remove patient from contact with poison if appropriate, for example gases, corrosives.
- Assess vital signs: pulse, respiration and pupil size. Inspect the patient for injury.
- Ensure a clear airway. If the patient is breathing but unconscious he or she should be placed in the coma position.

SUPPORTIVE MEASURES

Examples of drugs producing specific unwanted effects in overdose are shown in Table 57.1. Effects produced by drug overdose requiring supportive measures include:

- *Cardiac or respiratory arrest* — may result from a toxic effect of the drug on the heart, depression of the respiratory centre or from metabolic disturbance. In some circumstances recovery is possible even after prolonged resuscitation.
- *Cardiovascular complications* — including hypotension and arrhythmias. A low blood pressure should be treated if it is accompanied by poor tissue perfusion or low urine output. Arterial dilation and peripheral venous pooling can

Table 57.1 Complications of acute poisonings

Complications	Cause	Examples of poisons
Cardiac arrest	Direct cardiotoxicity Hypoxia Electrolyte/metabolic disturbance	Many
Central nervous system depression		Many
Convulsions	Direct neurotoxicity	Tricyclic antidepressants Theophylline
	Hypoxia	Many
Hypotension	Myocardial depression	β-Blockers Tricyclic antidepressants Dextropropoxyphene
	Peripheral vasodilation	Many
Arrhythmia	Direct cardiotoxicity	β-Blockers Tricyclic antidepressants Verapamil Digoxin
	Hypoxia Electrolyte/metabolic disturbance	Many
Renal failure	Hypotension	Many
	Rhabdomyolysis	Narcotic drugs Hypnotics Ethanol Carbon monoxide
	Direct nephrotoxicity	Paracetamol Heavy metals
Hepatic failure	Direct hepatotoxicity	Paracetamol Carbon tetrachloride
Respiratory depression	Direct neurotoxicity	Sedatives Hypnotics Narcotics

result from depression of the vasomotor centre and produce a low central venous pressure. This should be raised to between +10 and +15 cm water (measured from the mid-axillary line) by intravenous infusion of a colloid solution, for example dextran polymers. If blood pressure is low with a normal or raised central venous pressure, this suggests myocardial depression. Inotropic drugs such as dobutamine (Chapter 8) should then be used. Disturbances of cardiac rhythm should only be treated if they are severe; however, correction of metabolic disturbances, for example hypoxia, hypercapnia, potassium and pH is mandatory.

• *Convulsions* — may be due to a treatable under-lying cause such as hypoxia, hypoglycaemia or hypocalcaemia, or may be a direct toxic effect of the drug on neuronal function. Diazepam, intravenously or rectally (Chapter 21), is the treatment of choice. Artificial ventilation with neuromuscular blockade (Chapter 28) is used if the fits cannot be controlled.

• *Renal failure* — is usually a consequence of prolonged hypotension. Other causes include a direct nephrotoxic effect of the drug and renal damage produced by the products of toxic muscle necrosis (rhabdomyolysis).

• *Hepatic failure* — usually results from the direct toxic effects of specific agents such as paracetamol.

- *Impaired temperature regulation* — hypothermia is common, due to depression of metabolic rate with reduced heat production and to increased heat loss from cutaneous vasodilation. Rewarming reduces the risk of serious ventricular arrhythmias. By contrast, aspirin can produce hyperthermia by uncoupling cellular oxidative phosphorylation.

PREVENTION OF ABSORPTION OF POISONS

There are three principal methods of preventing further absorption of the drug:

(1) *Emesis* — can be used in a conscious patient who has not ingested a corrosive agent. Stimulation of the pharynx can be tried in children but is often ineffective. Ipecacuanha is a plant extract containing emetine and cephaeline which irritate the stomach and stimulate the medullary vomiting centre. Most patients vomit within half an hour. Prolonged vomiting sometimes occurs and there are doubts as to its effectiveness in removing drug from the stomach.

(2) *Gastric aspiration and lavage.* This should not be considered in unconscious patients without protection of the airway by an endotracheal tube to prevent aspiration of gastric contents. A large bore orogastric tube is used to initially aspirate gastric contents, then to lavage with aliquots of water at body temperature. Its effectiveness is unproven.

(3) *Activated charcoal* — is a formulation with a large adsorbent area which is given as a suspension in water. About 10 g of charcoal is required to every 1 g of poison which makes it impractical for poisons that are usually ingested in large quantities, for example paracetamol. An initial dose of charcoal can prevent drug absorption if given within 4 h of drug ingestion. Repeated administration over 24–36 h achieves further adsorption of drug in the small intestine. Drug is continuously being transferred in both directions across the gut wall, with the concentration gradient normally favouring net absorption. If drug in the bowel is adsorbed by charcoal, net transfer into the gut will enhance elimination of poison from the body. Constipation is the major unwanted effect of charcoal.

ELIMINATION OF POISONS

There are three principal methods of enhancing elimination of the drug:

(1) *Activated charcoal* (see above).

(2) *Renal elimination*: forced diuresis with intravenous infusion of large quantities of fluid has been advocated in the past if most drug is eliminated unchanged by the kidney or if renally excreted metabolites are toxic. The drug should be mainly present in extracellular fluid and be minimally bound to protein. However, renal elimination is most effectively manipulated if the drug is a weak electrolyte. Altering urine pH produces ionization of the drug which impairs reabsorption from the renal tubule by reducing its lipid solubility (Chapter 2). Weak acids are more readily excreted in alkaline urine (alkaline diuresis) while the converse is true for weak bases (acid diuresis). Alkalinization of the urine can be achieved with sodium bicarbonate or acidification with ammonium chloride. A major potential disadvantage of forced diuresis is serious disturbance of fluid or electrolyte balance but if urinary pH is manipulated only a modest increase in urinary flow rate is required.

(3) *Haemodialysis or haemoperfusion.* These are reserved for the most severely poisoned patients. Large amounts of drug must be present in the plasma for the techniques to be successful. Haemodialysis relies on diffusion of the drug across a semipermeable membrane from blood to the dialysis fluid. Haemoperfusion involves adsorption of drug from blood as it passes down a column containing activated charcoal or a resin.

SPECIFIC ANTIDOTES

Antidotes are only available for a minority of drugs commonly involved in poisonings. Some important examples are given below.

COMPETITIVE INHIBITORS

- Atropine acts at muscarinic receptors to block the parasympathetic effects of organophosphorus insecticides.

- Naloxone acts at opioid receptors to reverse the effects of narcotic analgesics.

- Flumazenil is an antagonist at benzodiazepine receptors. It is rarely needed, since fatalities are uncommon after overdose with this class of drug.

CHELATING AGENTS

- Desferrioxamine for ferrous ions.
- Dicobalt edetate for cyanide.
- Dimercaprol for gold, lead, mercury and arsenic.
- Penicillamine for copper and lead.
- Sodium calcium edetate for lead.

COMPOUNDS WHICH AFFECT DRUG METABOLISM

- Ethanol acts as a competitive substrate for alcohol dehydrogenase in the treatment of methanol poisoning, preventing formation of the toxic metabolites formaldehyde and formic acid.
- Acetylcysteine provides the substrate for conjugation of the cytotoxic oxidative metabolite of paracetamol when the natural ligand glutathione is exhausted (see below and Chapter 56).

ANTIBODIES

- Digoxin can be neutralized in severe poisoning by specific antibody fragments. The antibodies are raised in sheep and cleaved to remove the antigenic crystalline (F_c) portion of the molecule while retaining the specific antigen binding fragment (F_{ab}).

SOME SPECIFIC COMMON POISONINGS

PARACETAMOL

Paracetamol overdose can be fatal, with about 200 deaths occurring each year in England and Wales. Metabolism of paracetamol takes place in the liver, mainly producing non-toxic conjugates. A small amount is oxidized by the cytochrome P450 system to an active metabolite which conjugates with the thiol group on glutathione (see Chapter 56). When hepatic glutathione is exhausted (which occurs readily

in overdose) the metabolite denatures protein in the liver and kidney to produce hepatic necrosis and sometimes renal tubular necrosis.

Gastric aspiration and lavage is recommended within 4–6 h of a potentially serious paracetamol overdosage. In the first 24 h there are few symptoms apart from nausea, vomiting, abdominal pain and sweating. Within 24 h after a large overdose, liver damage begins, producing right upper quadrant pain and tenderness. The patient usually becomes jaundiced by 36–48 h and can progress to severe or even fatal liver failure. The most sensitive measures of liver damage are the prothrombin time or the International Normalized Ratio (INR) and the plasma unconjugated bilirubin. Renal failure is seen in about a quarter of patients with severe liver damage.

Antidotes used in paracetamol poisoning replace glutathione as a thiol donor in the liver. Since antidotes are most effective when given early, blood should be analysed for paracetamol if there is any suspicion of poisoning. Glutathione cannot enter liver cells from the blood, so a substitute is given. Methionine can be given orally as an initial measure, but intravenous N-acetylcysteine is the preferred treatment (although there is some evidence that it is more effective after oral administration, perhaps due to higher concentrations reaching the liver). Treatment used to be confined to the first 15 h after overdose, but recent evidence suggests that liver damage can be reduced even when the antidote is delayed for up to 20–30 h. It can also be useful in patients with established liver damage to reduce its severity much later after ingestion. A graph is available (Fig. 57.1) to

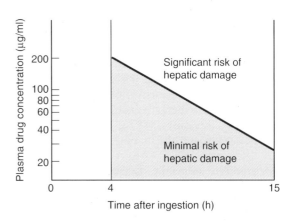

Figure 57.1 Graph showing relationship between plasma paracetamol concentration and the risk of liver damage.

indicate the risk of liver damage for a given plasma paracetamol concentration if the time of ingestion is known. The plasma concentration before 4 h is unreliable since absorption and distribution are still occurring. After 15 h, high plasma concentrations must be inferred by extrapolation of the graph. Treatment is only necessary if potentially toxic paracetamol concentrations are detected. Toxicity occurs at much lower plasma paracetamol concentrations if the patient has been using drugs such as alcohol or phenytoin which induce liver cytochrome P450 (Chapter 2).

SALICYLATES

Although salicylate poisoning is becoming less common, there are still some 150 deaths each year in England and Wales. Aspirin is rapidly hydrolysed to salicylic acid after absorption but further metabolism is rate-limited. Symptoms of toxicity are nausea, vomiting, abdominal pain, tinnitus, hyperventilation and sweating. Agitation frequently occurs in adults but children become comatose. The metabolic chain of events produced by aspirin is shown in Fig. 57.2. The severity of salicylate poisoning can be reliably predicted from the plasma drug concentration.

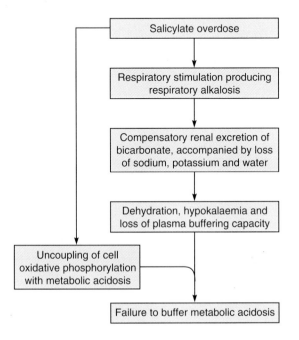

Figure 57.2 The metabolic consequences of salicylate overdose.

Gastric aspiration or emesis for up to 12 h after the overdose is widely practised since aspirin tends to remain in the stomach. However, activated charcoal may be better for reducing absorption and enhancing elimination. Correction of fluid, electrolyte and acid–base balance is fundamental to successful management; a fluid deficit of 3–4 l is not unusual in severe poisoning. Forced alkaline diuresis is no longer advocated to enhance salicylate elimination; simple alkalinization of the urine to raise the pH above 7.5 is effective and safer. In severe poisoning, haemodialysis is the treatment of choice.

TRICYCLIC ANTIDEPRESSANTS

Approximately 400 deaths per year occur in England and Wales from overdose with tricyclic antidepressants. Symptoms are due to anticholinergic effects and actions on the heart. Anticholinergic effects delay gastric emptying and therefore gastric lavage or oral activated charcoal will be useful up to 12 h after overdose. Drowsiness and confusion is followed by coma in more severely poisoned patients. Cardiac depression can produce hypotension and arrhythmias such as ventricular tachycardia.

Electrocardiographic monitoring is recommended for at least 24 h. Arrhythmias frequently respond to correction of acidosis. If this is not successful, phenytoin or direct current shock can be used, avoiding drugs which depress cardiac contractility.

OPIATE ANALGESICS

The triad of signs characteristic of opiate overdose are respiratory depression, pinpoint pupils and impaired consciousness (Chapter 20). They can be reversed rapidly by naloxone which is a competitive antagonist at μ opioid receptors. After a response to an initial intravenous bolus dose, it is often necessary to give repeated boluses or a continuous infusion because while the half-lives of most opiates are long, that of naloxone is very short. The effect of naloxone in poisoning produced by buprenorphine is often incomplete, and non-specific respiratory stimulants (Chapter 12) may also be needed. Organophosphorus insecticides can produce similar signs to opiates, but naloxone will have no effect.

Drugs of Abuse

A number of therapeutic drugs may be used as drugs of abuse because of their effects on the nervous system, for example hypnotics and anxiolytics (Chapter 21) and opiate analgesics (Chapter 20). This chapter covers other drugs which are encountered in clinical practice primarily because of their abuse potential.

CNS STIMULANTS

Several drugs which have central stimulant properties are abused and produce dependence. Those more commonly encountered are considered here. A comparison of some of these compounds is shown in Table 58.1.

Table 58.1 Comparisons among dependence-inducing drugs

	Dependence		
Drug type	Emotional	Physical	Tolerance
Morphine	++	++	++
Barbiturate	++	+++	+
Amphetamine	++	+	+
Cocaine	++	+	o
Cannabis	+	o	o
Alcohol	++	+	+
Tobacco	++	+	o

+++, Very severe; ++, severe; +, slight; o, absent.

COCAINE ("coke", "Charlie", "crack", "snow")

Mechanism of action and effects

Many of the psychic effects of cocaine may relate to inhibition of catecholamine reuptake into nerve terminals. The initial effect is a short-lived euphoria with tactile hallucinations. Tolerance does not occur.

Pharmacokinetics

Cocaine is used as intranasal snuff or by intravenous injection to obtain a rapid onset of effect and to avoid inactivation by first-pass metabolism (Chapter 2). In the "free base" form it is smoked as "crack" which produces an intense psychic reaction. Cocaine is metabolized by plasma esterases and the half-life is very short.

Other effects

- Severe emotional, but not physical, dependence occurs. It develops particularly rapidly with "crack". A rebound irritability, excessive sleeping and depression can follow withdrawal after prolonged use.

- Toxic psychosis, with delusions and sensations of great stamina, occurs with chronic use.

- Overdosage produces fear, convulsions, hypertension, cardiac rhythm disturbances and hyperthermia. If severe, death can occur from respiratory depression and circulatory collapse.

- Cocaine snuff produces necrosis of the nasal septum due to its vasoconstrictor action.

AMPHETAMINE, METHAMPHETAMINE ("speed", "uppers") AND 3,4-METHYLENEDIOXY METHAMPHETAMINE (MDMA, "Ecstasy")

Mechanism of action and effects

Indirect sympathomimetic effects (Chapter 4) and inhibition of monoamine uptake produce central sympathetic nervous stimulation, which is most marked in the reticular formation. This results in euphoria similar to that experienced with cocaine. Depletion of neuronal amine stores produces tolerance to repeated dosing. The D-isomer (dexamphetamine) is twice as potent as the L-isomer of amphetamine in its central stimulant activity.

Pharmacokinetics

Although amphetamine is sometimes used intravenously, absorption from the gut is rapid and complete. About half is then excreted unchanged in the urine, and the rest is metabolized in the liver. The half-life of amphetamine varies according to urine pH; if the urine is acid then ionization increases excretion (Chapter 2) to produce a short half-life. By contrast, if urine pH is high, then the half-life is considerably longer. Metabolites of amphetamine are believed to contribute to the psychotic effects seen with long-term use.

Other effects

These are similar to cocaine apart from weight loss and the gradual onset of tolerance.

CANNABIS ("dope", "pot")

Mechanism of action and effects

The psychic effects are due largely to tetrahydrocannabinol (THC) which produces euphoria and heightened intensity of sensations. These may be accompanied by hallucinations. Recent memory is markedly impaired and complex mental tests are less well executed. The derivative THC has an antiemetic action which has been used to prevent the nausea and vomiting associated with cancer chemotherapy (Chapter 55).

Pharmacokinetics

Cannabis can be smoked as marihuana which consists of crushed leaves and flowers of the cannabis plant or as resin scraped from the plant, known as hashish. Metabolism of THC is extensive with some active metabolites. Its high lipid solubility produces a large volume of distribution and a correspondingly long half-life.

Other effects

- Vasodilation and hypotension.
- Tachycardia.

HALLUCINOGENIC AGENTS

Examples: lysergic acid diethylamide (LSD) ("acid"), psilocybin ("magic mushrooms").

Mechanism of action and effects

The actions of LSD and psilocybin are similar. Visual hallucinations are frequent and auditory acuity is accentuated. Time appears to pass rapidly and emotions are altered with either elation or depression. The overall experience can produce a "good" or a "bad" trip. The actions on the brain are probably related to 5HT receptor blockade and anticholinesterase actions.

Pharmacokinetics

Oral absorption is good and the half-life is relatively short.

Other effects

- Serious psychotic reactions.
- Nausea, dizziness, weakness, ataxia, tremor.
- Emotional dependence is frequent but physical dependence is not.
- Tolerance.
- Overdose produces sympathomimetic effects including mydriasis, hyperactivity and tachycardia.

TOBACCO

Mechanism of action

Addiction to smoking involves several factors, both pharmacological and non-pharmacological.

Some 300 chemical compounds are present in tobacco smoke. The actions of nicotine are believed to be of major importance, but are not solely responsible for the effects of smoking. Nicotine produces dose-related responses. At low doses, cardiovascular chemoreceptor stimulation enhances sympathetic nervous system activity (Chapter 4) which may contribute to central nervous system stimulation. At higher doses, there is direct stimulation of the N_1 receptors on autonomic ganglia (Chapter 4). At even higher doses nicotine acts as a ganglion blocking agent. Initial stimulation of nervous tissue is therefore followed by depression.

Pharmacokinetics of nicotine

Nicotine is absorbed from the mouth in its unionized form, which is found in the alkaline environment of cigar and pipe tobacco smoke. Acid cigarette smoke ionizes nicotine which can then only be absorbed in adequate amounts from the larger surface area of the lung. Nicotine is metabolized in the liver and has a short half-life.

Effects of tobacco

Smoking tobacco products produces both short- and long-term adverse effects. Short-term effects include:

- Reduced activity of cilia in bronchi which decreases clearance of lung secretions.
- An increase in carboxyhaemoglobin concentration in blood, which reduces oxygen carrying capacity. This may be important in patients with ischaemic heart disease, increasing the chance of provoking angina.
- Decreased appetite, with weight gain on stopping smoking.
- Emotional dependence to nicotine and the physical act of smoking is powerful. Physical withdrawal is less marked.

Long-term effects of smoking include:

- Premature cardiovascular disease. The overall risk of death from coronary artery disease is doubled in smokers compared to non-smokers. That risk falls over the first 5 years after stopping smoking to a value close to that of non-smokers. Peripheral vascular disease and stroke are also increased. Contributory effects include increased plasma fatty acids and enhanced platelet aggregability.

- Chronic obstructive lung disease. Increased mucus secretion leads to chronic bronchitis. Progressive destruction of the supporting tissue in the bronchioles produces emphysema and airways obstruction.
- Increased risk of lung cancer. Inhalation of tobacco smoke is a major contributory factor and explains the greater risk in cigarette smokers. Giving up smoking reduces the risk progressively over about 10 years of abstinence. The constituent of tobacco smoke responsible for altering DNA structure and initiating the cancer process remains controversial but the relationship between smoking and lung cancer has been confirmed by numerous epidemiological studies.
- Peptic ulceration is twice as common in smokers.
- Smoking during pregnancy has several effects, the most important of which is an increased risk of a low birth weight child.
- Smoking induces a number of the cytochrome P450 isoenzymes (Chapter 2) and increases the clearance of drugs such as theophylline (Chapter 11) and imipramine (Chapter 23).

ETHYL ALCOHOL

Mechanism of action and effects

Alcohol is a general CNS depressant. There is initial depression of inhibitory neurones producing a sense of relaxation, followed by progressive depression of all CNS functions. Mental processes that are modified by education, training and previous experience are affected first, while relatively "mechanical" tasks are less impaired. Despite subjective impressions, there is no increase in mental or physical capabilities unless anxiety previously reduced performance. All effects are closely related to blood alcohol concentration:

- 30 mg/100 ml produces mild euphoria and the risk of accidental injury is increased.
- 80 mg/100 ml is the legal limit for driving in the UK. The risk of serious injury in a road accident is more than doubled.
- 100–200 mg/100 ml, speech becomes slurred and motor co-ordination is impaired.
- >300 mg/100 ml often produces loss of consciousness.

- >400 mg/100 ml is frequently fatal due to respiratory and vasomotor centre depression.

Tolerance to the effects of alcohol is seen in chronic alcoholics.

Pharmacokinetics

Although some ethanol is absorbed from the stomach, the majority is absorbed from the small intestine. High concentrations of alcohol (above 20%) and large volumes inhibit gastric emptying and delay absorption, as do foods high in fat or carbohydrate. Peak blood concentrations therefore depend on the dose and strength of the alcohol and on the timing of meals. Once absorbed, distribution is fairly uniform and the ready passage across the blood–brain barrier and high cerebral blood flow ensure rapid access to the CNS. The effects on the brain are more marked when the concentration is rising, suggesting a degree of acute tolerance.

Metabolism occurs mainly in the liver (Fig. 58.1), more than 90% being oxidized by alcohol dehydrogenase at a fixed rate which averages $10 \, \text{ml} \, \text{h}^{-1}$. Acetaldehyde is produced and then further metabolized by aldehyde dehydrogenase (Fig. 58.1). Intracellular accumulation of acetaldehyde is responsible for many of the unpleasant effects of a hangover. Small amounts of alcohol are metabolized via the microsomal ethanol oxidizing system, the activity of which is increased by enzyme inducers such as alcohol itself (unlike alcohol dehydrogenase) (Chapter 2). Only 2–5% of alcohol is excreted unchanged, some in exhaled air which is the basis of the breathalyser test.

Disulfiram is a drug which inhibits aldehyde dehydrogenase leading to acetaldehyde accumulation. Typical "hangover" effects of flushing, sweating, headache and nausea occur if it is taken with alcohol. It is sometimes used as an aid to abstinence. Certain other drugs such as metronidazole (Chapter 54) and tolbutamide (Chapter 43) can produce a similar effect.

Other acute effects of alcohol

- Peripheral vasodilation from depression of the vasomotor centre.
- Diuresis due to inhibition of ADH secretion.
- Gastric irritation, which depends on the concentration of alcohol and can lead to blood loss. CNS effects may contribute to vomiting after acute alcohol "binges".
- Changes in blood glucose. Alcohol initially impairs tissue uptake of glucose producing mild hyperglycaemia. However, hypoglycaemia can also occur. Gluconeogenesis is inhibited by the high concentration of NADH produced during metabolism of alcohol (Fig. 58.1). Hypoglycaemia usually arises several hours after alcohol intake and can cause brain damage.
- Increased sexual desire but with reduced performance.
- Inhibition of hepatic drug-metabolizing enzymes occurs after acute intake of alcohol, with subsequent induction of enzymes during chronic intake. This predisposes to drug interactions, especially with warfarin (Chapter 10) and anticonvulsants (Chapter 24).
- Increased blood pressure, possibly due to increased sensitivity of blood vessels to catecholamines.

COMPLICATIONS OF CHRONIC ALCOHOL ABUSE

There are no reliable estimates of the number of alcoholics in the UK, although more than two

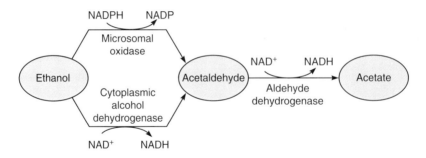

Figure 58.1 Metabolism of ethanol.

million people in the UK may be heavy drinkers. The distribution curve for alcohol consumption is continuous but skewed at the upper end, and the risk of alcohol-related problems rises with the average alcohol intake. The number of hospital admissions for alcoholism has risen by 25 times in the last 35 years and is becoming increasingly common in women.

- Dependence on alcohol is difficult to define; psychological dependence is common but physical dependence also occurs.

- Withdrawal symptoms occur after sudden cessation in dependent persons. If mild, these are confined to anxiety, agitation, tremor, sweating, nausea and retching. The most severe form of withdrawal is delerium tremens. Insomnia, hyperactivity, perceptual disturbance, tachycardia and hypertension are common. Severe delerium tremens produces confusion, paranoia and visual hallucinations. Generalized convulsions can occur at an early stage. Chlormethiazole (Chapter 21) is the sedative of choice to reduce symptoms of withdrawal but dependence to this drug develops if treatment is prolonged. Benzodiazepines (Chapter 21) can be given as an alternative, especially for fits.

- Neurological complications are produced by a combination of alcohol toxicity and nutritional deficiency (especially B group vitamins) which is commonly present in association with heavy alcohol intake. Peripheral neuropathy, and dementia are among the consequences.

- Liver damage. Reversible fatty infiltration commonly occurs. Cirrhosis is produced by more prolonged abuse, but individual susceptibility varies widely. Women are at twice the risk of men at any level of alcohol intake. Cirrhosis reduces the first-pass metabolism and systemic clearance of drugs eliminated by hepatic metabolism (Chapter 60).

- Pancreatitis, probably related to raised serum triglycerides.

- Metabolic abnormalities often give a clue to heavy drinking. Macrocytosis of red cells reflects a toxic effect of alcohol on the red cell membrane. Hyperuricaemia is produced by competition for renal tubular secretion between uric acid and organic acids which result from impaired glucose metabolism; this predisposes to gout. Raised liver enzymes and increased serum lipids (in particular triglycerides) are other features. The latter may be due to utilization of the co-enzyme NADP to metabolize alcohol rather than lipids.

- Cardiomyopathy which predisposes to atrial fibrillation and heart failure.

Although the majority of the long-term effects of alcohol are detrimental to health, modest intake (possibly particularly as wine) may be advantageous. The regular intake of alcohol up to recommended maximum levels (14 units per week in women and 21 units per week in men) may reduce the risk of atherosclerotic cardiovascular disease. This effect may be due to a rise in the protective HDL cholesterol fraction and reduced oxidation of LDL cholesterol (Chapter 51). These changes may be due, at least in part, to constituents of alcoholic drinks other than ethanol.

Drug Prescribing

Prescribing, Compliance and Information for Patients

About 80% of prescribing of medicines takes place in the setting of general practice (primary medical care). On average, men visit their general practitioners 3.5 times each year and for women the figure is 5. A little over two-thirds of consultations end with the issuing of a prescription. Prescribing is particularly frequent for elderly people, who are likely to continue treatment for long periods of time. It is also more common for women than it is for men.

DUTIES OF THE PRESCRIBER

There are certain legal requirements which must be met when a medicine is prescribed. The minimum are:

- The patient's name (surname and initial) and address. In the case of children up to 12 years, the patient's age must be specified.
- The name of the drug is obviously essential, although endless arguments have raged as to whether the generic name (the officially accepted chemical name) or trade name (a ''Brand'' name approved for use by a specific pharmaceutical company) should be used. One advantage of the generic name is that it is likely to indicate the nature of the drug. Thus, all β-adrenoceptor blocking drugs end with either -olol or -alol, for example atenolol, labetalol, metoprolol and sotalol.

Similarly, tricyclic antidepressants end with -tyline or -pramine, for example amitriptyline, nortriptyline, clomipramine, imipramine, lofepramine. By contrast, the trade names for these drugs give little idea of the active ingredient: Tenormin, Trandate, Lopressor and Sotacor; Tryptizol, Allegron, Anafranil, Tofranil and Gamanil. Another problem with trade names is that they rarely give any indication when there is more than one active ingredient. Thus, Parstelin contains both tranylcypromine and trifluoperazine. The generic names for many compound preparations have this indicated by the term ''co-'', for example co-amilofruse indicates the presence of both amiloride and frusemide while co-proxamol contains both propoxyphene and paracetamol.

Another advantage of generic prescribing is that pharmacists can dispense any product which meets the necessary specifications rather than having to buy in a specific brand. This helps to simplify stock holding and avoids unnecessary delays when dispensing for patients. A further major advantage is that generic prescribing is usually cheaper than that by trade name (Table 59.1). In recent years there has been an increasing tendency for doctors to prescribe by generic name (50% of prescriptions in many health regions). It is likely that economic arguments have been the chief factor leading to this change.

TABLE 59.1 Comparative (net ingredient) costs of prescribing by generic and brand names*

Propranolol (non-proprietary) 80 mg tablets, 20 = 15 p
    Inderal (Zeneca) 80 mg, 20 = 78 p
    Half-Inderal LA 80 mg, 20 = £3.70

Ampicillin (non-proprietary) 500 mg caps, 20 = 95 p
    Penbritin (Beecham) 500 mg caps, 20 = £3.21

Naproxen (non-proprietary) 250 mg, 20 = £1.34
    Naprosyn (Syntex) 20 = £2.43

*Source: *British National Formulary*, 1994, volume 27

Despite these advantages, generic prescribing can create problems. It is possible that the patient may be confused or concerned if a different brand of the same medicine is issued when a prescription is renewed (tablet sizes may differ as can their colour and whether or not they are scored). For drugs with a narrow therapeutic index, for example anticonvulsants, oral anticoagulants, oral hypoglycaemic agents and theophylline preparations (especially modified-release ones) a change to one which has a greater bioavailability could lead to toxicity, whereas one with a lesser bioavailability can lead to loss of therapeutic control. Recent stringent control both by the Medicines Control Agency and by pharmaceutical companies has substantially reduced the number of drugs for which a potential problem exists within the UK (Table 59.2).

TABLE 59.2 Drugs for which differences in bioavailability between manufacturers are important and have been demonstrated

Carbamazepine
Chloramphenicol[†]
Digoxin*
Glibenclamide*
Griseofulvin*
Nitrofurantoin*
Phenindione
Phenylbutazone[†]
Phenytoin
Theophylline (SR)
Tolbutamide*
Warfarin

*No longer thought to be a problem in the UK.
[†] Rarely used.

- Dose: this is an essential item on all prescriptions and should be written in terms of grams (g), milligrams (mg) or micrograms (which should not be abbreviated).

- The route of administration should be identified: oral, rectal or by various forms of injections, for example intravenous, intramuscular or subcutaneous. Considerable confusion can arise with intravenous administration of drugs since numerous systems exist for their delivery. Drugs can be given by direct injection into a vein or infused, for example, through the side-arm of a continuously running intravenous drip, via a motor-driven pump or added to intravenous infusion fluid. It is particularly important when prescribing drugs for intravenous administration to make clear the precise intentions to other medical or nursing staff who may be administering them.

- Sometimes drugs are administered once only while others must be given on a regular basis, in which case the frequency or times of administration should be specified, for example twice daily or 9 a.m. and 9 p.m.

- Duration of therapy can be specified in a number of ways, one being to complete the box near the top of the prescription sheet. Alternatively, it can be written on the prescription or the total number of tablets/capsules can be specified. An increasing tendency is to dispense medicines in original (patient) packs with tablets individually packed by the pharmaceutical company. The duration of therapy is vitally important in the case of controlled drugs such as opiates for which the total amount to be dispensed must be written in both figures and in words.

- Other essential items on prescriptions include the doctor's signature and the address of his or her place of work. The latter is effectively waived for hospital prescriptions since it is assumed that the medical practitioner is based at the hospital in question.

- Finally, the prescription must be dated.

In recent times there has been an increasing use of computer issued prescriptions. Details of the specific requirements are essentially similar to those outlined above. The reader is referred to the section on prescription writing in the *British National Formulary* for more intricate details.

ABBREVIATIONS

Directions should preferably be in English without abbreviation. However, there are a number of abbreviations which are widely accepted. They include the following for route of administration: o or po = oral, iv = intravenous, im = intramuscular, sc = subcutaneous and pr = per rectum. Others such as intrathecal must not be abbreviated because of the potential seriousness of inappropriate administration: intrathecal vincristine, for example, has led to the death of several patients. Besides the abbreviations already listed for quantities, ml or mL are acceptable. Quantities of less than 1 g should be written in milligrams, that is 400 mg rather than 0.4 g, whereas quantities of less than 1 mg should be written in micrograms, that is 500 micrograms, rather than 0.5 mg. If decimals are unavoidable a zero should precede the decimal point when there is no figure, for example 0.5 ml not .5 ml.

Concerning timing of doses, od (*omni die*) is acceptable but there is nothing wrong with saying once daily! Om (*omni mane*) stands for in the morning, and on (*omni nocte*) for at night. Ac is short for *ante cibum* (before food) and pc for *post cibum* (after food). Twice daily can be abbreviated to bd (*bis die*), thrice daily to tds (*ter die sumendus*) and four times daily to qds (*quater die sumendus*).

COMPLIANCE

The term "compliance" is used to describe the extent to which a patient takes his or her medicine. It is frequently assumed that once a prescription has been given, the patient will automatically comply with the doctor's instructions. There is, however, abundant evidence that this is often not the case. Indeed, many prescriptions are not even taken to the pharmacist for dispensing and the very substantial proportion which are collected are not taken in the manner intended. Prescriptions are sometimes not presented to a pharmacist because of cost or because the doctor failed to discuss the "hidden agenda" for which the presenting complaint was a front.

The degree of patient compliance is affected by many factors which include the duration of treatment. Less than 50% of patients comply fully with long-term therapy such as that for high blood pressure or psychotic illness. The frequency of dosing is a major influence. Few patients like taking their medicines with them to work. Thus, compliance with twice daily regimens tends to be better than that for more frequent administration. There is, however, relatively little to choose between the extent of compliance with once and twice daily dosing. Side-effects can also reduce the likelihood of a patient complying with therapy but at times can be turned to advantage. Thus, giving all of the dose of tricyclic antidepressant at night means that the side-effect of sedation can be used to aid sleep. In addition, giving the patient advanced warning of the likely side-effect of dry mouth with this compound may earn their trust and encourage him or her to continue therapy.

A proportion of non-compliance is due to patients forgetting whether or not they have taken their medicine on a particular day. Use of calendar packs can be helpful in this situation. The patient's health beliefs are also critically important (the majority of pregnant women will take prophylactic iron since they know that it will benefit the fetus). Compliance can sometimes be improved by involving the patient in monitoring his or her disease and its control by therapy, for example home monitoring of blood pressure, blood sugar in diabetes mellitus, or peak flow measurements in asthmatics. Finally, there is evidence to suggest that supplying patients with accurate information can improve their level of satisfaction and that satisfied patients are more likely to take their medicines.

INFORMING PATIENTS ABOUT THEIR MEDICINES

It is almost incredible to think that at one time doctors were reluctant to allow the name of a medicine to be shown on the container in which it was dispensed. However, paternalistic attitudes amongst the medical profession have been slow to disappear. Several surveys carried out in the early 1980s showed that patients felt that neither doctors nor pharmacists gave sufficient explanations about the medicines they receive. This situation was summarized by Leighton Cluff in the USA in his phrase "Better instructions are provided when purchasing a new camera or automobile than when a patient receives a life-saving antibiotic or cardiac drug". Indeed more than 60% of patients prescribed a medicine in the previous month remember being told little or nothing about it. Patients are particularly keen to know when and how to take their medicine, about side-effects and what to do about these, precautions to take such as possible effects on driving; problems with alcohol or other drugs, the name of the medicine, the purposes of treatment, how long to take it and what to do if a dose is missed.

In recent times there has been agreement both within the UK and more recently in Europe that manufacturers of pharmaceuticals should produce printed leaflets about medicines when these are dispensed in original (patient) packs. Field studies have shown clearly that patients who receive leaflets about their medicines are better informed and more satisfied than others who have not been given this information. However, leaflets are complementary to, and not a substitute for, discussion with the medical practitioner, pharmacist, practice nurse, etc. A data sheet, which contains essential prescribing information, is approved by the Medicines Control Agency for each licensed drug. It is planned that the *Data Sheet Compendium* (published by the Association of the British Pharmaceutical Industry) and a similar compendium of information leaflets will be lodged in public libraries. Furthermore, there are now available a significant number of books on medicines published and available in book shops. A good example is the *BMA Guide to Medicines and Drugs*.

60

Drug Therapy in Special Situations

PRESCRIBING IN PREGNANCY

Exposure of the fetus to drugs is undesirable, and should be avoided whenever possible. The placenta provides a potential barrier to entry of drugs from the maternal circulation, but lipophilic agents will cross readily, particularly if of low molecular weight. Drugs can be metabolized in the placenta which will further limit fetal exposure and the blood from the umbilical veins is partially shunted through the fetal liver which increases metabolism. Important problems associated with maternal use of drugs include:

- Teratogenesis: this is discussed in Chapter 56. The greatest risk is during the first trimester of pregnancy when fetal development is rapid, and even brief exposure can have profound effects.
- Pharmacological effects in the fetus following placental transfer of drug can be potentially serious. Warfarin-induced anticoagulation (Chapter 10) may predispose to cerebral haemorrhage during delivery; by contrast heparin is effective in the mother and does not cross the placenta. Non-steroidal anti-inflammatory drugs (Chapter 31) prevent closure of the ductus arteriosus after delivery; this is a prostaglandin-mediated action which is impaired by inhibition of cyclooxygenase. Amiodarone (Chapter 9) impairs iodine incor-

poration into thyroxine and maternal use can cause neonatal goitre.
- Interference with uterine contraction: the prostaglandin analogue misoprostol (Chapter 48) can produce uterine contractions and lead to abortion. Conversely calcium antagonists (Chapter 6) can inhibit or delay labour by reducing uterine contraction.

DRUGS IN BREAST FEEDING

There is surprisingly little information about the secretion of drugs into breast milk. Data are inconsistent and the risks for many drugs uncertain. Most drugs penetrate in quantities too small to be of concern. Several factors influence transfer including the characteristics of the milk (which changes in the first few days of lactation), the physicochemical properties of the drug and the amount of drug in the maternal circulation. In general, drugs licensed for use in children can be safely given to the nursing mother. Drugs known to have serious toxic effects in adults should be avoided. If drugs have to be used, compounds with short half-lives are preferred since they are rapidly eliminated. The feed should also be timed to coincide with the trough blood concentration in the mother whenever possible to minimize neonatal exposure.

PRESCRIBING FOR CHILDREN

Both the pharmacokinetics and responses to drugs are often different in children compared to adults. There are also considerable differences between the neonate and infant as the child develops anatomically and physiologically.

- Absorption: in the neonate slow rates of gastric emptying and intestinal transit may delay drug absorption, yet it may eventually be more complete due to prolonged contact with the intestinal mucosa.
- Distribution: neonates and young children have a low body fat content and high total body water. These will influence the distribution of both lipid- and water-soluble drugs. The newborn have a lower plasma albumin concentration which also has a lower affinity for drug binding. In addition, the higher plasma concentrations of free fatty acids and bilirubin will compete with drugs for plasma protein binding sites (Chapter 2). The overall effect is reduced plasma protein binding which increases the apparent volume of distribution of the drug but also increases the proportion of drug available for metabolism. Drugs which are strongly bound to albumin should not be used during neonatal jaundice because the drug will displace bilirubin from protein binding sites and increase the risk of kernicterus.
- Metabolism: the liver is relatively large in the young child compared to body size, but in the neonate the drug-metabolizing enzyme systems are immature. Therefore, first-pass metabolism and hepatic drug clearance are low in the neonate. When the enzyme systems mature, these processes will be more extensive in the young child than in the adult.
- Elimination: renal function in the neonate and very young child is much less developed than in the adult. Glomerular filtration rate in the newborn is about 40% of the adult level and tubular secretory processes are poorly developed. Elimination of drugs such as digoxin (Chapter 8), gentamicin and penicillin (Chapter 54) will therefore be delayed.

Overall, in children the larger volume of distribution and faster hepatic elimination mean that weight-related doses of metabolized drugs will need to be higher in children than in adults.

Conversely, smaller doses will be needed if the kidney is the major route of elimination. In neonates, inefficient metabolism means that smaller weight-related doses of all drugs will be needed. Prescribed doses are most accurately judged by considering both age and body surface area. The latter is a better guide to appropriate drug dosage than weight.

PRESCRIBING FOR THE ELDERLY

The elderly comprise a heterogeneous group who show considerable variation in "biological" age. Changes occur in both the pharmacokinetics and pharmacodynamics of drugs with increasing age.

PHARMACOKINETICS

Some aspects of these changes are discussed in Chapter 2:

- Drug absorption is unchanged by ageing, although bioavailability may be increased due to reduced first-pass metabolism.
- Older people have a lower lean body mass and a relative increase in body fat. The apparent volume of distribution of water-soluble drugs will therefore be smaller in the elderly and a lower loading dose of a drug like digoxin (Chapter 8) may be needed. Conversely, lipid-soluble drugs may be eliminated more slowly due to their larger volume of distribution.
- The size of the liver and its blood flow decrease with age. Although enzyme activity probably shows little change, the overall capacity for drug metabolism, particularly phase 1 reactions, is reduced. This is particularly important for lipid-soluble drugs which undergo extensive first-pass metabolism such as nifedipine or propranolol (Chapters 6 and 7).
- Increasing age is also associated with a progressive reduction in glomerular filtration rate. Elimination of polar drugs and metabolites will therefore be slower; this can produce toxicity when drugs have a low therapeutic index, for example lithium (Chapter 23), digoxin (Chapter 8) or gentamicin (Chapter 54). Because the elderly have a lower muscle mass than younger people, the plasma creatinine concentration (which is

dependent on lean body mass) is a poor guide to the level of renal glomerular function. It frequently remains within the "normal" laboratory reference range even when renal function is substantially reduced.

PHARMACODYNAMICS

The response to drugs can also be influenced by age:

- The density or numbers of receptors can be reduced with age; for example β-adrenoceptors are decreased in number which reduces the response to agonist drugs.
- Altered structure and function of target organs can also influence the effects of drugs. For example, baroreceptor function is impaired in the elderly and vasodilator drugs are more likely to provoke postural hypotension. The high peripheral resistance and less distensible arterial tree found with increasing age also respond less well to arterial vasodilators.

These changes in elderly people reflect the ageing process itself. However, they are often complicated by the presence of chronic disease (frequently involving multiple pathological processes) and variation due to both genetic and environmental influences. As a consequence of these changes, and the frequent use of several drugs, the risks of unwanted effects are higher in the elderly. For all these reasons it is usual to start drug treatment in the elderly with the smallest effective dose. Rational prescribing should also seek to minimize the numbers of drugs used.

PRESCRIBING IN RENAL FAILURE

Many drugs and their metabolites are excreted by the kidney and accumulate in renal impairment. There are several ways in which renal impairment may influence the handling of drugs:

- Metabolism in the liver can be altered in uraemic patients. Most oxidative metabolism is unchanged, but other processes such as reduction, acetylation and ester hydrolysis are impaired. Metabolism in the kidney is impor-

tant for the 1α hydroxylation of vitamin D and the degradation of insulin, both of which can be impaired in renal failure.

- Distribution of drugs can be affected by changes in fluid balances in renal failure. However, a more important influence is altered protein binding. Circulating concentrations of albumin are decreased in severe renal failure with proteinuria. In addition, retained endogenous metabolites change the affinity of drug-binding sites both on plasma protein, and also at tissue-binding sites. The greater concentration of free drug leads to increased elimination (by filtration and/or metabolism) so that the active unbound drug concentration may be unchanged. However, total plasma concentration of the drug (which is measured in most drug assays) will be lower, and assay results may be misinterpreted leading to an inappropriate increase in drug dose. Examples of drugs displaying this problem are theophylline (Chapter 11) and phenytoin (Chapter 24). Tissue binding of digoxin (Chapter 8) is reduced in renal failure so that a lower loading dose should be given to compensate for the reduced volume of distribution.
- Elimination of drugs by the kidney is only significantly impaired when the glomerular filtration rate is reduced below $50 \, \text{ml min}^{-1}$. For some drugs, clinically important accumulation will not occur until much lower filtration rates. Changes in tubular handling of drugs in renal disease is less well established.
- Altered pharmacodynamic responses to drugs are also found in uraemic patients. Drugs acting on the CNS in particular produce enhanced responses, possibly due to increased permeability of the blood–brain barrier.

Usually a reduction in drug dosage in renal failure will only be necessary if a high proportion of the drug is normally eliminated by the kidney and also the compound has a low therapeutic index (Chapter 56). Drugs which do not have dose-related unwanted effects rarely need large dose modifications.

A further important consideration is the avoidance of drugs which have toxic effects on the kidney. Use of these in renal impairment can sometimes produce an irreversible decline in renal function.

PRESCRIBING IN LIVER DISEASE

Changes in both pharmacokinetics and drug responses can occur in liver disease. The severity of the liver disease is important, but also whether the disease is decompensated, for example jaundice, hypoproteinaemia or encephalopathy.

PHARMACOKINETICS

The rate of absorption of drugs is little affected. However, several other aspects of drug handling may be altered:

- First-pass metabolism: is considerably reduced in conditions such as liver cirrhosis due to reduced enzyme activity and the presence of extensive porto-caval anastomoses.
- Enterohepatic circulation: will be impaired in conditions giving reduced formation or elimination of bile.
- Systemic clearance: may be reduced for drugs which are eliminated by hepatic metabolism, especially high clearance drugs where the elimination rate is dependent on effective liver blood flow.
- Distribution: if plasma protein synthesis is reduced, then the plasma albumin concentrations will be low. An elevated plasma bilirubin can also displace many drugs from their protein-binding sites. The effect will be to increase the volume of distribution. Examples of drugs which can be greatly affected are lignocaine (Chapter 9) and propranolol (Chapter 6).

PHARMACODYNAMICS

- The reduced ability to synthesize vitamin K-dependent clotting factors makes patients with chronic liver disease more sensitive to the anticoagulant effects of warfarin (Chapter 10).
- CNS-depressant drugs such as morphine (Chapter 20) or chlorpromazine (Chapter 22) have an enhanced effect in liver failure. This is due to a change in the sensitivity of neuronal tissue and can provoke encephalopathy in susceptible patients.
- Diuretics which produce hypokalaemia (Chapter 15) can precipitate hepatic encephalopathy in chronic liver disease.

Prescribing in liver disease should therefore be carried out with care; drugs which are extensively metabolized by the liver should be given in smaller doses. Those to which altered responses have been shown should be used only with close monitoring of the patient.

Index